Merry Christmas 2015

The Best of All Worlds

A Family Doctor's Path to Integrative Medicine

By Dr. Andrew Lenhardt

...

By Andrew Lenhardt, MD

Get free articles at drlenhardt.com

I know you're going to enjoy Dr. Andy's book. Let me know when you find "me."

Enjoy...

DISCLAIMER

This publication contains the opinions and ideas of its author. It is intended to provide useful and informative material on the subjects addressed in the publication. It is sold with the understanding that the author and publisher are not engaged in rendering medical, health, or any other kind of personal professional services in the book. The reader should consult his or her medical, health, or other competent professional before drawing inferences from the book.

The case histories included in this book are based on the author's experience with his patients. Names and certain personal information have been changed.

The author and publisher specifically disclaim all responsibility for any liability, loss, or risk, personal or otherwise, that is incurred as a consequence, directly or indirectly, of the use and application of any of the contents of this book.

ACKNOWLEDGEMENTS

There is a long list of people that have helped me with this book. I am grateful to all of the patients I have seen over the past 15+ years of clinical practice. I learn as much or more from them as they learn from me. I was originally going to write a short e-book designed for family practice residents so I could share with them some of my insights. I wanted them to learn from the successes and failures I have had in my work. Denise Sandell convinced me to broaden the scope of the book so I am thankful for her place in my life at just the right time. My primary editor Debbie O'Brien has been a tremendous asset and I can only imagine the messy product this would be if it weren't for her. Haley Bridger helped me early on in the editing process with the big picture and some of the ideas in the book. Amanda Aratilian worked with me as an intern over a summer and helped pull together much of the information in the "Lost Ones" chapter. Julian Flynn has been incredible with my blog drlenhardt.com and has helped coordinate the e-publishing. Thank you also to Ranee Flynn who helped with development of the book, the cover and marketing. Mory Bahar has helped with many aspects of the book's development, marketing and social media.

No person has made more of a difference in shifting my awareness than my wife Mary. Every day I am thankful that I have such an amazing, talented person in my life. My son Will has taught me some of the most important lessons of my life. He brings me great joy. A special appreciation goes to Edward Colley who is the person behind all of the illustrations in the book. So many times in my life, an experience has exceeded my expectations and the pictures he created easily fit into that category.

Table of Contents

INTRODUCTION

My goal as a physician has been to find the best of what the world has to offer in terms of wellness and prevention, no matter what the source. This book is a distillation of my experience after many years of clinical practice as a primary care physician. Whether you are a patient frustrated by the limitations of mainstream American medicine or a physician interested in using both traditional and non-traditional options, this is a crash course in integration. This book will provide an overview of the most important trends in health, pulling them together cohesively and illustrating that, in order for medical care in our country to improve, we must move American medicine toward a more balanced approach.

We have, in some ways, overspecialized and need to pull systems back together toward the whole. We are also coming to understand that man is more than just the sum of his physical parts. There is an interconnectedness of systems not always acknowledged in today's highly specialized medical establishment. Pharmaceuticals, miraculously life-saving in many instances, are now thrown at every symptom, with little discussion of more natural options. An optimal approach would be more proactive, with a focus on individualized care that considers all aspects of the mind, body and spirit.

In a relatively short period of time, there have been dramatic changes in our health systems, food supply and environment. These have mostly taken place silently and are unknown to the majority of Americans. These changes are primarily to our detriment, insidiously undermining our state of health and wellbeing.

The options available to Americans for maintaining good health are constantly expanding, but choosing the right practitioner, optimal diet or most effective supplement can be overwhelming. The standard approach for the majority of Americans is to see an "allopathic" provider—most often a medical doctor (MD)—but also sometimes a doctor of osteopathic medicine (DO). The primary care doctor is usually consulted first regarding medical issues. There are other disciplines, however, and more people are seeking alternative approaches to maintain health or regain good health. Scattered like chicken feed are osteopaths, chiropractors, naturopaths, herbalists, acupuncturists, massage therapists, shamans, faith healers, medical intuitives, Aryuvedic practitioners, and others.

I have been in medicine for over 20 years and currently work in the metro Boston area as an MD in family practice. I have personal experience with massage, yoga, acupuncture, homeopathy, osteopathy, kinesiology and many of the more typical allopathic approaches. I have always been open to alternative approaches to health, even going back to my early training.

I remember several experiences in medical school that, in some fashion, set the course my life and medical practice would eventually take. The first day of medical school, we were given a gift from Pfizer, one of the largest pharmaceutical companies. It was a book describing medical treatment options with an introduction added by the company. Even then, I had no interest in being influenced by that segment of American medicine. I slipped the book into the trash at the first opportunity. In the second year of medical school, we had to do a project summarizing a subject within health and wellness. I chose acupuncture. Because of a lack of research studies, I had difficulty at that time finding solid evidence for the benefits of acupuncture.

That same year, as we were preparing to start our clinical rotations, we had a single lecture on meditation by a man named Jon Kabat-Zinn. He was an expert on mindful meditation and, by then, had written two very successful books: *Full Catastrophe Living* and *Wherever You Go There You Are.* (I would later mindlessly leave behind the second book on a plane, apparently not utilizing his principles very effectively.) Mr. Kabat-Zinn ran a center at our medical school where people were taught the principles of meditation. He had success especially with people diagnosed with hypertension, often achieving similar blood pressure control to pharmaceuticals. I was completely engaged during his lecture. I listened intently to everything he had to say about meditation and its potential benefits for wellness. Even then, I imagined incorporating it into my future medical practice. Leaving the lecture hall, I expected the students around me to have had a similar experience. All I heard, however, was how useless the lecture had been. There was a steady flow of negative comments about how the hour was a total waste of time and had no place in the medical school curriculum.

After I had been in practice a couple of years, I received a book called *The Zen of Listening* as a Christmas gift. This book had more impact on my practice than any medical textbook. Applying its principles has enhanced the therapeutic relationships with my patients and improved my communication with the people I see in the office every day.

In my time in medicine, I have gradually come to appreciate what traditional medicine does very well and also what it does not do so well. One of the primary goals of this book is to give people some of the best mainstream options, but also to shed light on some of the good alternative options. My search for answers outside of the standard approaches taught in medical school and residency has been born of necessity. If my goal is to achieve care for the whole patient, there are times I will stick with the mainstream approach, because that is what I feel is best. There are other times when I will seek different options. But the world is ever more complex. Healthcare is changing rapidly with new developments every week. It will likely get harder and harder for us to step off the hamster wheel, take a deep breath and try a different approach.

One of the strong arguments for a new paradigm in healthcare is the fact we spend a lot of money in America with a relatively poor return on investment. In 2013, the United States budgeted 24 percent of the 3.8 trillion dollar federal spending to cover healthcare costs.[1] For perspective, 23 percent of the budget went to defense, 24 percent to pensions and three percent to education. The World Health Organization did an overall assessment of countries' health systems back in 2000.[2] The United States ranked 37th. Our cultural rival France was ranked number one and that that alone would lead some to discount the rankings out of hand. A summary published in February 2013 from the Institute of Medicine and the National Research Council[3] ranked the United States last among 17 countries studied in terms of overall health.

Most would agree that life expectancy is one of the most important measures of how well a healthcare system is doing. The United States is relatively low by that measure and, even more significantly, we have had a consistent decline in ranking compared to the rest of the world.

United States World Ranking in Life Expectancy

1980 18th

1990 21st

2000 26th

2010 29th

American men are living about four years less than men in top-ranked Switzerland and American women are living five years less than women in top-ranked Japan. A relative decline in life expectancy can be related to the overall health system and can also reflect many other factors, including poor lifestyle and a degradation of the food supply.

More statistics will be reviewed in "The Cost of Doing Business" chapter. Overall, it is obvious that our quasi-capitalist model of healthcare, with a strong emphasis on pharmaceuticals and technology, is not providing excellent care relative to what we spend. Being able to get an MRI or a CT scan within a few days is impressive, but it does not necessarily predict better outcomes.

An exquisite example of where new technology is not the answer is in the development of the three-dimensional CT scan. For years, there were reports that new technology was being developed that would take the place of the more invasive colonoscopy for colon cancer screening. Eventually, the 3D CT scan became available and it promised to be as reliable as colonoscopy at identifying polyps. The technology is amazing and does live up to that standard. I will review in "The Others" chapter why this breakthrough technology has not been implemented on a wide scale.

The health journals I read almost always report on new drugs being developed for any number of chronic health problems. The FDA approved 39 new medicines in 2012.[4] At least 10 of the drugs received approval for "fast-track" status. This volume of new medications reflects how central pharmaceuticals are to the current American healthcare system. The majority of these new pharmaceuticals, however, will likely have little or no impact on basic health and do nothing to improve the most important measures of wellness. This will be discussed in more detail in the *Polypharmacy* and *The Cost of Doing Business* chapters toward the end of the book.

More and more, the general public is craving providers that will meld traditional mainstream medicine and complementary options. There is growing momentum toward a broader, more open-minded and comprehensive approach to wellness. Mainstream physicians can benefit from stepping out of their small box and acknowledging that other practitioners are helping people be well. The vogue term for this is Integrative Medicine. There have been many pioneers in this area including Andrew Weil, MD, Deepak Chopra, MD, and Mark Hyman, MD.

There is a tremendous amount of resistance, however, in the current health-care system. Some of this exists because alternative options are unlikely to have documented evidence of their efficacy. The gold standard in medical research is the double-blind, placebo controlled multicenter trial. Yet most of the clinical questions a doctor or nurse practitioner (NP), nurse or physician's assistant (PA) try to answer in any given day are not answerable in terms of that standard.

I will also argue that evidence-based medicine is not, and cannot be, the centerpiece for medicine as it stampedes into the future. Much of my time in family practice residency was spent reviewing studies to try and achieve the best evidence-based answer to a particular clinical question. When evidence-based answers are easily gleaned in the flow of daily practice, it is optimal. It is not practical, however, to have evidence guide the majority of our clinical decisions. Most of the questions I want answered have no evidence-based answer. Or more precisely, they have no reliable evidence-based answer.

By one estimate, 85 percent of biomedical research is done by the pharmaceutical industry, and as the federal government struggles with debt, that percentage should continue to grow. The drug companies clearly have bias and, in my opinion, undue influence on the information available to practicing physicians. I feel that medicine would do better to move away from pharmaceuticals as the first option for most symptoms and diagnoses.

There is other resistance to the status quo of today's medical establishment that is fundamental to being a human being. It is much easier to assume you have the answers than to be totally honest and admit there are things you do not know. If hard pressed, medical doctors would have to admit that they do not have a solid understanding of many chronic disease processes. Mainstream providers have a lot at stake. The current system rewards them well financially. It rewards them with extremely high levels of prestige. Doctors are among the most well-respected professionals. People come to doctors with problems and expect to be given reliable answers that are in their best interest. In my experience, some physicians have a simple view when it comes to evaluating a patient: if they do not know the answer or cannot figure out the underlying cause or causes, then it must not be that important. If pressed, they may also assume a complicated person's symptoms are psychosomatic and send the patient to a psychiatrist.

The current system of medicine tends to be compartmentalized. If we see a patient with many problems, several specialist opinions are often sought. The neurologist will try to figure out their headaches. The cardiologist will work up the palpitations. An endocrinologist will treat the underactive thyroid. The primary care physician (PCP) is really the provider in the best position to pull it all together, since the piecemeal approach often misses some underlying systemic cause for the condition.

There are many underlying problems that can affect a wide range of organ systems. The simplest of these would be poor hydration, since most people do not drink enough water. Not hydrating well can contribute to fatigue, headaches, lightheadedness, palpitations, angina, kidney stones, constipation and dry skin, etc. Here, as in many other situations, the simplest solution is often the right solution.

Many of the other systemic problems get little or no attention in mainstream medicine. Physicians are not trained in these areas and, in fact, most of them never even come up once during seven or more years of medical training. Because of this, there is resistance and, often, overt hostility to any ideas out of the norm.

There are a few key ideas that I believe are essential in understanding many chronic disease processes. They all have in common that the mainstream medical community gives them little or no credence. They do, however, get a lot of attention in the alternative world. They are "holistic" in that they potentially affect people in a wide variety of ways, causing many symptoms and leading to many diverse diagnoses. I would put on this list chronic infections, systemic yeast overgrowth, gut flora imbalance or dysbiosis, food sensitivities/intolerances, genetic methylation cycle anomalies, iodine deficiency, magnesium deficiency and undiagnosed thyroid disorders. Key contributors to these systemic problems are the poor quality of food consumed, excessive stress, lack of sleep, and exposures to innumerable toxins, chemicals, pesticides and hormones. In the chapter "A Perfect Storm," I will review these contributors in more detail. The vast majority of Americans have no idea what they are putting in their bodies every day and are probably too stressed and overworked to care very much. It is estimated that more than 5,000 substances are added to processed foods, and none of them are currently tracked or regulated.

Many people, in my opinion, have chronic undiagnosed infections. This would include chronic Lyme disease, but there are likely many other chronic illnesses related to a chronic infection. I suspect that chronic infectious agents will be identified one at a time until some tipping point when the medical world will be forced to acknowledge a new paradigm. A person's microbiome is their unique composition of bacteria, viruses, funguses and other micro-organisms. The interplay of our immune system with our individual microbiome is central to a new approach to chronic illness.

We know that a healthy diet is crucial for long-term health and wellness. So far, however, we have been moving from one simplistic view of diet to another. Each simple view has some element of truth to it but is unsophisticated and limited in scope. People have been told for years that there is a simple formula for weight loss. To lose weight, you only have to burn more calories than you consume. People were told for many years that dietary fat intake was the problem, an idea now entrenched in American culture. People have an idea that if they eat a lot of foods high in fat and cholesterol they will be at a high risk of cardiovascular disease. This has led to people being told to avoid eggs, shellfish and nuts. Dietary improvement is a common theme in the book. There are many new ideas and concepts introduced that will help each person change their food intake and improve many aspects of their health.

The wide world of supplements is also considered in the course of this book. The superscript notation NS in the text signifies Natural Standard and refers the reader to Appendix B for an excerpt of a database from naturalmedicines.com (formerly health.naturalstandard.com), a website that publishes documented research on complementary and alternative supplements and therapies.

The chapter "Lipitor vs. Guggulipid" reviews cardiovascular health. The general public has a faulty understanding of serum cholesterol levels. The average person thinks that if they have high cholesterol levels on a blood test, their arteries are filling up with plaque and they are at high risk for a heart attack. They also think that if they have low cholesterol numbers, they are more likely to have clear arteries. Cardiovascular disease is much more complicated than that. Personally, I would rank blood cholesterol levels somewhere between eight and ten on the list of individual risk factors. Active involvement in a church and having a tight bond with a pet are probably more important.

We are bombing away with statin drugs to lower cholesterol, since these are thought to be the miracle drugs of our time. But when the numbers are analyzed, the benefit is relatively small. This goes against the standard dogma and is viewed as heresy by most cardiologists. Some doctors have fallen under the spell of pharmaceuticals, believing they are the answer to all of our problems.

History may show that the 20th-century medical establishment looked toward science, technology and pharmaceuticals as the answer only to realize their limitations. We need a broader, more inclusive approach to wellness that harnesses and optimizes the human body's stunning potential to prevent and fight disease. If we move in this direction, in the next hundred years we may discover the balance between nature and technology that promotes true health in body, mind and spirit.

Relatively early in my clinical practice I found that many of my patients with chronic health problems were not being served well. They would see me and other allopathic providers but continue with complicated issues that were poorly understood. I could not accept this and became more frustrated over time. This frustration has led me to explore alternative options as a way to improve the care for those lost in the system. I expected to add some minor refinements to my practice and instead discovered a wide variety of important issues crucial to my treatment of the chronically ill. This book represents that path to an integrative model.

1

Trust Your Gut

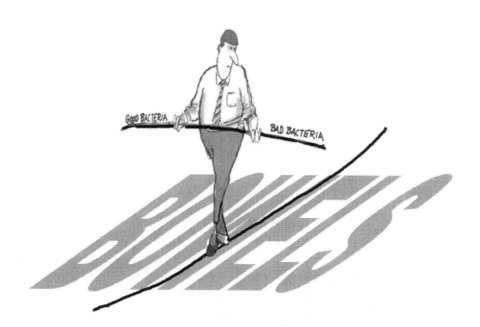

I have been asked several times over the years if I had courses in nutrition during my medical training, though I suspect those asking already knew the answer: No. In four years of medical school and three years in a more progressive family medicine residency, there was never a course or program dedicated to diet and nutrition. This is a staggering oversight. Though diet seems to be perceived by the modern establishment as a simple subject, somehow beneath the physician who is trying to manage complex medical diagnoses, it should be obvious that our bodies are made of the stuff we eat and drink. Nutrition, then, is an essential part of overall health and wellness. Thankfully, there are now many good resources available that elucidate the major impact of diet and nutrition on people's lives. You could pick up and read a hundred or so pages of *Conscious Eating* by Gabriel Cousens, MD, just to scratch the surface. Even I had trouble slogging through the tome as it was more complex than I bargained for, confirming that diet, though little understood, is far from simple. American medicine focuses primarily on the areas that maximize profit. It has evolved away from the interventions that can prevent and reverse disease. With dietary changes, improved nutrition and an appreciation of our microbiome, we have the opportunity to dramatically improve health and cure a wide variety of chronic illnesses. This should be the cornerstone of American medicine going forward.

David

David is a healthy 38-year-old male I usually only see at his annual physical. He works in IT, has a girlfriend who may be "the one," and takes good care of himself. He wears the cool, dark European prescription glasses that typically increase a person's perceived IQ by at least 10 points. The healthy male physical can be a straightforward visit with not much to talk about. If a person has no chronic medical problems, no complaints and an optimal lifestyle, there's not always a lot to discuss. Politics? Sports maybe?

David is in excellent health now, but that wasn't always the case. When he was around eight years old he started to have abdominal cramping and diarrhea. He initially was told by his pediatrician to avoid dairy, but that made no difference. He eventually saw five other doctors by his recollection, including allergists and gastroenterologists. He vividly remembers having a barium enema as an adolescent and says the experience was "horrible." He had other testing done and the results were all normal. The solution, even though the doctors did not have a clear understanding of the cause for his problem: prescription medication. He was put on Zantac with no improvement. The pseudodiagnosis irritable bowel syndrome (IBS) was invoked and he was sent on his way.

As an adult, David's symptoms became more intense when under stress and he was able to opt out of the military because of the gastrointestinal problems. He managed his way through life, eventually coming to me as a patient. I saw him for years and really didn't have much to offer him. My understanding of IBS, like that of most doctors, was somewhat limited. For the early part of my career, I would just tell people that it was very common with little or no understanding of what was causing the problem. If I could keep those people off unnecessary prescription medications for a while, that was the best I could do. Today, my views on the subject are more enlightened. I now have a framework of reference with options to improve and often to cure most people with chronic gastrointestinal symptoms.

I hadn't seen David for over a year when he came in for a physical in early 2010. I checked in with him about his health and especially about his IBS issues. He told me his girlfriend was very "holistic." Now, that can mean that she has yogurt twice a day or that she studied with Buddhist monks in the foothills of Tibet for 10 years, or anything in between. It usually means that the person has a broader view of wellness beyond the mainstream. A year or so before David came in for his check-up, his girlfriend noted that he had diarrhea after eating pasta. She recommended he stop consuming wheat. Shazam! In a very short period of time, his bowel problems resolved. After 26 years of symptoms, a non-medical person figured out his problem in 10 minutes after a nice dinner.

At his visit, David did have a new complaint to discuss. He said he had a tendency to get itchy, red eyes. He could come up with no particular pattern to the eye problem and it did not seem seasonal in nature. We went through some of the more common causes of allergies including mold and dust mites. We reviewed his home and work environments to try and identify any obvious causes. The standard approach to this would be to start allergy eye drops and possibly send him to an allergist for allergy testing. Because of his food intolerance to wheat, I reviewed his diet in more detail. He ate a lot of raw food. He avoided cow's milk—a psychic leftover from when doctors told him as a child that cow's milk was bad for him—and instead used soy milk in his coffee every morning.

Soy has become one of the great shams perpetuated on the American people. For years, soy was proposed to lower breast cancer in women as well as offer other long-term benefits. There were some vague ideas about soy being a staple in the Asian diet, Asian women having lower rates of breast cancer, and soy being a plant-based form of estrogen, a.k.a. a phytoestrogen. As is typical, it doesn't necessarily matter whether there is real benefit, it only matters that there is a perception of benefit. American businesses are very savvy on these matters and if they feel that an idea is prevalent enough, the opportunity for profit can't be too far away.

Yogurt sales, for example, are through the roof, although it's not clear that there is a large health benefit. There is a vague connection between yogurt and good bacteria. Mass-produced yogurt typically has a lot of sugar. The consumer zeroes in on the low fat content, but misses the fact that there is more sugar in most yogurts than in two servings of Frosted Flakes. Yogurt may actually be causing problems for many who cannot tolerate cow's milk.

In David's case, he bought into soy milk as almost certainly being better for his health than cow's milk. I think some of that comes from the assumption that Asians have more wisdom than we do. The Asian cultures have been around for thousands of years and we assume that they have figured out the answers to many of life's important questions. Americans are funny in that they can be supremely overconfident while at the same time be profoundly insecure. Deep down we think the Asians are smarter than we are and the Europeans more sophisticated. Of course, this cannot be admitted straight away because it would be unpatriotic. We're the greatest country in the world, right? Right? Damn right.

I discussed with David that maybe soy wasn't right for him either. I ordered a RAST panel (a series of blood tests to try and identify food allergies) that would ultimately come back with normal results. Soy is in the standard panel, along with wheat, cow's milk, eggs, nuts, shellfish and other food types that can commonly cause allergic symptoms. I also recommended he stop the soy milk since I have found that I cannot trust a negative RAST panel. Five years prior, I wouldn't have considered soy as a potential cause for red, itchy eyes. Now, I know better. Once your horizons broaden and your awareness expands, you see things as never before and there's no going back.

Unfortunately, his eye symptoms did not improve by avoiding soy. I sent him to an ophthalmologist for a more thorough eye exam. The itchy eyes eventually resolved spontaneously and we never had a good explanation for the underlying cause. Overall, I see more and more patients in my practice with health conditions that improve or resolve with dietary change, but this type of intervention can be a bit random. I will review later in the book ways we may be able to figure out more precisely whether an individual's issues are related to food allergies, sensitivities and intolerances. The testing can be reliable, but it's expensive and not covered by any insurance.

Steve

Gastroenterology is one area where mainstream medicine's approach to management can be lacking. The alternative world, on the other hand, can have a lot to offer. Some of the most common acute and chronic medical problems involving the gastrointestinal tract include esophageal reflux, irritable bowel syndrome, abdominal pain, and colitis.

Steve, a 46-year-old male, has visited the practice complaining of frequent acid reflux. He is 5 feet 11 inches tall and 225 pounds, married with two young children. He works as a roofer and says he doesn't need to exercise or go to the gym because he's doing physical work every day. His wife tries to get him to eat healthier, but this is a work in progress: he usually skips breakfast and grabs a cup of coffee on his way out the door, gets something off the lunch truck at his worksite, and eats a meat, starch and vegetable for dinner. Steve likes ice cream—Rocky Road to be specific—and enjoys some a few nights each week while watching TV. He has almost quit smoking, though under stress he'll smoke more. His wife won't let him smoke in the house, so he usually smokes in the truck. His routine is to come home and have a couple of Bud Lights, and if he's watching a game, another two. On the weekends, he can easily put away six or more.

Given Steve's chronic acid reflux problems, what are the management options? The modern cookie cutter approach to chronic acid reflux is to put patients on a prescription acid blocker indefinitely—either H2 blockers like Zantac, Pepcid or Tagamet or the stronger type called proton pump inhibitors (PPIs), which include omeprazole (name brand Prilosec or Nexium), pantoprazole (Protonix) and lansoprazole (Prevacid). Most providers will ask questions about caffeine, smoking, alcohol, acidic foods, fatty foods and other lifestyle contributors before issuing the prescription. The patient's symptoms typically improve after starting the medications, leaving them thankful for their doctor and this country's access to effective medications.

But my approach to reflux and other gastrointestinal problems has evolved over my years in medicine. I now try to avoid acid blockers, especially PPIs, as a long-term solution. The body has acid in the stomach for many good reasons: an acidic environment helps protect the body from pathogenic microorganisms and it allows for effective digestion and absorption of proteins, minerals and vitamins, especially vitamin B^{12}. PPIs, while providing some relief from symptoms, have been linked to an increased risk of osteoporosis in women. In fact, the reflux itself is not cured by lowering acid, so stomach contents may still be passing up into the esophagus when a person lies down. Acid-lowering medications actually deprive the stomach of the necessary amount of acid for digestion and this causes the stomach to *increase* its acid-producing cells. The problems with prescription acid blockers are spelled out in the book *Natural Alternatives to Nexium, Maalox, Tagamet, Prilosec and other Acid Blockers* by Martie Whittekin.

So, what are the alternatives? If there are no red flags requiring further evaluation, I will typically start by telling the person to chew their food more thoroughly and eat more slowly. This may not be the most scintillating piece of advice they ever hear, but the simplest solution is often the best solution. I have heard of a high-tech solution to this: a fork has been developed which beeps and chirps at the person if they are eating too much or too quickly. It can also be helpful for the person to avoid drinking a lot of water during the meal. It is possible that large amounts of water dilute the stomach acidity, interfering with the normal breakdown of food.

If the person with reflux can maximize their body's ability to process food efficiently, that and some dietary modifications are often enough to control the problem. If that doesn't work, I recommend taking a natural digestive enzyme supplement once, twice or even three times per day before meals. That will help a significant percentage of people with chronic reflux.

I'm not holding my breath for some controlled trial to determine how effective these strategies are because it won't likely ever happen. If we don't have a double-blind placebo-controlled multicenter trial with high statistical significance demonstrating efficacy, does that mean the strategy has no value? That standard, a basic premise of modern medicine, has become a convenient way to discount anything out of the mainstream. If nine out of ten people say that digestive enzymes significantly reduce their symptoms, that's usually good enough for me.

I use H2 blockers and PPIs in patients who don't respond to other treatments, but try to avoid this as a lifetime strategy. This may sound like a conspiracy theory, but it is distinctly possible that reducing stomach acid will interfere with how the body processes food, turning an acute problem into a chronic one. Long-term reliance on pharmaceuticals is a pharmaceutical company's dream come true. They exist to sell product. It may sound anti-capitalist to say so, but that's the way it is. Any benefit to a person's health and wellbeing is an incidental bonus.

For my patient Steve with chronic reflux, we discussed his lifestyle at each visit no matter what his chief complaint. The changes he made were incremental over a couple of years. With dietary modifications, reduced coffee intake and some weight loss, his symptoms improved. Eventually, he only needed to take an acid blocker a few times per month when the symptoms flared.

Babies and Reflux

Acid reflux is not just an adult problem. It is very common for infants to have esophageal reflux. This will typically peak between the third and fourth month of life and then resolve by six months. There are simple strategies that can help minimize the baby's discomfort, including keeping the baby upright for 5-10 minutes after nursing or bottlefeeding. If the baby has persistent symptoms related to reflux, it is standard practice to use acid blockers like ranitidine. Again, my approach is generally that of a minimalist when it comes to pharmaceuticals, but I use them regularly, depending on individual circumstances.

I remember well a case involving a 4-month-old baby girl. The mom brought her in following three days of vomiting and lethargy. The baby was getting worse and worse. There was no cough or fever. There was no diarrhea, which would typically clinch the diagnosis of a viral gastroenteritis infection. I reviewed her chart since I was not her primary physician. It showed she was healthy except for a diagnosis of reflux made at a prior visit.

This infant had been placed on ranitidine, the generic for Zantac, because of the severity of her symptoms. As far as the mom could tell, the medication was working well. The reflux-related symptoms had resolved and the infant was comfortable during and after breastfeeding. For some reason, I double-checked the baby's dose of Zantac. The mom said she was taking 5ml every day. There were two strengths available of the medication and I uncovered that the baby was given the stronger version. There was some mix-up and she was supposed to be taking 0.5ml daily. The baby was getting 10 times the recommended dose. This explained her symptoms and indicated significant, possibly life-threatening, toxicity. I told the mom to stop the medication. In 24 hours the infant was much improved, and in 48 hours she was well again.

This illustrates an important rationale for keeping pharmaceuticals to a minimum. People can experience side effects, reactions and interactions from prescribed medications. Some of these are mild, causing low-level, insidious symptoms like fatigue that reduces a person's quality of life. Some are severe and potentially life-threatening.

Age and Acidity

Brenda Watson has written several books on health, wellness and disease, often with a focus on gastrointestinal issues. *Renew Your Life* is particularly thorough. She discusses how the acidity in people's stomachs tends to decrease with age. Thus, an older person may need a very different approach to reflux and heartburn than a younger one. The older person may have reflux, not because they have excessive acid, but because they have inadequate acid to break down their food. In the alternative world, there is much attention given to regulating a person's internal pH. There are providers that will actually give a person hydrochloric acid (HCl) supplements to improve their gastric symptoms. This is heresy to an established gastroenterologist.

Chronic Bowel Issues

It is very common to see people in the office with some combination of chronic diarrhea, constipation, abdominal discomfort, bloating and gas. Sometimes, like in David's case, these symptoms have been ongoing for many years. Some patients have daily symptoms and others will have flare-ups lasting weeks or months, with periods of quiet in between.

If someone comes in with chronic constipation, a typical approach is to increase water intake and start a fiber supplement. If that doesn't work, add a laxative. If that doesn't work, switch to a stronger laxative. If the patient is still constipated, set up a visit with a gastroenterology specialist. They will do a colonoscopy that is invariably normal and put the patient on a more elaborate regimen of stool softeners and stimulants and laxatives until—Ding!—the person cooperates and produces a nice, soft, formed stool. This is not an optimal strategy, however. A person should not have to take two over-the-counter products and a prescription-strength laxative to poop.

Any person that comes in with chronic bowel issues needs to be considered in context, of course. The person's lifestyle, age and family history are relevant. Doctors, NPs and PAs are always on the look-out for "red flags." These would include relatively severe symptoms of short duration or unexplained weight loss or bleeding. Some patients will have black stools, which usually comes up during a provider's review of systems. The average person does not realize that a black stool can be a sign of bleeding from the upper gastrointestinal tract. There are three typical causes of black stools which I try to go with the medical students I supervise: bleeding from somewhere north of the colon, iron supplements and PeptoBismol.

For most people with chronic bowel issues, the diagnosis will likely be IBS. Most providers will pursue lab tests including thyroid function (TSH), complete blood count (CBC) and liver function tests (LFTs)—which technically don't measure the functioning of the liver—and an anti-endomesial antibody test. The anti-endomesial test is intended to diagnose celiac disease. Celiac disease is the most profound condition of gluten intolerance, an autoimmune process that tends to be chronic and progressive.

The issue of gluten intolerance is another area where the mainstream and alternative worlds diverge. The majority of doctors will do the celiac blood test and, when normal, conclude that the person does not have any problems with gluten. The alternative world would say (and I have found this to be the case in my practice) that most people with gluten intolerance will have normal celiac screening tests. There are other ways to uncover gluten intolerance, but in my experience the easiest is to have the person avoid gluten for two or more weeks. If symptoms improve, gluten is probably an issue, especially if they try it again later and the fatigue or headaches or joint pains or rashes return. I would consider this conclusive enough to recommend the person avoid gluten in the future. Many doctors can't stomach this way of managing patients. It's too vague. As before, if we wait around for a strict, evidence-based answer, many people are going to be unwell that could otherwise be helped.

The first round of testing is almost always normal. I can't remember once diagnosing a person with underactive thyroid in that context (although the TSH thyroid test alone is not reliable enough to rule out thyroid dysfunction as a contributing factor). The person almost never has anemia. If they do, a small percentage can have colitis with inflammation of the colon and bleeding. There are different types of colitis, which broadly refers to an inflammatory condition involving the colon. When I was going through medical school and residency, graduating in 1998 and 2001 respectively, there were really only two types of colitis: Crohn's disease and ulcerative colitis. With colitis, as is often the case in mainstream medicine, the underlying cause is not well understood. It could be autoimmune or infectious or both. It could be related to something in the diet or something in the environment or both. There are pharmaceutical options, but no fundamental understanding of causation.

IBS and reflux are the two most common chronic gastrointestinal conditions by far, but giving someone a diagnosis of IBS is not necessarily doing them a favor. This area of medicine may have the strongest divergence between conventional and alternative approaches. There are medications that have been developed for IBS called anti-spasmodics (these include levsin and bentyl). They do not generally provide much relief, but the quickest way to shorten a visit that's going nowhere is often to give the patient a prescription. It is a concrete plan of action and most patients are content that someone is doing something to help them. The sequence of visits will often go something like this:

Visit #1: See PCP for chronic bowel problem. Get some basic information and have a basic work-up. Perhaps try lifestyle change and/or prescription medication.

Visit # 2 (one month later): See PCP for follow-up. Things are usually about the same. Referral to a gastroenterologist.

Visit #3 (one month later): See the gastroenterology specialist. If the patient has abdominal discomfort, a trial of an antispasmodic is initiated. If the person has constipation, the specialist will often recommend fiber, laxatives, and stool softeners. If the person predominantly has loose stools,

OTC Imodium may be recommended and the person will probably have standard stool studies, including for culture and sensitivities (C&S) and ova and parasites (O&P). Arrangements also made for CT scan of abdomen and pelvis and/or colonoscopy and/or Upper GI study +/- small bowel follow through, depending on the variety of the person's symptoms.

Visit #4 (one month later): See GI specialist again for follow-up. Testing appears normal. Antispasmodic not helping. Working diagnosis given for irritable bowel syndrome. Often the person is given some basic advice to try and control symptoms and improve their quality of life. The unstated presumption is that we're basically waiting around for the pharmaceutical industry to come up with some blockbuster IBS medication that will take care of the problem.

Reiki

Fortunately, I have not had problems with acid reflux or IBS. I have had a few acute episodes, however, presumably caused by an intestinal virus. These infections usually resolve on their own after a few days. A couple of years ago, I had some gastrointestinal infection with diarrhea and moderate cramping and abdominal pain. On the second night, I was lying in discomfort and unable to sleep. My wife woke up, put her hand on my belly for a few minutes and the pain resolved, never to return. My wife is a yoga teacher who also has training in Reiki. Reiki is a form of energy healing developed in Japan.

The word Reiki is made of two Japanese words—Rei which means "God's Wisdom or the Higher Power" and Ki which is "life force energy." So Reiki is actually "spiritually guided life force energy." There are 5 "ideals" associated with reiki. The Ideals were developed to add spiritual balance to Usui Reiki. Their purpose is to help people realize that healing the spirit by consciously deciding to improve oneself is a necessary part of the Reiki healing experience.

- The secret art of inviting happiness
- The miraculous medicine of all diseases
- Just for today, do not anger
- Do not worry and be filled with gratitude
- Devote yourself to your work. Be kind to people.

- Every morning and evening, join your hands in prayer.
- Pray these words to your heart and chant these words with your mouth

The founder Usui Mikao[5]

My first introduction to energy work was following a traumatic rib injury. I was mountain biking and got overly ambitious coming into a drop-off. There was a moment of low-level terror when I felt my center of gravity go up over the handlebars and I knew there was no way I could stop myself. I landed hard on a large rock, injuring the left side of my chest. I was in severe pain for a couple of weeks, as rib injuries often take four to six weeks to heal. I went to one of my wife's yoga classes (she was my girlfriend then) and she could see I was in pain. The downward dog position was rough. After the class, I told her about the accident. She suggested Reiki healing and told me that I didn't need to believe in anything. I was so desperate for relief that I promptly assumed a corpse pose and allowed her to do her healing thing. She simply put her hand on my ribs, closed her eyes, and started channeling Reiki to the area. Within minutes, the pain to my ribs disappeared. I was astonished that I felt completely healed. Until that moment, I would never have believed such a thing possible.

The most dramatic demonstration of Reiki, however, came many years later, after my son had won a goldfish at a fair but before he had named it; change his water to the water; change he turned over and swam away to the fish turned over and swam away. One day, hoping to be a good and dutiful husband, I put the fishbowl in the sink to change his water. I ran the clean water in from the faucet, flushing out the old water in the process. I was distracted by something and then checked back and the goldfish was floating at the top. I put my finger in the bowl and the water was hot. Oops. I considered mouth-to-mouth resuscitation, but figured he was a goner either way. Maybe 10 minutes after that, my wife came into the kitchen and I showed her the sorry fate of our little fish. She put her hands on the outside of the bowl and after a few minutes, he turned over and swam away. We finally had a name for him: Lazarus.

To this day, I have no fundamental understanding of Reiki and don't have the time or inclination to go through Reiki training so I can become better informed. Some practitioners would say we cannot draw any firms conclusions from a sample size limited to three cases. By the normal standards of evidence, this is absolutely correct. I would propose, however, that mainstream providers need to stretch out of their comfort zone enough to consider that there are approaches that have value that may not have been studied adequately. Each option needs to be considered individually. Of the hundreds and thousands of mainstream and alternative options for the hundreds and thousands of health conditions, some are spectacularly worthwhile (like exercise and an optimal diet) and many are completely worthless. The worthwhile options are not limited to those that have been rigorously studied.

Digestive Enzymes

I have alluded to the fact that gastrointestinal health is, in my opinion, the area where mainstream medicine seems to have lost its way. As my understanding of gastrointestinal health has broadened, I have seen dramatic benefits for many patients who would otherwise languish. Consider the following cases.

I remember seeing a woman who had watery diarrhea every day for 10 years. By a strange coincidence, Pam had worked in the office of a gastroenterologist for much of that time. She had the $10,000 work-up—including labs, colonoscopy and CT scans—and tried every medication available.

I had seen her several times for other issues and, at the end of the visit, she would typically bring up her chronic diarrhea. On some level she had accepted the problem, but the symptoms had too much impact on her quality of life to be completely ignored. At one visit, I recommended she take a digestive enzyme supplement twice a day before meals. I did not think it would make much of a difference, but I had seen a number of people benefit from the supplement, so I figured it was worth a try.

About three months later, Pam came in for a sinus infection. At the end of the visit, I asked her how her bowels were doing. She responded casually, "Oh, that's all cleared up." She went from two digestive enzymes per day to one per day and the chronic diarrhea was essentially resolved. I was only hoping for some small benefit to improve her quality of life. I still don't know the underlying cause for her chronic bowel problems, but she probably could see the top 10 gastroenterologists on the planet and not get a definitive diagnosis. In this case, the best we could do was to improve her symptoms. For her, that was a lot.

It is worth noting that not all supplements are created equal. I have had patients find one digestive enzyme to be ineffective only to find another, like Digest Gold, that leads to dramatic improvements. This happens often with probiotics as well. Culturelle and Align are the most popular probiotics in terms of sales, but have a relatively small quantity of good bacteria with minimal variety of bacterial subtypes. To fail either of these does not mean that probiotics in general would be ineffective for a particular individual for a particular health issue.

Food Intolerances

If digestive enzymes are ineffective, I typically recommend an elimination diet. Many people have an intolerance or a sensitivity to one or more food types. This is absolutely lost on mainstream medicine where doctors tend to be overly reliant on standard testing. (If the trained physician or nurse practitioner can't verify an issue with testing, then often it "doesn't exist.") For many patients, I have found food intolerances to be the underlying cause of excessive heartburn, burping, gas, bloating and unexplained chronic bowel symptoms.

The Big Four may be wheat, gluten, soy and dairy, but there are many food types and individual foods that can cause health problems. One of my priorities is to make things are simple as possible. People have busy lives. It is a lot for an adult working full-time with three young children to buy a book, read it, absorb the book's material and put its recommendations into practice. I imagine Mr. or Mrs. So and So, passed out at 9:45 p.m., only half way through the introduction of the book in their lap. Anything I can do to distill the information down to its essential elements will make a tremendous difference in terms of adherence. Elimination diets, which have been around for a while, can be cumbersome, but there are different ways to accomplish the same end result.

Gluten, in particular, has received a lot of attention in the past few years. There are those that think this is a fad, but I disagree. The growing number of Americans with gluten intolerance is a reflection of a real problem with our food supply.

Gluten is the protein in wheat, oats, barley, rye and spelt which makes bread dough sticky and gives soy sauce, ketchup, and ice cream their consistency. The symptoms of a gluten allergy can be blamed on any number of ailments and a less intense gluten sensitivity will often go undiagnosed for far too long. A blood test or intestinal biopsy can diagnose a gluten allergy, but a gluten sensitivity is a distinct form of celiac in both impact and mechanism. A sensitivity may lead to headaches, muscle and joint weakness, skin problems, brain fog and possibly even depression. First of all, the response to gluten alters the gut lining, irritating the cells until they become more permeable and let toxins escape from the digestive tract into the bloodstream. People with gluten sensitivity have a hard time breaking down the large molecules that then enter the bloodstream undigested. These molecules are identified by the immune system as invaders and elicit an immune response from the white blood cells. This chain of events began with the simple decision to eat pizza, or even a healthy sandwich, and ended, after a series of disrupted processes, with external signs and symptoms.

Just to keep things as complicated as possible, there is a new grouping of foods that may prove to be the more definitive culprit for health problems. It can often be difficult to sort out carbohydrate-related food sensitivities and intolerances. The person who stops bread, crackers and pasta may feel better because they have taken wheat, gluten, yeast, hops or sugar out of their diet. Some researchers are focusing on a group of foods with the clunky acronym FODMAPS. This stands for fermentable oligo-, di-, mono-saccharides and polyols, which are poorly absorbed short-chain carbs found in wheat, rye and other grains. FODMAPS are found in other foods, including asparagus, celery, watermelon, milk, onions, garlic, apples and many other seemingly healthy foods. More precise testing would help patients focus more easily on which foods to avoid.

Elimination Diets

The elimination diet can be accomplished either by stripping the diet down and then adding food types back one-by-one, or by eliminating food types one at a time and monitoring for changes. In the first option, going to the Paleo diet often works well. The parents of my patient Noah decided the Paleo diet was a good option after I talked about trying to avoid the Big Four. (Noah's case will be described a little later.) The Paleolithic diet attempts to recreate the way cavemen ate a million years ago. The diet primarily includes fish, grass-fed beef, eggs, and fruits and vegetables. It gives people a specific framework and if they follow the diet, they will automatically be avoiding the Big Four (trademark pending). Typically, within a week or two the person will have a sense if they feel better. If so, they can then reintroduce foods to try and identify the culprit.

In the other approach, I recommend avoiding the food types for at least two weeks each to see if there is improvement. For those with food intolerances or sensitivities, they will almost never test positive by the standard methods. Some of these people will have seen specialists and had RAST panels, allergy scratch testing, anti-endomesial labs or even colonoscopy.

I have found a newer test that may reliably diagnose food sensitivities. It is called Mediator Release Testing (MRT). The process I went through to evaluate the validity of the test offers some insights into the barriers to achieving a collaborative approach to health and wellness and shows us the inherent conflict between mainstream MDs and alternative providers. I read as much as I could find about the MRT testing, because in addition to finding simple options for people, I try to recommend options that are relatively inexpensive for the patient, especially if the test or the treatment options aren't likely to be covered by health insurance.

According to what I read, MRT testing seems like a relatively simple, reliable way to diagnose food sensitivities. It avoids cumbersome or radical dietary changes while offering the person a chance to clarify the dietary cause or causes for their chronic bowel symptoms. It also tests for chemicals added to food, which is a bonus. The test was developed by Oxford Labs in Florida, but I found a wellness center relatively close to me (in Stow, Massachusetts) where they draw blood for the test and have providers to interpret the results.

I made contact with the Certified LEAP Therapist (CLT) at the wellness center, a Licensed Dietician/Nutritionist (LDN) and a Licensed Acupuncturist. He emailed back that he had been using the MRT test for five years, since 2008. He gave me a basic review of the test and said a person could have "tremendous changes" in as short a period of time as two weeks. This CLT said it was particularly useful for those with Crohn's disease, migraines, fibromyalgia, asthma and allergies.

Now for me, at this point in my medical career, knowing what I think I know, it would not surprise me if food sensitivities played a major role in all of those conditions and more. My inclination is to refer people for the MRT test. I asked about pricing and that one stung a bit. For patients with Blue Cross/Blue Shield, the MRT testing was mostly covered and the cost to the patient would be $295. For other insurances, however, there was no coverage; the person would have to pay out-of-pocket for the full evaluation package with consultation visits, $795. That level of cost is prohibitive for many patients, especially since I can only give them my general sense that I think the test is probably of value. I will need a few patients with sufficient resources to take the plunge so I can get a better sense of MRT's worth.

Stan and IBS

The IBS diagnosis is a catchall for many different underlying processes within the gastrointestinal system. Stress is a common element in a vast array of acute and chronic medical problems. For those with IBS, more often than not, the patient will have symptoms flare up or worsen with stress.

Stress associated with IBS and inflammatory bowel disease (Ulcerative colitis, Crohn's disease) has been long known but a mechanism had not been determined definitely. In the same issue of Gut, investigators showed that the stress hormone corticotropin-releasing hormone (CRH) regulates intestinal permeability (leaky gut) through mast cells. The investigators even identified specific receptors on mast cells. This new information sheds light on the possible link of leaky gut and mast cells with IBS, IBD and celiac disease; since stress can increase mast cells in the bowel and these cells can release mediators that cause gut injury and symptoms, stress reduction [is] important.[6]

I remember well a 68-year-old, Stan, who came to me as a new patient a few years ago. He had a white beard, neatly trimmed. He was chatty and seemed very positive. I would come to find later that he always wore the same red baseball cap with the name of some financial company on it.

You can tell a lot by what a person wears. It gives insight into their personality, their interests and background, and people are just begging to share information about themselves for a wide variety of reasons. The person with a 26.2 sticker on their car wants to make it absolutely clear to as many people as possible that she ran a marathon. This subtle advertising is preferred. No one wants to come across as egocentric. Thus, you will probably never see a sticker that says, "I run marathons, how about you?" In New England, a commonly viewed bumper sticker is "Mad River Glen, Ski It If You Can" which, of course, means that the driver of the Jeep Wrangler can. There is a new sticker meant as a retort that says "No One Cares if you can Ski Mad River." More subtle than that is the "MV" sticker strategically placed on the back window of the car so as many people see it as possible. MV = Martha's Vineyard. They have a second house on the island, in case you were wondering.

Stan was likely proud of the fact that he had been in finance, now retired. He also may have been trying to cover up his thinning hair. Perhaps he was tight with his finances and couldn't afford to buy another hat. Maybe he was physically insecure and felt more comfortable covered up. (He often kept his coat on during the visit as we talked.)

The primary thing Stan wanted to talk about at that first visit was his bowels. He had chronic bloating, abdominal discomfort and loose stools going back most of his adult life. On his own, a number of years before at the recommendation of a friend, he had gone off gluten. He said within a few weeks he felt better than he had for many years. His bowel issues improved and he had less fatigue and greater mental clarity. He stayed off gluten for over a year and was doing reasonably well.

For some reason, at that point, he was referred to the head of a gastro-enterology department at a major teaching hospital in Boston. Some well-intentioned relative probably convinced him to see the best of the best. He saw the specialist and had further testing. They checked him out with just about every test available to the modern MD in an effort to explain his bowel symptoms. As part of the work-up, he was checked for gluten problems. His blood tests for celiac disease were normal. The specialist told him unequivocally that gluten was not his problem. Incredibly, Stan took his advice and went back to eating gluten.

By the time he came in to see me, Stan was back to feeling tired and bloated with loose stools. There are many lessons to be learned by this scenario. Most people think that the head of gastroenterology at a well-regarded medical facility is automatically the best source of information for all situations. The physician at the top of the food chain has a lot of ego invested in their exalted position and it is even more difficult for this person to acknowledge they don't have all the answers. *Newsflash: no one has all of the answers and everyone has limitations to their knowledge and experience.*

"What should I do now?" Stan asked me at our initial visit. I thought, Gee, I don't know… Stop consuming gluten might make sense! But, in an effort to be respectful and make a good first impression, I played it cool. After a thoughtful pause, I said, "Maybe you should once again eliminate gluten from your diet." He did and his health is once again much improved.

Noah

There is a family of five that I see in the office, the Tilton Family. The oldest son, Noah, is extremely polite and well-mannered like the rest of his family. He is thoughtful and mature in the ways of life that matter most. As with many healthy people, I would typically only see him for annual well visits and for the occasional cough, cold or sore throat. In August of 2012, however, he came in complaining of two weeks of gastrointestinal symptoms. Each day was a little different. He experienced ongoing nausea, but also had episodes of vomiting with frequent belching, excessive gas and some abdominal pain.

Noah couldn't really be specific about times of day when the symptoms were worse. He sometimes didn't feel well in the morning on an empty stomach. He could feel nauseous after eating as well. A vague history like this is often frustrating to doctors. There can be an unreasonable expectation that the person should be taking notes every day to give a perfect history. Any doctor only need have a medical problem for more than a few days to realize how difficult it is to piece together a reliable history.

On review of systems, Noah was having soft, formed stools. He did not have diarrhea, fevers, headaches, rashes or other symptoms, except some mild fatigue. He had not been on recent antibiotics. There was no recent travel or camping or exposure to well water. There had been no changes to his basic healthy kid diet. In terms of family history, his younger sister had problems with cow's milk that seemed to clear up by the time she was three. My recommendation was that Noah avoid milk and dairy for at least five days. After that, if things didn't improve significantly, my plan was to start a probiotic.

The mom called to report some improvement, but Noah still had symptoms plus worsening fatigue, weight loss and some behavioral changes. His normal outgoing personality had changed and he was more quiet and subdued. He would often tell his parents that he just wanted to go to bed or lie down. The parents asked me about seeing a specialist.

When Noah saw the pediatric gastroenterology specialist, things were the same overall or maybe worse. Noah was also experiencing muscle aches, joint pains and now diarrhea once or twice per week. He had lost 10 pounds. The specialist noted a rash with small red bumps and redness to the trunk, upper extremities and the areas around the nose. She noted in her assessment and plan that she was concerned that there may be some underlying medical issue that was contributing to his multiple symptoms. She ordered a wide range of laboratory studies and started Noah on twice-a-day omeprazole to suppress acid in the stomach.

The lab tests—including complete blood count, complete metabolic profile, thyroid panel, celiac test and tests for inflammation—were normal, so the specialist ordered a colonoscopy and an upper GI study (where the person drinks a radiopaque liquid and then has a series of x-rays to visualize the esophagus, stomach and sometimes the small intestine). These tests were normal as well.

I saw Noah and his parents for a follow-up visit after that and discussed with them that a food sensitivity or intolerance would not always show up in standard testing. This was an issue we had touched upon before and they were receptive. They really did not want their son on long-term prescription medication if it could be avoided. I was diplomatic, but confessed that acid suppression didn't necessarily make sense to me for Noah's collection of symptoms. We talked about Noah going on an elimination diet, so they started the Paleo diet as a project for the whole family (no soy, gluten, wheat or cow's milk).

Within five days of changing his diet, Noah started to improve. By three weeks, his symptoms were nearly completely resolved. His personality returned to normal. He had more energy and a better appetite. His mother said it was "night and day." The skin changes were lingering but steadily improving as well. The plan, at that point, was to reintroduce the foods one-at-a-time to clarify which ones were making him sick. His parents gave him dairy and, within 24 hours, his symptoms returned. They eliminated it again and Noah improved. After a week, they reintroduced whole grains and Noah's gastrointestinal symptoms came back, but they were milder than before.

The pediatric gastroenterologist did not accept food intolerances as the cause for Noah's symptoms. She was convinced the prescription medication was the reason for any improvement. Yet, the family came to find that Noah could not tolerate cow's milk or gluten. The plan going forward was to avoid those food types as much possible and reintroduce them occasionally, maybe every 3-6 months.

After the initial period of improvement, Noah's health once again started to decline. He had fatigue and bloating and light stools. His parents were worried and brought him in for a follow-up. Light stools can be a sign of a liver problem, so I ordered laboratory tests including a liver panel. All of the tests came back negative. It turned out they had taken him off his probiotic supplement, which I hoped was the reason for the return of some of his symptoms. He went back on the probiotic, but things did not improve much.

About a month later, I saw Noah's youngest sister for her 12-month well visit. His sister was vigorous and healthy with no issues. I asked how Noah was doing. The dad said that he was doing great. I was relieved to hear it and assumed that the probiotic had, in time, regulated his system. The father went on to say that their family had a strong faith and thought the Lord had healed him. Apparently, Noah was about the same up until two days before the family came in for the sister's well visit. He had gone to Easter services at church and, during the blessing, he abruptly felt better. After the services, the parents noticed that Noah looked hale and alert. Noah said that God had gotten him better and he was back to normal. I didn't care where the wellness came from—traditional or alternative medicine, physical or spiritual means—as long as Noah was well, that was all that mattered.

I didn't see Noah in the office for over six months after that, but then, in the early part of 2014, I was on call over a weekend. I got paged from the Tiltons. I talked to Noah's parents on the phone and they said Noah wasn't doing well. He had an upset stomach and was going to the bathroom all the time to urinate. Over the past couple of months he had grown progressively more lethargic and experienced steady weight loss. The mom said he "looked like a skeleton." I recommended they take him to an Emergency Department for evaluation. The first set of blood tests showed signs of severe dehydration and a blood sugar over 500. The high sugars had overwhelmed his kidneys causing frequent urination so his body could purge the excessive glucose. He had developed autoimmune type 1 diabetes.

They saw a group of pediatric endocrinology specialists and went through the process of intensive education in the areas of carbohydrate counting and insulin requirements. By the time Noah came in to see me for a follow-up visit, his health had improved, but everyone in the family seemed a bit shell-shocked. He required multiple insulin injections per day with frequent blood sugar checks to avoid the high and low sugar numbers. It seems clear to me that his long course of gastrointestinal problems was the precursor to his autoimmune diagnosis. If we had a more sophisticated understanding of the interplay between the gastrointestinal system and his immune system, we may have been able to prevent Noah's diabetes.

Jon

Forty-one-year-old Jon has experienced many years of gastrointestinal symptoms. Married, with a son and daughter, he works as an assistant principal at a school. He does not smoke or drink. His diet is reasonably health. His wife is a nurse and she keeps him on the straight and narrow as well as she can. He's a guy, though, so this is not always easy for her.

Jon has esophageal reflux and has been on the acid blocker omeprazole for many years. The degree of reflux, as with many people, is out of proportion to his lifestyle. If a person is a 280-pound smoker, drinking six cups of coffee per day and having pepperoni pizza for dinner, it's obvious why that person has acid reflux. Most doctors, though, have no easy explanation for why a person with no discernible lifestyle factors would have regular symptoms requiring daily pharmaceutical therapy.

Jon has also been diagnosed with the old favorite IBS as well as a relatively rare condition called cyclic vomiting syndrome. Modern medicine is excellent at coming up with terms for various collections of symptoms, but not always as good at figuring them out. Jon would get flare-ups that lasted from a few days to a few weeks where he would vomit first thing in the morning and then have persistent nausea during most of the day. He would have a lot of burping and sometimes soft stools. He would also have bright red bleeding occasionally.

Jon has been followed by gastroenterology specialists for most of his adult life and has had several upper endoscopy procedures (where, under sedation, a fiber optic scope is guided down the esophagus and into the stomach). His scopes have shown inflammation of his esophagus and small intestine, namely esophagitis and duodenitis. He has had an anoscopy procedure by a colon and rectal specialist (where a small scope is inserted into the anus to visualize the rectal tissue) and a full colonoscopy.

We could say Jon's case is a great success because he has received a high level of care from well-trained and dedicated individuals using the most up-to-date modes of testing and evaluation. Cancer has been ruled out. He is on medication that, to some extent, controls his reflux symptoms even though it has been more difficult to control his flare-ups of nausea and vomiting. If the advertisements are to be believed, the strong acid blocker is significantly reducing his risk of esophageal cancer. He is able to work and has a relatively high quality of life. He skis at Stowe a few times every winter.

We could also say that the medical community has failed him. We could say that the doctors that see him have no real understanding of what is going on with him. Instead, he has been medicated in place of any real solution. It is the illusion of success. There is something fundamentally wrong with his gastrointestinal system and he needs a different approach if he is to be truly well.

Dan

Dan, a 12-year-old I see in the office, is one of the all-time characters. He and his twin brother, Eddie, loved Power Rangers and Star Wars when they were young. They would watch reruns on TV Land of the old *Emergency* show with Gage and DeSoto. They have grown up since then and now watch *The Jeffersons* and *All in the Family*. Dan and his brother are as different as fraternal twins can be. They are at opposite ends of the growth curve, for one thing. Eddie, the tallest boy in his class, is filled out. Dan is short and wiry. Eddie will eat just about anything, including olives, radishes and Brussels sprouts. Dan eats chicken fingers with Red Hot sauce, pizza, and occasionally a roasted carrot if he's in the mood.

The brothers started seeing me around the time they were six years old. By that time, Dan had suffered chronic constipation for several years. He would have a bowel movement about once every four or five days. He had already been working with pediatric gastroenterologists. If he took a strong prescription laxative, like Miralax, the bowel would be softer and slightly more frequent, but nothing would enable the desired soft, daily bowel movements. After years of seeing him, on a whim I recommended that his mom start him on a probiotic. She called two weeks later to say his bowels had almost completely normalized. He still has a limited diet but, amazingly, his chronic intractable constipation had mostly resolved with a simple, twice-a-day children's probiotic.

The picky eater is typically viewed as an annoying kid, maybe spoiled, but definitely a behavioral problem. Many, if not most, kids who are picky eaters are not spoiled or difficult, they have Sensory Integration Dysfunction. Kids that are "tactile defensive"(react to tags against their neck or don't like certain fabrics for pants) often can't deal with certain textures or smells of foods. If you see a picky eater offered a food and they are repulsed to the verge of retching, that is probably a sensory issue. Asking them to eat a slice of tomato is like asking a regular person to eat an earthworm or a slug.

Gut and Bowel Health

In order to talk about true bowel health, we need to talk about the health of a person's internal microbial flora. I think it will become clearer over time that maintaining a proper balance of not only good bacteria but good viruses and good funguses is one of the most essential elements of long-term health and wellness. Many people have been working in this area for years. As with most medical breakthroughs, the mainstream world is only slowly coming around. I now see gastroenterologists recommending probiotics more often. They, like others, are beginning to recognize that the bowel plays an integral part in overall health and is not simply a closed system that should be micromanaged based only on whether the person has heartburn and regular bowel movements.

In an excellent article on this topic, "Gut Microbiome-Host Interactions in Health and Disease," James M. Kinross and co-authors note that scientists have "established the importance of the gut microbiome in the disease pathogenesis for numerous systemic disease states, such as obesity and cardiovascular disease, and in intestinal conditions, such as inflammatory bowel disease."[7] They note that each individual has his or her own microbiome which tends to remain relatively stable over time. In most mammals, the gut microbiome is dominated by four bacterial phyla that perform these tasks: Firmicutes, Bacteroidetes, Actinobacteria and Proteobacteria. They speculate that, with investigation, we could potentially identify an individual's "core microbiome" which could then be used as a reference point for the health of the person's internal flora at any given time. The current probiotic supplements may not have the quantity or the diversity of flora needed to have a maximum impact in terms of prevention and treatment. In the future, we may be able to develop individualized probiotics delivered either orally or rectally to the colon. In the final chapter, *The Path to Righteousness*, I will describe the optimal probiotic and give a prime candidate that meets those criteria.

A still more advanced approach would include a broader, more complete evaluation of the micro flora in the body. It would not be confined to bacteria only, but would include parasites, viruses, yeasts and fungi. The internal environment of microorganisms probably starts in utero and the gut is populated shortly after birth. Interaction with the mother introduces bacteria to the newborn, and breastfeeding provides nutrition not only for the baby but also for the developing microbiome. Breastfed babies have lower rates of gastroenteritis, upper and lower respiratory tract infections, acute otitis media (ear infections), urinary tract infections, and other more serious systemic infections. In some instances, breastfed infants develop fewer symptoms to the same microbe that would cause disease in the bottle-fed infant.

A study came out in January 2013 on the use of "fecal implants" to help cure a person of Clostridium Difficile colitis.[8] This condition, nicknamed C. Diff, is the poster child for the negative impact of oral or intravenous antibiotics. Some individuals that go on antibiotics for a bacterial infection (or more often a presumed bacterial infection) will have their good flora wiped out so effectively that the medication will actually cause a secondary bacterial infection. The analogy I will use with patients is a scenario where all of the predators in Sub-Saharan Africa except lions are wiped out in an instant. The lions would then have no competition for prey. Their numbers would increase over a few generations. Research has shown that bacteria can double their population in about 10 minutes. This is how a pathogenic bacteria like C. Diff can quickly multiply causing an infection in the colon.

Any disruption to the development of a "normal" diverse microbiome could contribute to the development of acute or chronic medical issues.

This would include antibiotics and steroids, but there are other potential scenarios that may have a more profound influence. For years, some have believed that the excessive use of antibacterial soaps and detergents interferes with our natural immunity. The "hygiene hypothesis" proposes that excessive hygiene has increased our susceptibility to allergic diseases by suppressing the natural development of the immune system. This potentially explains, at least in part, the increased rates of allergies, asthma, eczema and even possibly autism. This also suggests that a reduction in microbial exposure as a result of improved health measures has contributed to an immunological imbalance in the intestine, and has increased the incidence of autoimmune diseases such as Inflammatory Bowel Disease. *The Autoimmune Epidemic* a book by Donna Nazakawa that will be reviewed in more detail later, refutes the hygiene hypothesis. The author believes the problem lies in the opposite scenario: our poor immune systems are being bombarded with so many foreign toxins, chemicals and drugs that they are, if anything, overstimulated and overexposed.

Diets

Every week a new diet comes out. We hear that carbs are the work of the devil one day and that carbs are essential for us another. Protein is all the rage now, even though Americans consume more animal protein than the inhabitants of almost any other country on Earth, except for the beef-crazy Argentinians. Today's marketing gurus are adding the word "protein" to the covers and boxes of as many food items as possible because research suggests this will increase sales. Atkins was all the rage for a while. Then it was South Beach. These books sell millions of copies because everyone is trying desperately to find that one diet that is right for all.

A couple of years ago, my friend's wife introduced me to the book *Integrative Nutrition* by Joshua Rosenthal. This was a breakthrough in many ways. It was the best reference I had come across, to that point, linking diet to a person's day-to-day health. Many people have irritability, body aches, headaches and fatigue related to the foods they are eating. This gets little or no attention in conventional medicine, leaving the average person with no insight into why he or she can feel so different from day to day. The book also introduced the idea that there is no optimal diet for all people.

Human beings are an incredibly diverse group with countless variations in genetics, ethnicity, culture, geography, etc. Some people respond well to the basic tenets of healthy eating: balanced diet with limited carbohydrates, whole grains, lots of fruits and vegetables and minimal processed foods. For others, though, this basic approach to nutrition and diet just does not work.

Everyone knows people that eat and eat, never exercise and stay thin. Unfortunately, there are more people that eat very little, are heavy and gain weight. Some would say all of these overweight people are just lying—they have cream puffs and ring dings hidden under their beds and they don't really only eat one meal per day. Sure, there are people that eat terribly and are obese as a result. I believe many others are working against a stacked deck.

In a special edition of *Scientific American* in September of 2013, there were a number of articles about food. In an article entitled "Everything You Know About Calories Is Wrong," author Rob Dunn outlined a number of major fallacies when it comes to the calorie = weight idea:

To accurately calculate the total calories that someone gets out of a given food, you would have to take into account a dizzying array of factors, including whether that food has evolved to survive digestion; how boiling, baking, microwaving or flambéing a food changes its structure and chemistry; how much energy the body expends to break down different kinds of food; and the extent to which the billions of bacteria in the gut aid human digestion and, conversely, steal some calories for themselves.[9]

Dunn notes that "protein may require as much as five times more energy to digest as fats," which supports a protein-rich diet for weight loss. The article emphasized the great variation among people, noting that, to truly help someone lose weight, we need to understand as much as we can about an individual's physiology.

In humans, two phyla of bacteria, Bacteriodes and Firmicutes, dominate the gut. Researchers have found that obese people have more Firmicutes in their intestines and have proposed that some people are obese, in part, because the extra bacteria make them more efficient at metabolizing food: so instead of being lost as waste, more nutrients make their way into the circulation and, if they go unused, get stored as fat.[9]

A more precise explanation of why the simple calories in, calories out equation doesn't work well for the general population is described very well in another article in the September 2013 *Scientific American*. The article distinguishes between two paradigms: *energy imbalance* where the only way to lose weight is to eat fewer calories and expend more calories, and *hormonal imbalance*. The latter "focuses on the complex physiology of the fat cells. Consuming carbohydrates raises levels of sugar (glucose) in the blood which, in turn, activates the release of the hormone insulin. Fat cells respond to insulin by holding on to their fat stores and even adding to them.[10]" The article notes that high fructose corn syrup in particular may lead to insulin resistance. I will expand on these ideas in the final chapter, "The Path to Righteousness." We may find that the notion of overeating causing obesity and then contributing to insulin resistance is fundamentally flawed.

The Plan and the Role of Inflammation

Lyn-Genet Recitas' book *The Plan* may explain why millions of people are overweight beyond even the hormonal imbalance concept. The revolutionary idea presented is that the majority of adults, especially those over 35 years old, have three or four or more food sensitivities that are causing internal reactivity and inflammation. Many people are eating foods they think are healthy for them but that are actually causing them to be obese. Some of the most common foods that cause trouble are oatmeal, turkey, tomato sauce, salmon and asparagus. Recitas takes the reader through a 20-day plan to try and identify the foods that are wrong for them. She states plainly that people can eat 1,200 calories per day of the wrong foods and gain weight or over 2,000 calories of the right foods and lose weight. This, for most with weight problems, would be a dream come true. If *The Plan* is right, then people just need to find the right diet for themselves as individuals and they will lose weight.

The author states her approach very clearly from the start: "There is no such thing as healthy. There is only what works for *your* body." The wrong foods cause an inflammatory response in the body that results in bothersome symptoms and ongoing health problems. There is also a compounding effect, where the tissues become more and more reactive with each exposure to the wrong food or other environmental trigger. She says that poor hydration and excessive sodium intake exacerbate the inflammatory response.

Recitas maintains that eating the foods wrong for any given individual can cause unexplained fatigue, arthritis, anxiety, depression, eczema, infertility and many other health problems. She also estimates that 80 percent of the women she sees do not have a normally-functioning thyroid gland. The author gives an unconventional approach to evaluating and improving thyroid function. I also think thyroid disorders are undermanaged and this will be addressed later in the context of David Brownstein's books.

My instincts tell me that *The Plan* is groundbreaking material that could have a major impact on health and wellness in America. It is possible, however, that even if Recitas is right on with her approach, most healthcare providers will dismiss the potential benefits and her book will disappear amongst the thousands of self-help books that come out each year.

Inflammation from the foods we eat is a relatively new concept and it will take some time before it is widely accepted. Gemma, one of my favorite patients, came in to a follow-up visit to discuss her asthma and chronic sinus problems. She was using inhaled steroids every day and needed an antibiotic every few months for sinus infections. I talked to her about the potential that something in her diet—dairy or wheat, perhaps—was contributing to her health problems. She brought it up to her pulmonologist and he scoffed. "No way," he told her, "that comes up for maybe one person out of a hundred thousand."

The importance of inflammation in other forms of chronic illness is already well established. Inflammation is an element in the development of cardiovascular disease. Cardiovascular disease, represented by heart disease and strokes, is the greatest cause of mortality in industrialized countries. There is research that the benefits of statin medication are derived, at least in part, from their anti-inflammatory action.

Inflammation is significant in the development of cancer as well. There are blood tests, including the erythrocyte sedimentation rate (ESR) and the C-reactive protein (CRP), that measure inflammation in the body. These are non-specific tests as the levels can be elevated in many acute and chronic medical scenarios including an active infection and cancer.

The Coca Pulse Test

A personal exploration into food choices involved something called the Coca Pulse Test. The test was recommended to me by a patient's parent interested in holistic options. The premise is that a person's pulse will go up after eating foods of which they are allergic. This test was relatively simple to do, but I had no way of knowing if it had merit.

I brought a pulse oximeter home from work. That machine monitors the pulse as well as the oxygen saturation percentage. My son and I went through an exercise where we each ate five different foods to see how our pulse would react. The foods were: steak, broccoli, cow's milk, an apple and a biscuit. I was curious how it would go, especially since my son had some bowel problems potentially related to cow's milk and gluten.

I ate a small amount of each of the five food types and checked my pulse at baseline (before consumption), at 30 seconds, and again at a minute. There was no significant change to the pulse for any of them. I then tested my son. We started with steak and his pulse went up by 19 points after 30 seconds—quite a dramatic, unexpected result. I waited for his pulse to come down and then tried broccoli. This time, his pulse went up 32 points after 30 seconds! I waited a few minutes for him to equilibrate and then had him eat the last three food types. With each of these there was no appreciable change to his pulse. I then wondered if the pulse response to steak had something to do with it being the first thing he ate. Maybe he was just hungry. I did the steak test again and his pulse response was exactly the same, going up by 19 points at 30 seconds.

This is pseudoscience at its best. Something seemed to happen during the Coca Pulse test, but I really don't know what to do with the information. I am skeptical that the rise in pulse correlates with a true food allergy. With no hope for answers through double-blind studies, we can only do our best and interpret results with caution.

Conclusion

In the end, all roads seem to lead to something like a Paleo Diet. There is variation among people, but Paleo is the most likely candidate for an optimal diet. The Gray Sheet was a sheet summarizing the dietary recommendations of Overeaters Anonymous (OA). It was developed in the 1960s and centered on the total elimination of all man-made sugars and starches with the idea that such foods cause people to crave carbohydrates more and more. The person becomes obese, fundamentally changing their internal physiology. This increase in adipose, or fat tissue, feeds the downward spiral.

The Atkins Diet and then the South Beach Diet focused on similar themes. Recitas' book *The Plan* would likely lead most people away from carbohydrates. *Wheat Belly*, developed by the cardiologist William Davis, MD, narrows the focus even further, indicting American wheat specifically as the root of all dietary evils. Even the alternative nutritionist I send people to, who has had major successes more often than not, will recommend a dietary overhaul taking the same foods and food types out of peoples' diets. There is no telling how great an impact there could be for Americans if Paleo/ Wheat Belly/Gray Sheet diets were incorporated. It is probable that the rates of obesity, diabetes, high cholesterol, sleep apnea and the associated cardiovascular risk would plummet.

These may be the best options, in escalating level of difficulty:

1. Cut out wheat and then dairy, or vice versa.
2. Cut out both wheat and dairy.
3. No flour, no sugar.
4. Do an elimination diet either by removing one food type at a time for at least two weeks each or by stripping down to a basic diet and adding them back every two weeks or so.
5. Follow "The Plan" as described in the book of the same name.
6. Gradually transition to Paleo with no processed foods also avoiding the low quality gluten-free carbohydrates.

With all of these options, however, a person still needs to find a dietary approach that works for them individually and one that they can stay with over long periods of time. To never have a piece of chocolate cake or a slice of pizza for the rest of our lives would be difficult. For some, doing no flour and no sugar two meals a day and low carb for the third meal with occasional indiscretion may be the best plan of all.

2

The Power of the Mind

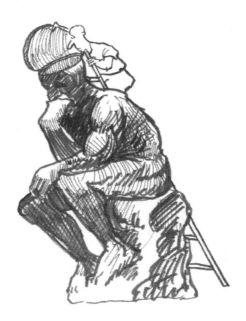

The most common mental health issues in the United States are insomnia, depression and anxiety. There is, of course, a spectrum when it comes to mental health, and most people have brief periods of time in their lives when they are depressed or anxious or cannot sleep. Psychiatrists tend to manage the more complicated psychiatric conditions like bipolar disorder and schizophrenia, but psychiatrists are in relatively short supply so most of these issues are managed by primary care physicians.

Mental health issues impact both children and adults, but pediatric mental health issues are often more complex because it can be difficult to figure out a patient unable to provide a thorough history or give insights into their experience. There is a very telling case involving a now 7-year-old little boy named Henry. His family tried conventional medicine, non-traditional options and just about everything in between. Trying to help him and watching the lengths his parents went to pursuing various options was, in its own way, an advanced exercise in integrative medicine. They were determined to do anything and everything to help him. This is a common element that leads people both into and out of mainstream medicine to get answers.

Henry

From a young age, Henry started having behavioral outbursts. The emotional fits would come on quickly. There would be disagreement on some issue and, before long, he would be unreasonable. A typical episode would escalate until he and at least one parent were very upset. As Henry got older, the episodes became more intense. He could practically destroy a room in five minutes, throwing things, tipping over lamps, pushing over chairs. Standard parenting approaches didn't work. The situation was tearing the family apart.

His older sister—often an innocent bystander swept up in the turmoil—was also affected. She started to have problems sleeping at one point and her teachers commented that she seemed distracted and upset at school. We must always remember the collateral effects of an individual's health issues on those around them, especially other family members.

As an experienced family physician, I found myself completely lost trying to understand what was happening with Henry. Technically, he met criteria for Oppositional Defiant Disorder (ODD), but there was much more to it than that. ODD, in itself, is classic for modern medicine. We have a label for almost everything as if being able to name something somehow gives us a deeper understanding of it.

The first child psychologist Henry's parents saw recommended a reward system. The mom set up a chart and tracked good behaviors with incentives. That did not work. The second psychologist watched Henry at his pre-school to try and find clues to what would set off these largely unpredictable outbursts. She could find no pattern. A parenting expert made standard recommendations about consistency, etc. It was another dead end.

The third psychologist went over the Standard Parenting Model once again. This model is embedded in most or all of the world's cultures. In this approach, the parent is the boss and the child is the subordinate. The parents must be firm and consistent. There is no room for negotiation or collaboration. The model assumes that a child will always look for ways to manipulate the parents if given the chance. Henry's parents were already familiar with these ideas and had done their best to be firm and consistent. It hadn't worked to that point, but after meeting with this child behavior expert, Henry's mom and dad made an effort to ramp it up a bit. This ended up having the opposite effect. The more inflexible they were, the more frequent and intense were Henry's emotional storms.

The first breakthrough for the family was finding the book *The Explosive Child*[11] by Ross Greene. Henry's dad talked about reading it and being blown away because it described Henry so well. On some level, Henry's parents felt like they were the only ones dealing with their issue. It helped to know there were many other families going through the same ordeal. That first night, Henry's dad stayed up until 3 a.m. finishing the book and taking notes. He even sent an email to Ross Greene thanking him for his help. In the book, Dr. Greene advocates for triaging a child's issues and avoiding power struggles whenever possible. The parents have to decide which scenarios are non-negotiable, such as those involving safety. For example, if the child is going to run into traffic, you wouldn't calmly try to negotiate with him.

On the other end of the spectrum are issues so minor that the parent makes an effort to just ignore them and let it go. In the middle are the important issues that come up on a regular basis. Dr. Greene encourages parents to negotiate and collaborate with the child. Being rigid and inflexible with a rigid, inflexible child is like pouring gasoline on a fire. The parents thought the book was going to be a framework guiding them out of the chaos. It wasn't that simple. It helped them minimize the power struggles, but that only went so far since Henry still had to be out in the world interacting with other children and adults that had not adopted the approach of *The Explosive Child*.

The next person the family saw was a locally-renowned child psychologist with over 30 years of experience. The first time they saw him, he was lecturing on good parenting at a school in their town. Henry's mom and dad went to see him for a couple of visits. They brought up *The Explosive Child* and the psychologist said he was familiar with the book. It turned out that he really didn't apply many of the principles, though. He had his own opinions about how to manage these kids. The parents found that there is a profound difference between having a professional, detached involvement in some issue and actually living with it. To understand this is crucial for anyone dedicated to being an effective practitioner.

If someone comes to my office with chest pain, it may be obvious to me that they are not having a heart attack. If I can understand the person's perspective, though, they will be genuinely relieved when I tell them they are not having a heart attack. In Henry's case, several mental health professionals said they had read the book *The Explosive Child*. The parents were at first optimistic, believing this meant each professional would understand Henry's tendencies. It became clear each time, though, that while the providers may have read the book, they had not absorbed the material because they had no true life context for the information. It was an academic exercise rather than a personal quest.

With a confident manner, the third child psychologist described to the parents what they needed to do: "Go to a hardware store," he said, "and get a good lock." The mom reported this to me later. "Put the lock on his bedroom door," he continued. "Whenever he's having a fit, put him in the room and lock the door. Don't open the door unless you hear the sound of breaking glass." He told them it might take months and months, but eventually Henry would change his behaviors. It was like trying to break a wild horse.

It seemed cruel, but at the time Henry's parents were desperate enough to try almost anything. They stuffed him in his room one night during an episode but without the lock. The dad talked about holding the door with all of his might as Henry tried to get out. That first time, Henry nearly destroyed the room. He pulled all of the bedding from the bed. He threw the lamps on the floor ripping the lampshades. He tipped over a bureau.

This eminent psychologist also advised the staff at Henry's preschool. The teachers were told to drag him into a small room and close the door when he got upset. Henry would scratch his own face bloody. He would punch himself in the head repeatedly. The school could not handle him and asked him to leave. The strategy from this psychologist made things worse for months and it was a major setback in every way. It took some time before the family was able to get back to the normal level of chaos.

One of the lessons Henry's parents learned was never to rely 100 percent on any one person's opinion. People will misrepresent their expertise and degree of success if they are being paid for their opinion and especially if you are paying out of pocket. People can have strong egos. For even the most highly-qualified professional, there is a limit to their knowledge and experience, though many are unwilling to acknowledge this. I will often tell people that I am only giving my opinion based on my current level of knowledge and experience. I have changed my thinking on many issues over the years. I often will have some sense that they are becoming confident in me as I am talking to them. My ego is grateful, but I don't want them to ever trust anyone's opinion completely, including my own.

Around the same time I was seeing Henry and his family, I was seeing another family in the office where the mom and the dad were engineers. They must have sensed I was open-minded, because at some point they started telling me about an alternative health practitioner they were working with named Gloria. They said that three of their four children had developed Lyme disease. They lived next to a wooded area, had dogs, and all had many tick exposures. The children could not be helped by mainstream physicians who refused to accept the possibility of Lyme disease as a cause for their chronic unexplained headaches, fatigue and joint pains.

The family ended up finding Gloria who worked with a lot of chronic Lyme patients. She had recommended a combination of supplements and antibiotics and, from the parents' perspective, the children all got better. Both parents were now believers. In my experience, engineers are often the most hardheaded, rational people when it comes to demanding proof. The fact that both parents were engineers led me to take their claims seriously. If the dad had been an energy healer and the mom an astrologist, it may have been more difficult to convince me.

By then, Henry was getting progressively more difficult at home. He fought his parents on just about every small task and transition. He resisted brushing his teeth, going to bed, getting up in the morning, putting on his clothes, eating breakfast, leaving the house, etc. Every day was one battle after another and it was tearing the family apart. At one of many follow-up visits, the mom said: "Just one day, that's all I ask. I pray all the time that he will cooperate for just one day. Is that too much to ask, for one day of peace?"

I was on the fence about whether to recommend the alternative provider to Henry's family, but then an episode clinched it for me. One of the sons in the engineers' family, Bud, came in to see me with a severe cough. During his visit, he had almost continuous paroxysms of coughing—in 15-plus years of seeing patients, possibly the worst I've seen. I suspected Bud had picked up pertussis. The pertussis infection has a melodramatic nickname, The Hundred Day Cough. Pertussis is typically very difficult to get under control. It can be extremely contagious and it has been estimated that ninety percent of vulnerable household contacts will get pertussis if exposed. Antibiotics are imperative because they decrease contagiousness, but they have only a minor impact on the symptoms. Most patients will be prescribed inhalers, codeine cough syrups, steroids and just about any other option with only limited benefit.

I put Bud on a standard antibiotic, Zithromax or azithromycin, and he didn't improve much. The cough was so bad he couldn't go to school. The family actually filmed his coughing fits and put it on *YouTube*. I really wasn't sure what to do, which is uncomfortable for any physician. The family contacted Gloria and she did her own evaluation. She recommended an antibiotic, Biaxin or clarithromycin, that was in the same class as the one I had already prescribed. Now, almost no doctor would prescribe a second antibiotic in the same class as the first; they would want to change course to, hopefully, get different coverage for other bacteria or to try and overcome the possibility of antibiotic resistance. I agreed to try the Biaxin and, bang, Bud started to get better. Within 4-5 days he was fine. In my clinical experience, this was a singularity, so I had to be impressed.

I discussed Bud's treatment (first traditional, then alternative) with Henry's parents and they eventually brought Henry to see Gloria for evaluation. In retrospect, it was a perfect storm of factors that brought me to refer the family to an alternative provider instead of another MD. It was a time when I was becoming more open to alternative approaches. I was desperate to help many patients, including Henry, who were not being helped by mainstream providers and, to the contrary, often were being harmed by their advice. I discovered I would need all of my open-mindedness to work with Gloria because her methods were far different from anything I had come across.

Henry went to see her and much of her evaluation focused on muscle testing. Most people have no experience with muscle testing, which falls under the area of Applied Kinesiology (AK). Apparently, it has to do with the merging of a body's energy field and the energy field of some other thing. Much of Gloria's testing focused on finding certain food types that were wrong for the individual. Muscle testing is controversial, of course, and most in the mainstream give it little or no credence. It would, for most people, be lumped in with shark cartilage and psychic readings as just another form of chicanery. An extensive discourse on the history of muscle testing can be found in David Hawkins' book *Power vs. Force* along with explanations of the underlying scientific principles. It is my guess that most of the people that trash this concept have not read this book.

Novak Djokovic, the number one tennis player in the world, presents a more compelling case for this testing. He was a good professional tennis player plugging along for years with some success. A story in the September 2013 issue of *Men's Fitness* magazine portrays him as "plagued by what other players saw as a lack of fitness, and worse, a lack of toughness." In 2010, Djokovic saw a holistic health provider, Igor Cetojevic, MD, in his home country of Serbia. Dr. Cetojevic did muscle testing that revealed certain food intolerances. Based on what "seemed like madness" at the time, the tennis player was told he was strongly intolerant of wheat and dairy, with a mild sensitivity to tomatoes as well. In the article, Djokovic is noted to have responded, "But Doctor, my parents own a pizza parlor!" Djokovic radically changed his diet based on these results. By his account, his health and energy level improved in a short time. Since then, he has risen to the number one world ranking with six Grand Slam singles titles.

Henry's dad described the experience with muscle testing at one of the follow-up visits. Gloria, the alternative provider, muscle tested the father first to show Henry that it was no big deal. She had Dad hold a series of foods in his lap and, with each one, reach his arm out to the side. They started with a box of Corn Flakes. Dad put his arm straight out and Gloria tried to push it down while he resisted. She went through five or six major food types, including wheat, eggs, cow's milk, soy and corn. Henry's dad tested "strong" on all of them.

She then took the testing a step further. She initiated "surrogate testing" where Henry would hold the food item in his lap and his father would stand next to him with his hand on Henry's shoulder. The dad would then put his opposite arm out to the side, which Gloria strength tested. The dad was essentially serving as a conduit for Henry, because kids don't always test predictably. On several food types, including gluten, cow's milk and salicylates, Henry (via his surrogate) tested as "weak." The dad said it had been easy to keep his arm rigid when Gloria tested him on those foods, but when Henry held them and the surrogate testing was done, so help him, he couldn't keep his arm up—the wispy, 60-year-old medical intuitive pushed it down easily.

Based on these tests, Henry's parents overhauled his entire diet. The mom drove five towns over to find a Whole Foods (a.k.a. "Whole Paycheck") grocery store and got high-end, gluten-free everything. They also took cow's milk out of Henry's diet. I think she spent about $500. Many people could never afford that bill, but at least they were lucky in that regard since the dad was an executive for a Fortune 500 company. At a visit with me, they reviewed the recommendations for changing Henry's diet. I had no idea what salicylate foods were, but they turned out to be a lot of fruits and vegetables, including apples. Henry usually had an apple at bedtime, so they nixed that too.

The parents were strict for a couple of months. Four-year-old Henry resisted the limitations of his diet at first, but then surprisingly got on board with what they were doing. He seemed to understand why it was important. On some level, he was frustrated and willing to make changes if they would help. Some changes were more difficult than others. Avoiding gluten, as anyone knows who has tried it, can be very difficult. The gluten-free rice pasta is reasonable, but the breads fall apart and are awful unless toasted.

Sadly, they didn't really see much improvement in Henry's behaviors. He would have good days and bad days, as before. It didn't seem to make any difference. We discussed the issue and I agreed that they should gradually add back many of the foods. Henry started eating gluten and cow's milk and apples once again and things were the same. Shortly after going back to a modified version with minimal gluten and no artificial colors or dyes (but otherwise "normal" diet), he seemed to be doing very well. For a few months his behaviors were better, but that just confused the parents more. They found that the most relevant thing from a dietary perspective was the simplest of all. Henry had to eat on a regular basis. One factor with the highest predictive value for outbursts was if he hadn't eaten enough. Some form of protein in the morning like eggs or turkey also seemed to help.

I have since sent a number of people to Gloria, the medical intuitive who did the muscle testing on Henry. I do believe that what she is doing is real and has a genuine impact on the health of many people. I tend to only send her the most challenging cases. These are people with a wide range of problems and I am hoping to find some systemic explanation rather than the more typical piecemeal approach where we manage each symptom or organ system independently. The majority of the people that work with her get better. Some people show dramatic improvement and within a month are almost completely well. Some people show slow, steady improvement over many months. A minority experience little or no lasting benefit. Like all of us, she has limitations.

I have seen dramatic improvements in the mental health of many other adult and pediatric patients after making changes to their diets. Some of these changes were recommended by me, some by Gloria, and others instituted by the patients themselves. Cases are peppered through the book that describe where the diet was the most important change the person made to transform their life from poor health to a more vigorous state of wellness.

After that evaluation, Henry saw a pediatric neurologist who really didn't provide any specific answers, but recommended a trial of a stimulant for Attention Deficit Disorder. Many kids with ADD will have impulse control issues. The medication really didn't seem to make any difference. Henry saw a pediatric psychiatrist who was unable to give him a specific diagnosis. These specialists with many years of experience could say what Henry didn't have but, amazingly, couldn't really pinpoint a specific issue.

Neuropsychological testing was recommended. This is a series of very intensive evaluations done by a psychologist specifically trained in the area. This testing measures a wide variety of cognitive and mental health domains that assess for cognitive deficits, learning disabilities, attention problems, anxiety, depression and other potential issues. The mom found one of the best psychologists in the area. It cost them over $3,000 out of pocket. Henry was on the low end of the Attention Deficit Disorder Spectrum with significant underlying anxiety especially in crowds and social situations.

The mom and dad were reading books and scouring the internet, searching for anything that might be contributing to Henry's behaviors. The parents got rid of all fragrances and airborne chemicals. They read that phthalates found in plastics could cause behavioral problems, so they got rid of all of their plastic kitchen paraphernalia and replaced it with glass. They put Henry on fish oil. They took him to an Aryuvedic doctor, Dr. Singh, who said to increase his physical exercise, massage him with a special oil every night before bed, give him different liquid vitamins and substitute homemade ghee for regular butter. They did all of those things and ten more that they couldn't remember, and Henry still had unpredictable outbursts.

Aryuveda is a branch of medicine from India going back over a thousand years. The dad said Dr. Singh spoke with supreme confidence, leaving no room for questions. I have learned to be skeptical of anyone who claims to have all the answers. Practitioners in the alternative world are not necessarily benevolent individuals working selflessly for the good of humankind. They are human beings with egos who want to make a good living the same as the Chief of Neurology at Cedar Sinai.

One thing that still surprises me is the expense of using alternative practitioners. Many charge $200 or higher per hour. This issue has contributed to Lyme practitioners being discounted by mainstream physicians. There are many doctors that have created practices solely to manage people with chronic Lyme disease. Chronic Lyme disease is controversial for many reasons and it does not help the cause when a Lyme doctor charges $2,000 for the initial 2-hour visit. That is the real charge for a provider in Manhattan. (Manhattan doesn't seem like a hotbed for Lyme disease. It's more of a hotbed for high living.) I don't begrudge these providers being paid well. If they are providing a unique high-quality service, they deserve compensation. People have to pay out of pocket for visits to most alternative providers, however, and the costs are often so prohibitive that I often cannot convince someone to go see them.

To further muddy the waters, it is common practice for alternative practitioners to recommend certain expensive vitamins or supplements and then, "Oh, what do you know, we just happen to have those exact items over here near the cash register. Suzie will help get what you need. Thank you." Cha-ching. Perhaps this conflict of interest is less important when people are in need of help.

Dr. Singh talked negatively about Henry with him sitting right in the room with his parents. His conclusion was that Henry had autism. He spoke with complete and utter self-confidence. He said a large part of Henry's problems stemmed from the fact that his mother had him at an advanced maternal age. It turns out that Henry's older brother, born 12 years earlier, was very similar when he was a young child. When the dad recounted that fact, Dr. Singh slowed his monologue for a few seconds, but then just started back up again as if the contradiction had never been uttered.

Dr. Singh charged Henry's parents $500 for the hour-and-a-half appointment, then recommended exercise, massage, Indian butter and $100 worth of vitamins that could be purchased from him right then. They took his advice that day, but it didn't make any difference as far as they could tell.

The family finally had a breakthrough after I referred them to a group of specialized occupational therapists at Project Chilld in Beverly, Massachusetts. Henry had an extremely thorough series of evaluations from the OT group, with screening just slightly less than the Apollo astronauts. It was clear, based on their objective findings, that Henry had Sensory Integration Dysfunction, specifically auditory processing and visual processing problems. Henry started intensive sessions with Project Chilld three days per week for over an hour each time. The parents started to see clear improvement in his attitude and behaviors. It helped with the daily battles over each transition.

Overall, several important elements helped Henry's family improve the behavioral health of their now 6-year-old. *The Explosive Child* book opened up new avenues for dealing with Henry in a more collaborative way. Aspects of the Standard Parenting Model also proved crucial. Today, Henry's parents have strict overall guidelines while allowing some daily flexibility.

Can you see how challenging it was to make an accurate diagnosis for Henry? Some said it was important to make a specific diagnosis for him so it would be easier to get treatment. Others said to avoid labels at all cost because they would impact how he was treated in the school system. A child with behavioral issues can be diagnosed with depression, anxiety or bipolar illness. Maybe the child sees a psychiatrist who has just seen three kids with bipolar and now hears that this new patient has erratic behavior. Before you know it, your child has been diagnosed with bipolar and medications are recommended.

A child can have learning disabilities that affect their success in school. We cannot get reliable histories from most young children, so it can be hard to figure out how efficiently they are learning. We also cannot easily remember how a child thinks, so adults impose their own tendencies on the child. Many will have sensory integration problems that interfere with their ability to process information in the brain. I have been in medicine in one capacity or another for about 20 years and still have limited understanding of sensory integration. The child psychiatrist was very honest and explained that he had minimal experience in this area. The child neurologist didn't even bring it up as a possible factor. The field of medicine is changing so rapidly it is hard for the most dedicated provider to keep up. There is no shame in even a specialist admitting there are developing fields that were not addressed during residency training 20 years prior. It is more important than ever for providers to be open-minded and honest about what they do not know.

The difficult child can have hearing problems that affect their focus and lead a parent to think he has Attention Deficit Disorder (ADD). ADD is controversial and, according to some, greatly over-diagnosed. Supporting this is the dramatic difference in the rate of diagnosis across the United States, with much higher percentages in the Northeast. Others would say it is under-diagnosed and that millions of adults have the problem but are undermanaged because the issue wasn't well understood when they were children. There are many good books around and excellent people working in these fields. The school system is invaluable and typically will bring a team together in an effort to figure things out. There can be a conflict of interest, however, because schools typically have budgetary constraints. Neuropsychological testing is intensive and can be a tremendous resource for evaluating this variety of potential contributors.

For Henry to succeed and be well diet was important, but his parents were unable to identify any specific food types (other than those high in sugar) that set him off. What they learned was that he needed to eat often and never go many hours without eating something healthy. If he had some form of protein in the morning, he was more likely to have a good day. He needed to be physically active. Henry did well with consistent long-term (one year plus) therapy for sensory integration dysfunction. There is a growing body of research linking bowel health to mental health, so to that end, I recommended that Henry start a daily probiotic. He was also ultimately put on a low dose of an SSRI medication for his anxiety. His parents struggled for a long time over whether to try medication. His father thought they had no choice and his mother felt it was absurd to use medication for such a young child. When Henry couldn't make it in school, the mom relented. Within a few weeks of being on the medication, Henry's anxiety and irritability were dramatically reduced. This ultimately was the final piece to the puzzle and he got better and better, developing more confidence. For Henry to succeed and be well, he needed a blend of the old, the new, the alternative and the mainstream. To this day, his parents are convinced he would not have improved without all these elements in place.

Insomnia

Insomnia is an incredibly common problem. Most people will have nights when they don't sleep well as a result of some stress in their lives. Chronic insomnia, however, is a different matter altogether. There are millions of people who regularly have trouble getting to sleep or staying asleep. The magnitude of this problem is reflected in the large number of pharmaceuticals, OTC options, herbs and supplements used to help people drop off. I try to only use prescription drugs either as an occasional option or a short-term strategy when possible. The prescription options include Ambien (zolpidem), Restoril (temazepam), Lunesta, Sonata, Rozerem, Trazodone and tricyclics like Elavil (amitryptiline). The more natural options include melatonin, valerian root, and even hops in its natural, non-processed form (not in its processed version as 4-5 beers before bed).

The first line of attack in helping someone to sleep better is to evaluate their sleep hygiene.[12] This refers to such basic principles as avoiding caffeine after noon and having a dark, quiet bedroom. Blackout window shades can be the most important single intervention. These suggestions alone will help some people, but many will need a different approach. A newer option, sleep restriction, may be more effective at control-alt-deleting a person's circadian pattern. In sleep restriction, the person estimates the amount of time they sleep and specifies the time they want to get up. They then, intentionally, stay up—delaying the time they will fall asleep. If the person is getting five hours of sleep and wants to wake up at 6:00 a.m., they try to stay up until 1:00 a.m. The person works back by 15 minutes every three days in an effort to reset their sleep cycle. The cited example would have the person up until 1:00 a.m. for three nights, then 12:45 a.m. for three nights, then 12:30 a.m. for three nights, etc.

The standard approach in mainstream medicine is to use one of the prescription medications, and there is a strong incentive to prescribe since getting a good night's sleep is so important. But there are many alternative options that one can invoke as well. Melatonin is, by far, the most commonly-used "natural" option. I have seen a wide variety of responses to melatonin over the years and still cannot predict who will respond and who will not. Using genetic tests like MTHFR could help differentiate who will respond to an option like melatonin and who would not. Valerian is an herb used to induce somnolence, but I have found it minimally beneficial overall. Kava Kava, an herb from the South Pacific, was used many years ago for anxiety and insomnia until reports of possible liver damage led to its disappearance.

Many relaxation techniques can also be extremely helpful, but the person has to be dedicated to the practice. The average busy American would rather throw back a pill than learn a deeper way of breathing. I will often recommend a very simple technique. When lying in bed trying to go to sleep, the person focuses on the ebb and flow of the breath. They take a regular breath in and then, on the breath out, try to release all tension in the body. With each exhale, they imagine themselves sinking deeper and deeper into the bed. This can be effective, especially for those that have difficulty falling asleep.

The most promising avenue may be working with a hypnotist and learning self-hypnosis, but again this requires an ongoing commitment of time and resources. It would be a hard sell to get some HMO to pay for eight sessions with the local hypnotist although, in the big picture, it could save a lot of money that would otherwise be used for prescription sleep medications. The person reviewing the claim would probably envision some wacky entertainer in a stars-and-half-moons jacket coaxing a group of audience participants to quack like a duck or sing "Happy Birthday, Mr. President" like Marilyn Monroe.

I asked one of my naturopath colleagues how he manages insomnia. He differentiated, as I would, between someone who can't *fall asleep* and someone who can't *stay asleep*. He said that someone waking up between 1:00 a.m. and 3:00 a.m. is awake during "liver time" (clearly, a different system of thinking). For this situation, he would do a series of 8-10 acupuncture sessions over four weeks using the points Liver 14, Lu 1, An Mian 1 and 2, and Spleen 6. He rattled off some other more natural options like Peace Pearls from Classical Pearls or Relaxin from Chi Herbs or the combination of a liver herbal formula such as Ease Pearls or Liver Chi. If, on the other hand, the person can't fall asleep, the options included calcium lactate, mintran or minchex (supplements) from Standard Process Labs. The naturopath also mentioned targeting the adrenal glands with different herbs and supplements.

As I've stated earlier, these naturopathic options typically have no overlap with my practice or any other MD's practice. It's time to work together, find the best options (whether from mainstream or holistic sources), and move forward to improve each patient's health.

Depression

Depression is another common complaint. Most people will experience depression or melancholy at some point in their lives but, for the purposes of this book, depression is used to describe a more chronic condition. The bible of psychiatric diagnoses for medical doctors in America is the American Psychiatric Association's *Diagnostic and Statistical Manual of Mental Disorders.* According to the Fourth Edition (DSM-IV), someone who is clinically depressed:

...suffers from a depressed mood or loss of interest in normal activities that lasts most of the day nearly every day for at least 2 weeks; this mood can last longer if untreated. Other than depressed mood or loss of interest, symptoms include at least four of the following: significant weight loss or gain, sleep disturbances, agitation or unusual slowness, fatigue or loss of energy, feelings of worthlessness or guilt, lack of concentration, or recurrent thoughts of death or suicide.[13]

A representative patient of mine is 28-year-old Susan. She works as an administrative assistant and lives a reasonably healthy lifestyle, but came in after several months of "feeling down" and being tearful. She lacked motivation, had low energy and was having trouble sleeping. She had had these episodes off-and-on for most of her adult life, with no apparent explanation. She was hoping to avoid medication but would consider it.

There are several non-pharmacologic options that would probably help her. Vigorous exercise would almost certainly help, but she was tired and unmotivated. I remember seeing a card that said: "If you want me to start running, I'm going to need some motivation…Like a clown waving a bloody knife and chasing me." Most people cannot afford to rent a malevolent clown on a regular basis. Therapy would probably help, and for many people that can be most effective. Others are fundamentally disinclined to therapy and sit there waiting for the therapist to work their magic. It is possible that there was some dietary contributor to Susan's difficulties and many holistic providers would emphasize diet and nutrition. But again, the depressed person may not have the motivation to pursue dietary change. We could have the answer right in front of us, but the person in need may not have the capacity to walk through that door.

St. John's Wort

The alternative world has used an herb called St. John's wort for many years, more widely in Europe than America. A review of the literature shows conflicting results in terms of its success. I have had a number of people try it over the years; some think that it helped and others weren't convinced. In 2002, the National Center for Complementary and Alternative Medicine (NCCAM) and the National Institute of Mental Health Office of Dietary Supplements (ODS) conducted a study to help determine the benefits of St. John's wort. The study seems to be well designed as a double-blind, placebo-controlled trial and includes a concurrent study using a widely used antidepressant, Zoloft (generic name sertraline), that was also compared to placebo for efficacy. The NCCAM director at the time, Stephen Strauss, MD, commented on the mission of his Center with reference to the St. John's wort study:

Our commitment is to apply exacting scientific methods to studying popular complementary and alternative medicine practices and to publish the results of such studies in critical peer-reviewed journals, so that the public and practitioners can make the most informed decisions about them… This study represents one of our first downpayments on this commitment.[14]

The study found that all three groups (St. John's wort, Zoloft and placebo) produced similar levels of improvement and the final conclusion was that "the overall response to sertraline on the primary measures was not superior to that of placebo, an outcome which is not uncommon in trials of approved antidepressants."[14] In fact, this apparent lack of efficacy occurs in up to 35 percent of trials of antidepressants. The study noted that "an extract of the herb St. John's wort was no more effective for treating *major depression of moderate severity* than placebo."[14]

The busy medical provider often will only have time for a cursory look at study results. If he or she took a quick look at the trial results and believed the source for the study was reliable, it might be enough to discount St. John's wort as ineffective, period, end of story.

I have reviewed and then re-reviewed this study and there is another element that may be important, especially in evaluating the mainstream's willingness to faithfully consider alternative options. There is a contradiction in the study right on the summary page that is hard to miss. The director of the ODS, Paul M. Coates, PhD, noted that, "St. John's wort is taken by many people for the relief of mild to moderate depression."[14] The study, however, uses patients meeting criteria for "major depression," and this distinction is made several times.

On the face of it, we can glean several things from this study. First, and not surprisingly, there was a placebo effect for those with depression. St. John's wort and Zoloft (sertraline) were no more effective than placebo. It is mentioned that this is a recurring theme with SSRI medications even though millions and millions of Americans currently take them for extended periods of time for depression. Unfortunately, the pharmaceutical industry buries studies they sponsor that do not show benefit and this is more true with SSRIs than almost any other class of medication. It has been estimated that the results of nearly half of all antidepressant trials have been suppressed by the pharmaceutical industry.[15]

Second, most who favor St. John's wort would use it for mild to moderate depression (as the Director of the Office of Dietary Supplements wrote). This study, then, cannot be used to make any reliable conclusions about St. John's wort because the appropriate patient population was not used. There were several other studies done by NCCAM around the same time with a similar theme. (The glucosamine study will be discussed in the Rheumatology and Chronic Pain chapter and the saw palmetto study will be reviewed in the Urology section.) In these studies, they evaluated a commonly used alternative option, but with an inappropriate patient population, ultimately coming to the conclusion that the alternative option was ineffective. The way the studies were organized, it's as if they were set up to fail. The NCCAM may not be the paragon of unbiased virtue needed to legitimately evaluate alternative options.

SSRIs

For many with depression, especially those with a chronic recurring pattern and a positive family history, medication is the standard approach. Almost all doctors will start with a class called Selective Serotonin Reuptake Inhibitors, or SSRIs. This group of medications includes Prozac, Paxil, Zoloft, Celexa and Lexapro. Several other medications commonly used include Effexor, Cymbalta and Wellbutrin. There was a meta-analysis done in 2010 published in the *Journal of the American Medical Association* (JAMA) that suggested that for the majority of people with mild to moderate depression there was SSRI benefit, but not significantly more than placebo.[16] (A meta-analysis is a special type of investigation where the results from many different studies are pooled together, usually to increase the statistical power. Sometimes, this can identify side effects and/or results that would be missed in smaller individual studies.)

The analysis suggested that for the ten percent of patients that met the criteria for "major depression" there was more definitive benefit. As part of the study, the limitations of the meta-analysis were reviewed. Because the conclusions potentially undermined one of the most fundamental tenets of mental health management in America, the study came under some intense scrutiny. In my review of the psychiatrists' reviews, it does seem like the meta-analysis was deficient in many ways and thus it is not clear if we can extrapolate across the population.

If there is any validity to the results, however, it puts the primary care physician in a delicate ethical position. It would seem that SSRIs may work in some circumstances because you have a vulnerable individual seeking help from someone they know and respect in the area of mental health. If the provider knows that it will likely make the person feel better, but suspects it is all or mostly placebo, should they prescribe anyway? I think most doctors would prescribe, arguing that helping the patient is the primary goal. If I cannot get the person to exercise regularly or be in therapy, I will typically offer citalopram. In my experience, I have found SSRIs less beneficial for depression, but extremely effective for generalized anxiety disorder. Either way, the placebo effect can be very powerful and is almost universally accepted, so some clinical research should focus on this effect. If the pharmaceutical industry is dominating the landscape of clinical studies, however, I'm guessing they are not motivated to expand our application of this mind-body benefit.

There are other, more natural, options that may be beneficial for depression, including SAMe[NS (see appendix B)], L-methylfolate[NS] and fish oil.[NS] One study showed that depressed people had lower levels of omega-3 fatty acids in their blood. The quick conclusion from this was that fish oil and other sources high in omega-3 fatty acids could potentially reduce a person's risk of depression. But this is a classic erroneous conclusion since we have no way of knowing what is cause and what is effect. The other possible explanation for the study result is that people who are depressed take relatively poor care of themselves. Being depressed would have the secondary effect of impacting a person's appetite and choice of foods. Depressed people may have lower levels of omega-3 fatty acids in their bloodstream for this reason.

Other studies have been done, however, that suggest there is real benefit for depression from omega-3s. *CNS Neuroscience and Therapeutics* summarized three studies in the summer of 2009:

In the adult unipolar depression study, highly significant benefits were found by week 3 of EPA [one of the primary omega-3 fatty acids used in supplements] treatment compared with placebo. In the children's study, an analysis of variance (ANOVA) showed highly significant effects of omega-3 on each of the three rating scales. In the bipolar depression study, 8 of the 10 patients who completed at least 1 month of follow-up achieved a 50% or greater reduction in Hamilton depression (Ham-D) scores within 1 month.[17]

There is a book that is designed to find a more holistic and balanced approach to improving mental health. *The Chemistry of Joy* by Henry Emmons, MD, contains an incredible amount of information on the relative importance of diet, vitamins, supplements and lifestyle modifications. The material can be somewhat overwhelming but, for the motivated individual, it is the most comprehensive source for non-pharmaceutical options I have come across. It uses Aryuveda, the centuries-old healing system from India, to identify individual personality types. These include Vata (light, quick and changeable as air), Pitta (passionate, determined and intense as fire), and Kapha (sturdy, solid and stable as earth). There are sections that then recommend specific lifestyle modifications based on each personality type. This individualized approach is likely a more robust, long-term solution, but also requires a much greater effort for the person trying to improve their mental health.

Individualized management of chronic mental health conditions through genetic testing should be the future of psychiatry. The most important anomaly is probably methylene tetrahydrofolate reductase (MTHFR).[18] Decreased activity of this enzyme will lead to low levels of L-methylfolate[NS] that is a precursor to many neurotransmitters including serotonin, melatonin, dopamine, epinephrine and norepinephrine. MTHFR defects also affect creation of BH4 that is required for adequate production of thyroid hormone.

A person can have a list of important genetic anomalies screened through the website 23andme. The $99 cost may be the best bargain in healthcare. This testing checks for MTHFR and other genetic anomalies implicated in mental health including COMT, CBS and VDR. The challenge after getting the raw data crunched through a website like geneticgenie.org is finding a provider that can review the results and make specific recommendations on optimal diet, vitamins and supplements.

I have been incorporating methylated B-vitamins into my depression management over the past year. For those with a genetic MTHFR anomaly and chronic depression, I have a growing number of patients that have responded better to L-methylfolate, methyl-B12 and B6 than a laundry list of prescription antidepressants tried in prior years. Many, however, do not respond to these supplements because they need a more complete evaluation beyond MTHFR. Amy Yasko, PhD, is an authority on these issues and has written many articles and books that can be referenced including *Feel Good*, a book intended for the general public. The book reviews methylation cycles[19] within cells. These cycles are often dysfunctional in chronically ill patients. Part of my path in integrative medicine going forward is an endeavor to become increasingly more sophisticated in my understanding of these complex biochemical cycles.

Anxiety

Anxiety is another extremely common issue for patients seen in primary care offices. From "livescience.com", the Top Ten Fears are:

1. Snakes
2. "Creepy Crawlies" like spiders and insects
3. "Scary Spaces" especially claustrophobia
4. "Other People" especially public speaking and crowds
5. Heights
6. The Dark
7. Thunder and Lightening
8. Flying on a Plane
9. Dogs
10. The Dentist

There is a long list of phobias including a smattering of some of the stranger ones: albuminurophobia (fear of kidney disease), Dutchophobia (fear of the Dutch), Ephebiphobia (fear of teenagers), or even Pupaphobia (fear of puppets).

In a medical encounter, the initial line of questioning often focuses on the duration of the issue, but it also surveys the degree to which the anxiety is impacting a person's life in terms of school, work and relationships. For the person with chronic anxiety, the SSRI medications are a good option. In fact, I have found over the years that while the benefit of SSRIs for depression is mediocre, these "anti-depressants" are extremely effective in treating chronic anxiety. My first option for medication is typically Celexa (generic citalopram).

It may be heresy for the millions that prefer to avoid medication, and especially those dedicated to "natural" options, that the SSRI prescription medication is the best option, but that is my experience. These medications are well tolerated with minimal side effects and, so far, show no known long-term negative impact. They can dramatically change a person's life for the better. If I see a person with chronic anxiety for follow-up and they have not responded to an SSRI, I'm actually surprised. Now, let's say that I could use an herb or something more natural than Celexa and it was equally effective. Assuming cost and side effect profiles are the same, is that preferred? This is a philosophical question that goes right to the heart of the matter. If the pharmaceutical is derived from a natural source, does that make it more acceptable? There are no pat answers to these questions and each person has to make up their own mind about how important it is to stay close to nature.

Natural Treatments for Anxiety

Of course, the alternative world has much to offer for anxiety and stress management. Chamomile tea[NS] is composed of a compound called matricaria recutita that binds biologically like the drug Valium (diazepam). Chamomile can also be taken as a supplement with 1.2% apigen. Apigen, the active ingredient in chamomile, has also been studied for its ability to inhibit cancer cell signal transduction and promote programmed cell death that decreases risk of cancer. The University of Pennsylvania Medical School conducted a study on patients with GAD (Generalized Anxiety Disorder) and found a significant decrease in symptoms after eight weeks of taking the supplement when compared to placebo. Lavender oil[NS], lavandula hybriola, also behaves like Valium, but can be used as an aromatherapy to treat mild anxiety, or internally, for mood imbalances and gastrointestinal distress. The amino acid in green tea[NS] known as L-theanine helps to curb a rising heart rate and blood pressure. A study done in 2003 with anxiety-prone subjects showed that 200 milligrams of L-theanine helped test takers remain calm. It would take 5-20 cups of green tea to get this dose of the amino acid, but the calming effects of one cup can be felt nonetheless.

It is possible that the most effective non-pharmacologic options for chronic anxiety are relaxation techniques. There is a woman in my area who teaches clients progressive relaxation similar to the relaxation response developed by Herbert Benson.

From the Massachusetts General Hospital website, where they also utilize the relaxation response:

In the late 1960s, in the same room in which Harvard Medical School's Walter Cannon performed fight-or-flight experiments 50 years earlier, Herbert Benson, MD, found that there was a counterbalancing mechanism to the stress response. Just as stimulating an area of the hypothalamus can cause the stress response, so activating other areas of the brain results in its reduction. He defined this opposite state as the "relaxation response".[18]

The relaxation response is a physical state of deep rest that changes the physical and emotional responses to stress (e.g., decreases in heart rate, blood pressure, rate of breathing, and muscle tension).

When eliciting the relaxation response:

- Your metabolism decreases
- Your heart beats slower and your muscles relax
- Your breathing becomes slower
- Your blood pressure decreases
- Your levels of nitric oxide are increased

If practiced regularly, it can have lasting effects. Elicitation of the relaxation response is at the heart of the BHI's research and clinical mind/body programs.[20]

The specialist near me, Sandra Bemis, is an expert on suggestion and self-hypnosis. She takes the person through a process where they learn, through reinforcement and trigger statements, to get into an "alpha state." Her approaches are effective for smoking cessation, weight loss, irritable bowel syndrome and stress reduction, but when I asked her which area was the most responsive to her techniques, she said anxiety. Her costs are also relatively low at about $75 per session. She usually works with people for six sessions and, assuming they do the exercises at home, the client can have a robust long-term solution. Imagine if we used this approach and it was effective for the majority of people. The cost savings relative to years of therapy sessions and/or long-term medication would be tremendous.

Obsessive Compulsive Disorder

A subset of chronic anxiety patients will have underlying Obsessive Compulsive Disorder. People usually will not bring up issues if they are potentially embarrassing. The person with OCD is typically aware there is something wrong but will almost never bring the issue up to a doctor. Like most issues, there is a spectrum of disease. The severe forms involve repetitive actions like checking the oven or the locks on the door 14 times before leaving the house. Any patient with severe "dyshidrotic" eczema of the hands should be questioned about excessive worrying about germs or "germaphobia" leading to hand washing all day. The most common presentation of OCD, however, is the person impossible to reassure. Every doctor has patients that are worried about some dread disease no matter how much time you spend with them. That is typically a form of OCD or Generalized Anxiety Disorder and the patient will need to be asked specific questions to tease out the diagnosis.

Bipolar

Bipolar illness tends to be more complex in management. A person diagnosed with this condition, and ultimately managed by a psychiatrist, will usually be managed with two or three different pharmaceuticals. The summary mentioned earlier suggests that omega-3 fatty acids could help not only unipolar depression but also bipolar. Our fundamental understanding of conditions involving mental health, including bipolar, is very limited at this time. We could potentially find ways to correct the underlying issue on a neurological level, rather than using pharmaceutical after pharmaceutical to control and suppress the secondary manifestations. It would be interesting to take a small group of bipolar patients and do a study where half are managed by psychiatrists and half are managed by naturopaths or some other non-traditional provider.

ADD

Attention Deficit Disorder (ADD) and Attention Deficit Hyperactivity Disorder (ADHD) get a lot of attention. The usual approach, as mentioned previously, is stimulant medication—amphetamine-based drugs like the "speed" that was sold on the streets in the 70s and some of the weight loss drugs used to suppress appetite. These are widely abused on just about every college campus in America. I have heard anecdotally that a college student preparing for an exam will pay up to $20 per pill for one of these stimulants.

Some time in the early 2000s, I heard of a program from England called DORE. The system involved a series of assessments leading to the development of individualized exercises designed to establish new connections in the brain. These exercises were highly successful in improving learning disabilities, including dyslexia, dyspraxia and ADD/ADHD. It is still utilized in the United Kingdom. DORE came to our area, but was not supported by insurance companies. It was unsustainable with not enough people willing to pay out-of-pocket, so they shut down the operation in the U.S. In a reasonable health system with resources allocated in the most efficient manner, we would use DORE to "cure" a high percentage of children so that they would not need medications for much of their lives.

As in most areas, we really need a new approach, a new paradigm for addressing mental health. We need to take into account factors that get little or no attention, including a person's diet and nutrition. One excellent source for alternative approaches is William Shaw, PhD, through Great Plains Laboratories. On his website, a number of tests are listed that can help clarify other reasons why a child has focus problems. These include an organic acids test (for intestinal yeast and bacterial overgrowth), hair testing for heavy metals, tests for copper/zinc imbalance, and others for food allergies and intolerances. Dr. Shaw contends that "two thirds of children diagnosed with AD(H)D have undiagnosed food allergies that generate most, if not all, of their symptoms."

The child with focus problems and/or hyperactivity at risk of getting a lifelong diagnosis of ADD/ADHD is typically better off with an initial focus on sleep, diet, electronic screen time and other psychosocial factors. The child often needs an assessment for an auditory processing problem as that variant of sensory integration dysfunction tends to go undiagnosed. Neuropsychological testing can help clarify mood disorders, learning disabilities and other related factors. Only those that have refractory difficulty in school, after all of the primary areas are addressed, would be considered for medication.

The stimulant medications, if used selectively, can be incredibly effective. I have seen many students do very well in school with improvement in their behavioral issues as well. I have seen many adults become more productive and self-confident on stimulants.

If we could introduce a program like DORE that utilizes the amazing plasticity of a young brain, we could potentially resolve many problems, including learning disabilities, anxiety and ADD. Voilà a robust, long-term solution that dramatically lowers healthcare costs and improves the quality of lives. Of course, this would require much upfront investment and a different approach by providers, many of whom are maxed out and don't have the time for involved discussions or complex psychosocial histories. We would need ancillary providers as experts and many, including psychopharmacologists, are already in place.

Orthomolecular Psychiatry

One day, a patient brought in an article written by Carl C. Pfeiffer, PhD, MD, a proponent of a field called orthomolecular psychiatry. The field focuses on a more individualized approach to chronic mental health conditions. To follow this paradigm, a provider would try and identify the optimal diet, vitamin, nutrient and medication regimen for the patient. This unorthodox approach has been rejected by mainstream psychiatrists. The standard mainstream approach to mental health issues is to use a small group of prescription pharmaceuticals with little or no discussion about diet or other lifestyle contributors. With a paucity of research, it would be difficult to reliably evaluate the merits of orthomolecular psychiatry.

The article from Dr. Pfeiffer reviewed a supplement called deanol,[NS] or DMAE. This substance is a precursor to acetylcholine, a neurotransmitter in the brain. According to Dr. Pfeiffer, deanol has been found to have benefit in a variety of neurological and psychiatric conditions including Alzheimer's disease, learning disabilities and attention deficit disorder. My patient said she had used this "natural substitute for Ritalin" with clear benefit and no side effects.

I was able to find a study from 1975 involving 75 children who had issues with learning and hyperactivity. The children were given either 500mg of deanol, 40mg of methylphenidate (a relatively high dose of the stimulant in Ritalin) or placebo. Both of the drugs demonstrated significant improvement in behaviors and other outcomes. Deanol could be an effective option for ADD and ADHD with fewer side effects and no abuse potential. In our current system, however, with limited emphasis or research on non-pharmaceutical options, it is difficult to recommend the option with confidence.

Mind and Matter

It's clear that mental health can be strongly impacted by the foods we eat and the overall health of the gut. Where we have relied on pharmaceuticals to alleviate all symptoms—whether manifested in behavioral problems, emotional problems, or simply a lack of sleep—we'd do better to ask the following questions: Could dietary changes and exercise alone resolve my issues? Are there natural alternatives or therapeutic options that would offer long-term improvement? Is it worth pursuing genetic testing for abnormalities like MTHFR and COMT to try and find the optimal lifestyle changes and supplements? The answer to these questions is yes. We need to move beyond our current model if people are to be truly well in mind, body and spirit.

3

Hardwired

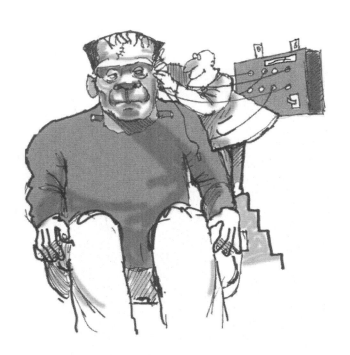

It is important to question our assumptions. We will see a case later in the book of someone with severe allergies, asthma and sinus problems cured by acupuncture. We will also see a case later in the book of bedwetting in a child cured by simple dietary changes. By the current thinking, autism is something to be managed, but not reversed. I have had several experiences in my clinical practice that challenge this notion. One mom I see in the office would not accept that her daughter Ella's condition was untreatable:

My daughter was diagnosed with Pervasive Developmental Disorder [a clinical term applying to autism] shortly after her first birthday, though we had suspected that she was on the spectrum before then. The diagnosis was devastating for me, as I could only think about what her future would hold, the difficulties and isolation she might be faced with. I have a background in alternative medicine, and I decided that I would try everything holistic that I could to improve her quality of life. I had no idea at that time if anything would work, nor did I fully understand everything that would be involved in the years to come.

I started to learn everything I could about dietary interventions and autism. I read online and scoured the bookstores looking for information. I had personal experience with milk intolerance since childhood, so we first switched her to goat milk instead of cow's milk. We tried a gluten-free diet [and] saw minimal improvements, but I felt certain that I had not yet found the right combination. I started her on a high-quality probiotic, and started reading about the SCD (specific carbohydrate diet) and GAPS [Gut and Psychology Syndrome] diets. At the age of two, we started her on the SCD diet and saw excellent results. She would regress and go through die off and then have periods where her eye contact and interactions improved. Her sleep was still very poor, but she was more affectionate and seemed to be less in her own world all the time.

I am a craniosacral therapist, and had been using the therapy on her since her birth. I had read in *The Impossible Cure* how craniosacral helped to recover another autistic child in conjunction with homeopathy, and I began to integrate homeopathy into her regimen. I found another book called *Beyond Hope* that helped with determining the best remedies and dosages and used the craniosacral therapy to check her progress. My focus at that point was to detox her liver from candida toxins and to help chelate heavy metals from the vaccinations she received before the age of one (I stopped vaccinating her after receiving the PDD diagnosis, though I had noticed a significant change in her craniosacral patterns after the first set of vaccines).

Her progress on the SCD program was stalling and she was complaining about body aches and pain in her genitals, which caused me to suspect that she was not processing oxalates well (SCD is a high oxalate diet). I switched her back to a gluten-free, casein-free diet that was low in oxalates and also excluded soy and corn. I also started her on olive leaf extract, which served as an antifungal, antibacterial and antiviral therapy. I gave her Candex [an alternative antifungal treatment] at night to help with the yeast in her intestines, and found her a constitutional homeopathic remedy to strengthen her overall system. She would still show signs of improvement and regression, so I added in digestive enzymes before all meals to help her system break down foods properly. I also added magnesium[NS] at night to help her sleep and help with constipation. With these changes, she began to show great improvements.

We did IgG testing to rule out food sensitivities and tweaked her diet to exclude these. She received therapy at preschool and Applied Behavioral Analysis (ABA)[21] therapy three days a week at home. I had been giving her a multi[vitamin] and fish oil[NS] for a few years, and now removed these as well, at which point her stimming[22] virtually stopped.

At the age of five, her neurologist told me she no longer qualified for the autistic diagnosis, and she now presents as a typical kindergartener. We keep her on the gluten-free, casein-free diet, and keep her away from her food sensitivities, but she can now tolerate oxalates, soy and corn. I have also continued with the probiotic, olive leaf[NS] and magnesium, but discontinued [the digestive] enzymes with success. She regresses mildly when she is sick, or if she ingests any artificial colors in her foods. She stims when she is very excited, but other than that she is delightful..., funny, compassionate and intelligent, and I find peace in knowing that she has a bright future ahead of her.[23]

I played a minimal role in Ella's success story. I was supportive of the process, but served mostly as an interested observer getting updates at her well visits. I learned more about autism management from Ella and her mother than I could ever find in a medical textbook. It was apparent to me from her path what it takes to reverse underlying autism. It takes a dedicated individual or team doggedly sorting out the most effective traditional and complementary options. Ella's improvement was achieved by addressing the important ideas in this book: improving the diet, tending the microbiome, correcting flora imbalance and yeast overgrowth and using selective vitamins, herbs and supplements.

Autism rates have been steadily increasing over the years no matter how you define the condition. It is coming to dominate much of pediatric neurology. I am coming to believe that many cases of autism can be treated using some of the principles above. Prevention, at the deepest level, would be even more powerful. The majority of children with autism have problems with methylation. Most will have genetic MTHFR (methylenetetrahydrofolate reductase) anomalies and, if this test is more widely performed, there is a chance we could identify those parents at the highest risk of having a child on the autism spectrum. I can imagine a pregnant mother and infant child positive for MTHFR being treated with methylated B vitamins like L-methyl folate preemptively. Other genetic testing would help clarify other relevant anomalies. Studies to sort this out would be relatively simple to do with a huge potential benefit.

Adult Neurology

While autism is the big-name diagnosis in pediatric neurology, some of the most common diagnoses in adult neurology include headaches, seizures, and neuropathy (nerve pain). People may come in to a medical office concerned that they are having transient ischemia attacks (TIAs), also called "mini-strokes." These TIAs mimic the symptoms of a stroke, but without permanent damage to the brain. Other neurology patients have actually had a stroke or cerebrovascular accident (CVA). Still others have suffered memory loss or other cognitive decline. People are often worried that short-term memory loss is a prelude to Alzheimer's or some other forms of dementia. Parkinson's disease is another relatively common diagnosis in the specialty. Neurology is a field that is prime for prevention and proactive approaches. Headaches, in particular, can be managed in a cursory way with medications, or time can be spent trying to identify an individual's triggers.

Headaches

Consider Bonnie, a 35-year-old woman complaining of headaches for five days. She had mild nasal congestion and wondered if allergies or a sinus infection might be the cause. There was a focus of the headaches around the right eye. On review of symptoms, she had intermittent stomach upset, but no vomiting, fever or other changes. She seemed prone to headaches, averaging one or two a week, and would get a few migraines each year with vomiting and extreme light and sound sensitivity. In terms of family history, she at first said one aunt had migraines, but that no one else had headache issues. When asked more specifically if anyone in her family had "chronic sinus headaches," she reported that her father often got "sinus headaches."

I discussed with Bonnie that she probably did not have a sinus infection. The paradigm I use for explaining headaches comes from the book *Heal Your Headache* by David Buchholz. This book, recommended to me early in my career by a patient suffering from chronic headaches, forever changed my understanding of the underlying causes for headaches. It explained that there is a common thread to all headaches and that, like many things, there is a spectrum. Many people have a genetic predisposition to headaches. These can be mild "tension" headaches, on the low end of the spectrum, or full-blown migraines, with a person crawling into bed utterly debilitated.

Bonnie was probably in the middle of the spectrum at this visit. She had a unilateral focus with moderate intensity and mild gastrointestinal symptoms. It is not commonly known that migraines and other non-sinus headaches often present with nasal congestion. It is logical, then, for someone to have pressure around the eye with nasal congestion and to think it must be a sinus problem. In one study of people who said they had "chronic sinus infections," 95% of them actually were on the migraine spectrum with no sinus issues whatsoever.

The difference between someone with a mild "tension" headache across the forehead and someone with a full migraine is typically which triggers are involved. Each person has different triggers. Some of them are minor and others are major, but they tend to be additive. The list of potential triggers is very long and, surprising to most people, includes bread, cheese, dairy, yogurt, onions, peas, bananas, citrus fruits and many others.

I will typically ask about the most common triggers: stress, lack of sleep, menstrual changes, under-hydration, caffeine, artificial sweeteners, processed lunchmeats and alcohol. For some people a few triggers are key. I remember some of the outstanding victories over the years. I've had a few female patients whose headaches significantly improved when they stopped using Splenda. I had a young male patient who was having migraines after workouts. We figured out that it probably was the combination of dehydration from exercise and the banana and yogurt smoothie he downed afterward. My favorite was picked up by another doctor in our office. A 20-year-old male was having regular headaches which, after some time, were linked to the baloney sandwich he ate every day at lunch. When he stopped eating baloney the headaches went away.

A major player in headaches is MSG (monosodium glutamate). For many years I thought of MSG as something in Chinese food, but I have come to understand otherwise. A mother of one of my pediatric patients sent me an email about how common MSG is in foods and I was dumbfounded. Moms are tenacious and, if their child is ill, do much of their own research, often providing me with excellent information. The various ways free glutamate is labeled on foods include: anything with the word glutamate, yeast extract, anything "hydrolyzed," gelatin, soy protein, whey protein, carrageenan, bouillon and broth, stock, maltodextrin, citric acid, pectin, anything "enzyme modified," anything containing "enzymes," malt extract, milk powder, soy sauce, anything "protein fortified," corn starch, corn syrup, dextrose, rice syrup, anything "enriched," xanthum gum and others. This potentially helps me explain some patients with persistent headaches despite my initial recommended changes to lifestyle.

If I cannot clear up a person's headaches, and testing like an MRI of the brain is negative, they will often see a neurologist. If the neurologist is also unsuccessful, there is another option that I have been utilizing more lately. There is a small subgroup of chiropractors that specialize in the upper cervical vertebrae. I have read there are only about 400 of these subspecialists in America. I have seen people with chronic intractable headaches (and many also have neck, dizziness and inner ear issues) cured by a chiropractor who does this type of spinal manipulation.

Neuropathy

Neuropathy is a broad term for pain from a nerve source. The most common situation for nerve-related pain is a person with a pinched nerve. Every week I see at least one person with numbness, tingling and burning, sharp, shooting pain down an extremity. Most of these cases are caused by a pinched nerve in the neck or lower back. The majority of pinched nerves are caused by a protruding intervertebral disc.

Over the years, I have developed a cookie-cutter approach to these patients that seems to work well. I almost always recommend an oral steroid, prednisone, as the first option. I will say to people that of all the options—heat, ice, anti-inflammatories, Tylenol, muscle relaxers, narcotics, physical therapy, chiropractor, acupuncture and massage—the prednisone is by far the one with the greatest potential immediate benefit. For some, a short course of prednisone gets them out of the acute phase and then we can work on a more long-term, preventative approach with exercise and strengthening, either on their own or as directed by a physical therapist or chiropractor. It is difficult for me to assess the success of acupuncture because so few patients have seen an acupuncturist for this issue. If insurance covered the sessions, I might have a larger sample size. Acupuncture is incredibly variable from practitioner to practitioner. I learned a few years ago that each acupuncturist takes an individualized approach to a given problem, which may explain the wide range of responses to treatment I have seen.

There is a different form of neuropathy, called peripheral neuropathy, that is typically a chronic, slowly-progressive condition. It most often affects the toes, feet and then legs symmetrically. The number one cause is diabetes. The next two most common causes are B12 deficiency and long-term heavy consumption of alcohol. The B12 deficiency can sometimes be a window into a larger systemic problem. The question for me is usually why is someone not absorbing enough B12 into his or her system? It is relatively uncommon for an American (other than vegetarians) to have a diet lacking in vitamin B12 as it is found in fish, meat, chicken, eggs and milk, among other foods. It is more and more common that they are B12 deficient because of malabsorption. This can also be a sign that they have genetic anomalies within methylation cycles like MTHFR. Standard approach is to put them on B12 tablets or start B12 monthly injections, case closed. It would be better, however, to view the B12 deficiency in a larger context. If the patient has other signs of malabsorption, we may be able to achieve a greater impact on their health by sorting this out. The person may have a food intolerance or sensitivity issue. They may even have some chronic infectious process or flora imbalance affecting their bowel function. They may be taking a strong prescription acid blocker like Prilosec.

As will be discussed below, many with B12 deficiency will be in the low normal range on their lab tests. Sometimes a trial of vitamin B12 is worthwhile to see if the person's neuropathy or other symptoms improve. Additional lab tests like mean corpuscular volume, methylmalonic acid and homocysteine can also help clarify if there is underlying deficiency. There are several forms of B12 available. Cyanocobalamin is the B12 option typically used and the only form known to most physicians, but it is not always optimal for each individual. Some, based on their individual genetics, have a much better response to methyl-B12, adenosyl-B12 or hydroxy-B12.[24]

There is a very effective option from the alternative world for peripheral neuropathy: alpha-lipoic acid. My preference is always to identify the underlying cause for any problems and pursue a cure, but this is not always possible. For those with nerve pain to the extremities, but no easily identifiable cause, I often use alpha-lipoic acid starting at 300mg twice a day. I sometimes work up to 600mg twice per day if needed.

The person with peripheral neuropathy who also has a wide variety of symptoms including headaches, fatigue, muscle pain, and joint pain, should be assessed for the possibility of chronic Lyme disease. The Horowitz book *Why Can't I Get Better? Solving the Mystery of Lyme & Chronic Disease* provides a questionnaire that can help put the overall picture in perspective. This will be explored later in the book. There is also the chance that underlying thyroid dysfunction is causing or contributing to chronic pain. This will also be reviewed later.

Strokes

Stroke prevention is one of the most important areas for primary care physicians. Uncontrolled hypertension is the number one risk factor for a stroke, so managing blood pressure aggressively is paramount. The current benchmark? In 2014, a national group loosened the standards for hypertension for people over 60 years old with the goal of a pressure below 150/90. Managing blood pressure appropriately could mean meditation, exercise, or uncovering and managing obstructive sleep apnea. It could mean spending twenty minutes reviewing a person's diet in detail. The person who has had a stroke or TIA deserves meticulous attention so that every possible contributing factor is brought to the light of day.

Yet we have to be careful with prescription medications, especially for the elderly, because the potential for side effects and harm steadily increases as a person ages. It is important for healthcare providers to listen to their instincts. Often, primary care involves determining whether a person's presenting symptoms fit neatly into a common diagnosis or not. Shoulder pain: rotator cuff or other? Elbow pain: lateral epicondylitis (the medical term for "tennis elbow") or other? Numbness and tingling in the hand/wrist: carpal tunnel or other? The more experienced a person is on any subject, the more finely tuned their instincts. A person who has played a hundred thousand hands of poker should trust the uncomfortable feeling that wells up from inside during a hand. When that happens, they are probably behind and should get away from it. There really isn't any need to calculate number of outs and the likelihood the other player will fill a flush. This internal sense can be more powerful and more reliable than the rational, conscious mind.

A crucial related aspect of primary care is the sense that something serious is going on and needs immediate attention. Early on in practice, every acute chest pain is potentially an acute myocardial infarction (or heart attack) and any unexplained weight loss is an occult malignancy. New primary care providers are more likely to overdiagnose serious problems and overtest to rule them out.

The deeper honed instincts, however, are often the failsafe. I remember seeing 85-year-old Stanley. It was a Thursday afternoon and he had been seen by another provider three days prior for a flare-up of gout. Stanley was put on the anti-inflammatory indomethacin at the highest dose, which I thought at the time was a bit risky for an elderly patient. He came in with his wife and daughter. If the patient comes in with one or more family members, I typically take the visit very seriously.

The wife and daughter said Stanley wasn't acting normally. They couldn't be specific, no matter how many questions I asked them. He just wasn't right. In speaking with the patient himself, he was pleasant and interactive with fluent speech. I did a thorough neurologic exam that was completely normal and non-focal. I reviewed with the family some of the potential explanations for the change in mental status. I recommended stat blood and urine tests and then uttered the fateful words that if those tests were negative we would get a head CT the next day.

The tests were negative and that night Stanley got worse, ending up in the ER. When the head CT showed an intracranial bleed, he was airflighted down to Massachusetts General Hospital. He had emergency surgery and survived, but was neurologically impaired for the next few years until he died. The instinctive part of my brain had worked it all out. I did a much more thorough neurological exam than usual and I brought up the head CT. I had a hunch what should be done, but for some reason did not take the next step.

Strokes and Cholesterol Levels

There is an assumption in mainstream medicine that higher cholesterol levels in the blood are associated with a higher risk of stroke. There is a corollary assumption that if you use a statin to reduce blood cholesterol levels, you will reduce a person's risk of stroke. In the chapter on cardiovascular health, *Lipitor vs. Guggulipid,* I will describe a hypothetical scenario where I do not prescribe a statin and then a patient has a cardiac event. The "Standard of Care" is violated and a mock trial is held where the cardiologists condemn my approach.

In 2013, the inevitable happened. I was seeing an 82-year-old male, Zeke, for a physical. He had well-controlled hypertension and was otherwise in good health with no issues or problems to discuss. He had a history of moderate hyperlipidemia and had been on a statin cholesterol medication for many years. I reviewed the lack of evidence for any benefit of risk reduction for statins in people in his age group. We discussed the potential side effects including muscle pain, premature cataracts and diabetes. Based on this discussion, he stopped the medication.

Five or six months later, he had difficulty getting words out one day. He went to the hospital and an MRI scan of the brain showed he had had a small stroke. There were no further incidents. A week after discharge from the hospital, he came to see me for a follow-up visit. He was as pleasant as always, but one of the first things he said to me was: "The doctor in the hospital said I had a stroke because you stopped my cholesterol medication." We had a calm, reasonable discussion about the issue. The hospital doctors had recommended he restart the medication and I agreed but not because I thought it was in his best interest. I felt vulnerable to some form of lawsuit if I went against the standard of care. For my own peace of mind, I did a search and reviewed the studies to make sure my advice had been sound. Indeed, there was minimal evidence that statins would have prevented his event.

I sent him a letter and cc'd the specialist in the hospital. The letter went on to include some of the statements from the studies:

- Cholesterol appears to be only a weak risk factor for ischemic stroke.
- The epidemiological evidence regarding the risk of ischemic stroke attributed to cholesterol is inconsistent and conflicting.
- A large study summarized that "there was no association between serum cholesterol and stroke."
- One study showed that the maximum dose of Lipitor (80mg per day) lowered the risk of stroke over five years by 2.2%.

At an 80mg dose, many patients would have muscle pain, some would develop diabetes and others might suffer memory deficits. For Zeke, I restarted his cholesterol medication and then noted at a follow-up visit a month later that his neurologist had quadrupled the dose from 20mg up to 80mg per day. That gargantuan increase in dose helped clarify for me that the neurologist truly believed that the statin would lower Zeke's risk going forward. If the specialist was only interested in CYA medicine, he would likely have left the dose alone.

Homocysteine

There is an issue in medicine that gets little or no attention yet may be a major player in an individual's risk of a stroke or cardiovascular event. When I was in residency training, I first heard of elevated serum homocysteine levels as a potential risk factor for cardiovascular disease. Research clearly showed that elevated levels of homocysteine in the blood put people at risk of blood clots, strokes and cardiac events. There was a hope that by using B-vitamins to lower homocysteine levels, we could reduce a person's risk going forward. It turned out that doctors could reduce blood homocysteine levels with treatment but this did not lower the person's risk. Because of this, doctors stopped ordering homocysteine levels and the issue was mostly dropped in clinical medicine.

In my practice now, if I see a patient with a potentially life-threatening blood clot or a premature cardiovascular event or a strong family history of these issues, I will sometimes add a test to their evaluation for MTHFR (methylenetetrahydrofolate reductase). Testing can assess whether a person has normal MTHFR genes from their mother and father. Research is clear that if the person has mutations to both genes, a homozygous state, they will not process folate normally and this can lead to elevated homocysteine levels. Current standard of care recommends against MTHFR testing because there is no hard evidence that managing an abnormal result (with B-vitamins) will reduce risk.

In my review of the literature, MTHFR and other methylation cycle anomalies (that can be tested through 23andme.com) may be among the most important manageable risk factors for stroke, heart events, blood clots, miscarriages, dementia, birth defects, autism, colon cancer and lymphoma, yet they get little or no attention. In my current state of cynicism regarding the American health system, I think it is possible that MTHFR is blown off because the potential for profit is relatively low. I think there is a relatively high likelihood that reducing homocysteine in these patients with some optimal combination of B-vitamins would lower risk. I often recommend supplements like Methylprotect, Methylife or Ben Lynch's version that have combinations of methylfolate, methylB12 and B6. These supplements and others like them are almost certainly safe and relatively inexpensive. For an issue of this importance, I feel it's imperative to use the best supplement available to manage the issue. I cannot wait around for a double-blind, placebo-controlled trial that will never come.

Memory Problems

People are very concerned about the potential for memory loss and dementia. I will occasionally see a person in their 30s or 40s with short-term memory problems and difficulty with word retrieval. The cause is almost always stress and/or lack of sleep. People whose lives are too busy are overwhelmed. Anyone with sleep deprivation will see an impact on their focus and ability to concentrate. I will spend some time discussing prevention with these patients to help put their minds at ease.

The older person with memory problems is, of course, a more typical patient encounter. In a study published in 2002 in the *American Journal of Epidemiology*[25], the researchers followed several thousand people over five years. At the end of the period, 194 out of 4615 subjects could be diagnosed with Alzheimer's disease. In evaluating factors associated with a lower risk of developing Alzheimer's, four characteristics popped up, including use of non-steroidal anti-inflammatories, drinking wine and drinking coffee. The variable associated with the lowest risk was regular physical activity.

There is a relatively standard approach to memory loss and dementia. The person in question will typically have a mini-mental status examination (MMSE) that measures different aspects of cognition and gives a score out of a possible 30 points. The patient will have a series of blood tests to look for reversible or other identifiable causes for cognitive decline, including kidney tests, liver tests, a thyroid test, B12 level and blood test for tertiary syphilis. MRI of the brain is standard. After that, if the person is felt to have a level of memory problem that is somewhere on the dementia spectrum, medication is considered. Aricept is almost always the drug of choice first-line, but the benefits are relatively small. The truth is that there are really no good medications for Alzheimer's disease and we'd be better off dedicating resources to preventing the illness. My #1 recommendation to a person at any age with memory and focus problems is the website Lumosity. My best guess is that the games in Lumosity help the areas of speed, memory, attention, flexibility and problem solving more than any medication that will be developed in the near future.

There is growing evidence for more aggressive supplementation with vitamin B12. The normal laboratory range for B12 is typically 200-1200. One of the great lessons for me in clinical practice is to not view laboratory results as simply black and white, normal or abnormal. Many people who would benefit from B12 supplements will have results in the 200-500 range. Another blood test that can push me toward earlier supplementation for a patient is the mean corpuscular volume (MCV). Most people with B12 deficiency will have fatigue and then changes to their red blood cells, reflected by an increase in the MCV. My sense from researching the subject is that a significant percentage of people would have memory problems and dementia prevented if their B12 level were maintained above 500 either through diet or supplementation.

The population is getting older, though, so there may be better pharmaceutical options in the future. Genetic testing is already available that can run part of a person's exome and give a likelihood they will develop Alzheimer's. Currently, with no effective treatment options, this is not necessarily information the average person wants to know.

It is not clear what the alternative world has to offer for the prevention or treatment of dementia. Gingko biloba[NS] has probably received the most attention over the past 20 years, but the research is murky at best. There is a new supplement called trehalose.[NS] This option came up at the Naturopathic Conference I attended. The speaker was discussing the pathophysiology of autism. He reviewed the difference between an acute insult to the body like an ankle sprain that leads to short-term inflammation, and a chronic, recurrent injury pattern that leads to scarring. In autism, there are likely multiple external factors and substances causing inflammation and scarring of the central nervous system. Trehalose may break up plaques in the brain with potential benefits for autism and Alzheimer's dementia patients. This is premature as a solution, but it may have more value as a path to reverse the process than as a treatment itself. As is common in our country, if trehalose has value, the pharmaceutical industry may develop a prescription medication for use at some point many years into the future. It would be fabulously expensive and not go generic until I'm 100 years old.

Bill

Sixty-five-year-old Bill has Parkinsonism. He has seen many specialists over the years, including a cluster of neurologists. He has many of the classic signs of Parkinson's disease, including loss of facial expression and stiffness to his extremities, but does not have some of the other signs, like a pill-rolling tremor. Because Bill had chronic joint pain, unexplained fatigue and sweats, the first time I saw him in the office I wondered about the possibility of chronic Lyme disease. I thought maybe he had chronic Lyme and Parkinson's as separate issues. For the 10 years prior to seeing me, he got progressively worse. He had to quit his job at the post office while in his 50s. He had to live with his elderly mother. The specialists he saw considered the possibility of Lyme disease absurd. They believed, like most physicians, that his negative Elisa blood test for Borrelia Burgdorfer (the bacteria that causes Lyme disease) definitively ruled out Lyme as a possibility. One of the specialists gave him the nickname "The Mystery Man." This was acknowledging that they really couldn't figure him out. To admit that you don't know what is wrong with a person is always a good start for a healthcare practitioner. It is certainly better than pretending you understand more than you do. Every day, people are getting half-baked, dubious advice because their physician won't admit that they just don't what's going on.

I arranged for Bill to see an alternative practitioner that works with chronic Lyme disease. Over a year's time, on a regimen of antibiotics and immune-stimulating supplements, with changes to his diet, he slowly but steadily improved. His joint pain resolved and his fatigue diminished. His Parkinsonian symptoms stabilized. His neurologist was able to gradually decrease his Parkinson's drugs. She had no explanation for his improvement. Parkinson's patients don't improve very often. They typically need more and more medication to achieve less and less benefit. For over seven years his neurologic status has remained the same.

I have little tolerance in my work or in my life for people who feel they know the truth on some issue, period. What tends to happen to these people is they start with an opinion of some kind. The idea or belief may have come from a parent, if it's a political view, or maybe a preceptor, when they were a neophyte medical student. This idea may appeal to the person for any number of complex reasons. Over time, everything that supports their opinion gets reeled in and added to their internal basket of positive proof. Anything they hear or read that goes against their opinion is rejected quickly. As time goes on, they have a basket getting more and more full with evidence that their opinion or belief is correct. The contrary information has been sloughed off, so there really is no basket of evidence to contradict. When the supporting basket is overflowing, that person has undeniable, near complete confidence that what they believe is the truth. This is why you can have two equally intelligent, reasonable individuals with opposite opinions, both utterly convinced that they are correct.

As time goes on, the amount of supporting information is insurmountable. It is unquestioned. Doctors have an idea like "Statins are one of the greatest developments in modern medicine." Every cardiologist reinforces this. The specialists want more and more people on the medications. It is all self-reinforcing. The longer it goes on, the more ridiculous any contrary opinion seems. It can get to a point where it is nearly impossible to change an entrenched idea.

Many doctors (wrongly, in my experience) assume the blood tests they order are foolproof, whether for Lyme disease or a number of other chronic problems. The patients I suspect of chronic Lyme will often see specialists in orthopedics, rheumatology, infectious disease and other areas. They are given no explanation for their fatigue, joint pain, headaches, cognitive deficits, sweats, etc. They receive no diagnosis and are given no meaningful treatment options. They are only told one thing definitively: they do not have chronic Lyme disease.

Bill is not completely well, but the current approach to his management has been significantly more effective than anything tried before. I see him on a regular basis for follow-up. He has improved but plateaued with persistent mild Parkinsonian signs. He has fatigue from sleep apnea, which is surprising since he is very thin. The alternative Lyme practitioner's approach likely helped him improve, but she probably gave him some degree of false hope. She implied at one of his earliest visits that he would be well within 3-4 months. When he came to see me with this unrealistic time course, I tried to temper it without being negative. Many providers knowingly or unknowingly are trying to work the mind-body connection through positive statements.

For a while, things were the same for Bill—improved, but he was still tired and unwell. In the spring of 2013, I talked with him about a relatively new test for Lyme disease. Advanced Laboratories in Pennsylvania developed a Lyme culture that first became available to health providers in 2012. This test was unique because no other lab had ever been able to culture the bacteria from a blood specimen. I had researched the test and my sense was that Advanced Labs was a legitimate group that had developed a reliable test. A good friend of mine with a PhD in molecular biology reviewed the test and his assessment ultimately was that the culture to polymerase chain reaction (PCR) approach they developed was legitimate. One of the problems with the test was cost. It was not covered by insurance companies and a person would have to pay $595 out of pocket.

I talked with Bill about the test and for a while he was unwilling to pay to have it done. I was honest with him that this was a new test, not cleared through the regulatory groups like CLIA. The Centers for Medicare & Medicaid Services (CMS) at the federal level regulate all laboratory testing (except research) performed on humans in the U.S. through the Clinical Laboratory Improvement Amendments or CLIA. I could not completely verify the reliability of a negative or a positive result. After a few months of mulling it over and talking with his family about the cost, he called to say he wanted to do it.

I called an Infectious Disease group in the area hoping for advice on the new Lyme culture. The administrator referred me to their "Lyme test expert." When I heard that, I knew I was in trouble. The dreaded expert opinion can be onerous enough, but if his was going to be the last word on the subject in an area as controversial as Lyme disease, I feared the narrow mainstream judgment was at hand. I was not let down. If anything, the vigor of his response was more than expected. He wrote:

This sounds like a test for the banned list. The laboratory in question otherwise offers wellness testing. While B. burgdorferi [the causative agent for Lyme disease] can be cultured with some success from [a] biopsy of an erythema migrans rash, there is little reason to do so. This laboratory claims to culture B. burgdorferi from blood, where, in general, it is not found. It is difficult to fathom the intent of such testing. We should not be submitting testing to this laboratory, and clinical staff abetting this should be strongly counseled otherwise.

Bill's test came back positive. I don't think this is 100% reliable, but I think it is more likely than not that he has had Lyme disease for more than 10 years. I asked him what he wanted to do with the positive result. He has seen many different allopathic specialists over the years and I asked if he wanted to get a new opinion from a different infectious disease specialist. He decided to work with the alternative provider. She recommended antibiotics and a new supplement to improve immune function. I would love to say that Bill responded and his health improved. Subjectively, he told me he felt somewhat better, but not dramatically.

Each patient experience helps me sort out the best and the worst of mainstream and alternative approaches, but it will always be a work in progress. The issues are too complex and each person's situation is too unique for a standardized approach to be used.

4

Immunology and Chronic Infections

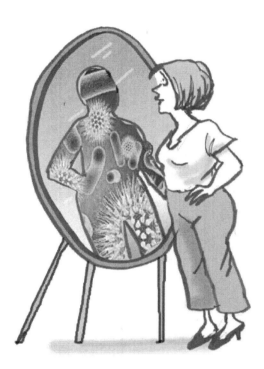

I went through one of our infectious disease specialists' schedule to check what he was seeing in the office. Out of 10 visits, he had two HIV patients, two patients with possible Lyme disease, two with MRSA (or Methicillin-resistant Staphylococcus Aureus) infections, one with hypogammaglobulinemia (a type of inherited immune deficiency), one with a liver abscess, one with epididymitis (an infection involving the tissue adjacent to the testicle) and one with multi-drug-resistant infections and immune compromise after kidney transplant. Out of this small group, some had acute infections that could be cleared with relatively short courses of antibiotics. The Lyme disease patients often see a specialist if the infection has become chronic and difficult to manage. Over the years, I've begun to appreciate just how many chronic illnesses may have their roots in chronic infection. "Superbug" bacteria, resistant to multiple antibiotic drugs, are a growing problem in American medicine. This may be from doctors' over-prescribing of antibiotics for viral conditions. It also may be related to the widespread use of antibiotics by the food industry to enhance the productivity of food stock like cows, chickens and pigs.

Acute Infections

One can summarize acute infections relatively easily. I often tell the medical students I work with that acute infections involving the ear, throat, sinus and lung are "viral until proven otherwise." There are many studies over the past 25 years showing that the vast majority of these types of infections will resolve with basic supportive care. Skin infections can be viral in the cases of shingles or the herpes simplex virus (HSV). More often they are bacterial and oral antibiotics are necessary. Urinary tract infections (UTIs) are almost always bacterial and traditional thinking says that antibiotics are necessary to treat the infection so it does not progress into the kidney or the blood stream. There is some question about the role of cranberry juice and cranberry supplements for prevention, or possibly even treatment, of UTIs. A full survey of the research into cranberry juice shows no conclusive support for or against it as an option, but even a definitive study would probably do little to change current practice. It is already an established idea in our culture that cranberry juice is worthwhile for UTIs, so it would be hard to put the genie back in the bottle. The naturopathic approach to UTIs will come up in the Urology section of "The Others" chapter.

It is interesting to contrast an MD's and naturopath's approach to managing acute infections. My general approach is to use antibiotics as infrequently as possible. The antibiotics usually don't make a difference and they can cause a wide variety of side effects. I focus my efforts more on reassuring the person that by enhancing the capacity of their own immune system, they should be well relatively quickly. This would include focusing on the basics of diet, hydration, whole food vitamin C from the diet or as a supplement (not ascorbic acid which is only one small part of the vitamin C molecule) and getting adequate rest. Diet may also play a role in our susceptibility to infection. The television actress who played Blossom, Mayim Bialik, said, "I've never had a sinus infection or been on antibiotics since cutting out dairy."[26] Based on what I understand now, her experience does not surprise me. In many ways, the naturopath's approach is similar, although most adhere to a strict model with no pharmaceuticals under any circumstance. They would often substitute a homeopathic option, ascribing much more closely to the *primum non nocere* dictum (first do no harm) that even the most cautious allopathic provider embraces.

I made contact with a naturopath from British Columbia at a 2013 conference. It was fascinating to hear his approach to some of the more common acute infections. In an email reply later, he also commented on the lack of benefit of antibiotics. He seemed to assume this would be a new concept for me. This speaks to the gap of understanding between allopaths and naturopaths, yet we probably have more common ground than either side realizes. There is such a wide variety of approaches among providers that it is difficult to generalize for any specific question of management.

At my first job, patients could call with just about any infection of any duration and they would, more often than not, get an antibiotic called in over the phone.

"Hello, this is Suzie Smith. I've had a sore throat since yesterday with a mild cough."

The nurse from that office would reply: "Oh, ok, I'm sorry you're not feeling well. We can call in that amoxicillin for you, no problem."

"Great!" Suzie is thrilled. "Thanks. You guys are such a great medical office."

I was right out of residency then and a relative purist when it came to these issues, so I was horrified at this flagrant overuse of antibiotics. The patient thought she was getting very attentive and efficient medical care even though she was never even seen by a doctor. She didn't have to miss work. It was probably cheaper for the insurance company to pay for a generic medication rather than an office visit. The pharmaceutical company that manufactured the amoxicillin made a bit of profit. The local pharmacy near my first job was probably making money left and right filling all the excessive antibiotic prescriptions. So if everyone is doing so well in this scenario, what's the problem? After all, this keeps our economy rolling along. The problem, of course, is in the overprescribing of antibiotics—this increases resistance and, over time, the antibiotics become less effective. We also destroy much of the person's healthy internal flora, the impact of which will be a common theme in this book.

When asked how he treated acute infections in his office, the naturopath from British Columbia said that, in his opinion, "the natural stuff is superior to antibiotics."[27] He used herbal antibiotics and immune modulators "such as andrographis[NS], hydrastis[NS], propolis[NS], echinacea root[NS] (NOT [the] leaf because [the] leaf doesn't work) and others."[27] He added that hydrotherapy is very effective for acute infections and that some naturopathic doctors or ND's use intravenous hydrogen peroxide, which really "kicks ass" in "acutes" [a.k.a. acute infections] or IV vitamin C. These options would never in a million years be considered by an MD in managing an acute infection. We have no training for any of them.

There is still the question of how much evidence supports these options. What we do know is that most acute infections resolve on their own with no treatment at all. If people on antibiotics get better, that does not mean that the antibiotic had benefit, since they might have felt better in two to three days anyway. By the same token, if a naturopath uses one of the above forms of therapy and people improve, we cannot reliably say that their option had benefit either without some more definitive evidence. In an ironic twist, maybe the naturopaths are overmanaging acute viral infections with herbs and IV treatments that incur cost with no firm evidence. Often, reassurance is the best management option. I believe in chiropractors, but for years I would comment to patients that the research shows that a person with acute back pain will be better 80% of the time within a week and 90% of the time within 2-4 weeks. Thus, the chiropractor is starting with a 90% success rate. I am much more inclined to send someone to a chiropractor for chronic back issues.

Echinacea

For many years, echinacea has been one of the most commonly used alternative options for the treatment of a wide variety of acute infections. There have been studies done to assess how effective Echinacea is in shortening the course of a viral upper respiratory infection. Overall, there seems to be some disagreement regarding effectiveness. In 2010, researchers from the University of Wisconsin conducted a randomized controlled trial[28] in which they studied the potential benefits of echinacea as a treatment of the common cold. The researchers randomly assigned 713 study participants, 12 to 80 years of age, into four groups to receive: no pills, placebo (blinded), echinacea (blinded), or echinacea (unblinded). All had cold symptoms. Participants received 2 tablet doses four times the first day, followed by one tablet four times daily for the next four days. (The echinacea tablets contained the equivalent of 675 mg of E. purpurea root and 600 mg of E. angustifolia root.) Participants who received echinacea (blinded or unblinded) had no significant improvement in either duration or severity of illness compared with those who received no pills or placebo. Although the authors noted that there were small trends in the direction of a benefit from echinacea—an average half-day reduction in duration—this was not deemed a significant enough benefit.

The University of Maryland website, however, came to a different conclusion: A review of 14 clinical trials found that echinacea reduced the odds of developing a cold by 58% and the duration of a cold by 1-4 days. However, some experts dispute these findings claiming there were several weaknesses in the analyses. Echinacea preparations tested in clinical trials differ greatly. It is important to choose a high-quality echinacea supplement and I would trust my naturopath colleague and get the root.

Zinc

Another option that is still in common use is zinc. I remember first hearing about zinc as a third-year medical student on my family practice rotation. At that time, zinc came out in lozenge form and my instructor thought then they would shorten the duration of a cold. Research after that did not support the benefit for lozenges, but for a while there was more support for Zicam, the zinc nasal spray. On the Mayo Clinic website, you can read that neither is likely worth the effort: "The highest quality randomized trials generally show no benefit. Intranasal zinc may result in permanent damage to the sense of smell. The FDA issued a warning against using three zinc-containing nasal cold remedies because they had been associated with a long-lasting or permanent loss of smell (anosmia)."[29]

More recently, I have become intrigued by another natural option, umck-aloba or umcka. There is research to suggest activity against viruses and bacteria, including the flu virus and resistant staph aureus bacteria. It seems particularly effective for acute bronchitis. If that is true it would be worth trying, since the cough of bronchitis tends to hang around for weeks. As with many of the other more natural options, we may not have definitive evidence or we may have a mix, some studies showing benefit and others showing a lack of effect. I have had positive feedback about umcka from a number of patients who assert that starting the herb at the onset of a cough or cold shortened the duration of symptoms. I'm glad they are getting better quickly, but how could we possibly know if the umcka helped them or not? There is a need for well-designed controlled studies to answer these important clinical questions.

The natural option with the strongest evidence according to the Natural Standard database is andrographis. This plant, native to South Asian countries like India and Sri Lanka, is often used for the prevention and treatment of the common cold and influenza. The leaf and the underground stem are used to concentrate the active parts of the herb.

The summary recommendation is a common refrain: maintain a healthy diet, exercise regularly, get enough sleep, and lower stress as much as possible to maximize the effectiveness of your immune system. If you get sick, consult a provider if the symptoms are severe, progressive, or in some way concerning. Otherwise, let if fly.

Chronic Infections

Connections to Chronic Illness

The issue of chronic infections causing chronic illness has been slowly gaining momentum over the past 20 or more years. I would predict that the fields of infectious disease and virology will take center stage in the future. There is already a long list of chronic conditions and cancers linked to chronic infections. These include liver cancer, stomach cancer, peptic ulcer disease, cervical cancer and others. Why would we think that those identified are the only chronic illnesses linked to chronic infection? We have probably only scratched the surface.

The link between chronic infections and chronic illnesses reinforces the importance of a healthy lifestyle. Adequate nutrition, hydration and sleep are necessary to maintain an optimal immune system. There is evidence that if people get fewer than six hours of sleep their cortisol (a.k.a. "stress hormone") levels go up by 50 percent. Management of stress—especially through exercise, meditation, yoga, proper breathing and other relaxation techniques—is essential, as is maintaining healthy bowel flora.

It is well established that a bacterial species called Helicobacter pylori, or H. pylori for short, plays a key role in the development of stomach ulcers and stomach cancers. This was confirmed when an Australian physician and researcher, Barry Marshall, drank a cup of the bacteria to prove a point. Soon after downing the concoction, he became severely ill from the ulcers that formed in his stomach and esophagus.[30]

Despite this demonstration, skepticism persisted for years. To this day, the eradication of the bacteria with a specific antibiotic regimen is underutilized in the prevention of recurrent ulcers. There is more to the story, though, because millions of people have H. pylori in their gastrointestinal tract and never get ulcers or stomach cancer. The interplay of these microorganisms and our immune system is in some way complex and in other ways brutally simple. If a person pursues an optimal lifestyle, their immune system will function at a high level and the impact of these pathogenic microorganisms can be minimized.

Lessons from HPV

We have developed intricate symbiotic relationships with these agents over millions of years and human beings coexist with the majority of these organisms to our mutual benefit. Some strains, however, can be pathogenic and cause illness, especially in a vulnerable individual. Mild strains of a common virus, the Human Papilloma Virus (HPV), cause the simple warts found on hands and feet. More aggressive strains, usually transmitted sexually, can cause cervical cancer.

The Pap Smear has been one of the major successes of modern preventative medicine. It is used to take a sample of the cells from the end of the uterus, or cervix, to check for cancerous and pre-cancerous changes. Due to these interventions, there has been a 75-percent decrease in the incidence and mortality of cervical cancer over the past 50 years in developed countries.

Some cancer-causing HPV strains are now targeted by the Gardasil vaccine for teenage boys and girls. The presence of another sexually transmitted virus, the Herpes Simplex Virus (HSV), with HPV can increase the risk of cervical cancer even more. More recently, it has become clear that oral/oropharyngeal cancers are primarily caused by strains of the HPV virus as well. This was not known for much of my medical career. The most likely scenario is that the person who develops oral cancer contracted it during oral sex, but there may be other means of developing the chronic infection. Gardasil has been shown to protect those immunized against the more aggressive strains of the HPV virus and will likely reduce the incidence of genital warts, cervical cancer and oral cancer.

Linking Seizures to Infection

It is well established that a parasitic infection can cause seizures. This is most common in Latin America in a condition called cysticercosis. The disease occurs after exposure to a pork tapeworm. The disease is spread via the fecal-oral route through contaminated food and water. After ingestion, the eggs pass through the intestine into the tissues and migrate preferentially to the brain and muscles. There they form cysts that can persist for years. In some cases, the cysts will eventually cause an inflammatory reaction presenting as painful nodules in the muscles and, when the cysts are located in the brain, seizures.

It is possible that the chronic seizures of others are caused by an unidentified infectious agent. Around 50 percent of people with seizures will have a normal Electroencephalogram (EEG). As with many issues in medicine, there really is not a complete understanding of why people get seizures. A minority will have a positive family history, so there can be some underlying familial tendency.

Syphilis

One of the granddaddies of all infectious agents is syphilis. This spirochete bacteria is typically sexually transmitted but can also be passed mother-to-child in vitro to cause congenital syphilis. There are not many syphilis cases around these days and I have not had one positive test in my 15+ years in medicine, but the infectious agent provides insights into chronic infections and chronic illnesses. If the infection is untreated and progresses to a more advanced stage, a person can have cardiac involvement, seizures or signs of dementia. Testing for syphilis remains part of the standard work-up for a patient with dementia. I have heard there is a tome written more than a century ago that describes the disparate presentations of syphilis, in detail, over hundreds of pages. Strangely enough, the book presents a perfect description of chronic Lyme disease when read in the modern era of medicine and infectious disease. Those who fail to learn from history are doomed to repeat it.

Lyme Disease

The causative agent for Lyme disease is a spirochete bacteria similar to the one that causes primary, secondary and tertiary syphilis. Lyme disease is a tick-borne illness that can present with a variety of symptoms. I work in an area of the country where Lyme disease is prevalent. A few years ago, I saw an 82-year-old female in the office. Grace complained of knee pain and unexplained fatigue over the prior couple of weeks. The knee pain seemed to her out of proportion to her mild, chronic knee pain attributed to osteoarthritis. She was also experiencing mild, intermittent headaches. Grace ran a horse farm and did yoga three times a week. She was frequently exposed to deer ticks but had no specific bite she could remember and no rash. We discussed some of the controversy regarding Lyme disease and I told her that, in my opinion, the lab results are never completely reliable to rule out the infection but this is especially the case early on in the course.

There is one scenario where I willingly overprescribe antibiotics: in an effort to reduce the likelihood of someone developing chronic Lyme disease. I try to avoid antibiotics in just about every other scenario of an acute infection. Because the tests for Lyme disease are unreliable, and because starting antibiotics early in Lyme disease is so crucial, I feel I have no other choice but to treat aggressively. I evaluate each case individually in terms of likelihood for Lyme disease. Most physicians, on either side of the Lyme controversy, acknowledge that it is primarily a "clinical diagnosis," which means one based on symptoms rather than a positive blood test.

I started Grace on empiric doxycycline and she started to improve. The headaches and the knee pain resolved over a week or so, but her fatigue did not improve. Grace came back to see me and I initiated a broader work-up. When the labs came back, she had anemia. This was a new finding as she had shown a normal hemoglobin level a month prior at an annual physical.

People often misunderstand anemia. There are three main types of blood cells: red cells, white cells and platelets. The red cells carry oxygen to tissues. The white blood cells fight infection and perform other functions of the immune system. The platelets clump together aiding in clot formation. Anemia is a reference to a decrease in the quantity of red blood cells. There are many different causes for anemia, some acute and some chronic. A normal hemoglobin level is typically over 12 for women and over 13 for men.

I discussed with Grace the possibility of a co-infection, Babesia, causing her anemia. A co-infection, in this context, would be some other infectious agent transmitted concurrently with the Lyme disease. Babesia is an intracellular parasite that can be transmitted by the same tick that transmits the bacteria that causes Lyme disease. The Babesia organism can take up residence and reproduce in red blood cells causing them to be consumed by the body.

Many years ago, I saw an elderly man in his 80s who came in for an acute visit. He looked horrendous and, within a second of walking in the room, I knew something was seriously wrong. He was extremely tired and appeared pale. I checked a hemoglobin level in the office and it was below eight, so he had lost about half of his red blood cell volume. My concern was for internal bleeding. We called an ambulance and he was admitted to a local hospital. They found that he had Babesiosis of uncertain duration. He required several blood transfusions and supplemental oxygen. He ultimately responded very well to antibiotics and regained his health relatively quickly.

For Grace, I remember her significant other, a kindly retired professor named George, trying to convince her to see an infectious disease specialist. In my experience, the ID specialists often rely on the Lyme blood test, so I wasn't sure she would get a clearer diagnosis, but I would never dissuade someone from seeing a specialist if that's what they wish. I started her on azithromycin and mepron and about a week later the Babesia test came back positive. Grace eventually regained her good health and got back to yoga and horseback riding.

Because of controversies around chronic Lyme disease, I have come to a place where I am at odds with the majority of specialists in my area. If I am concerned about chronic Lyme and the person sees an ID specialist near me, they are invariably told they do not have chronic Lyme. This is in contrast to the Lyme specialists scattered around the northeast that diagnose most of the patients they see with chronic Lyme. There's me in the middle, thinking the answer is probably somewhere in between. One of the foremost authorities on chronic Lyme disease is Richard Horowitz, MD. In 2013, he published a book called *Why Can't I Get Better? Solving the Mystery of Lyme and Chronic Disease.* In the book, he reviews the challenge of managing those with chronic Lyme disease. He uses the term "multi-system infectious disease syndrome" and has a 16-point approach to improving the health of his patients. This, in some ways, mirrors my own evolution as a provider trying to sort out complicated patients. Horowitz's points include:

1. Lyme disease and co-infections
2. Immune dysfunction
3. Inflammation
4. Environmental toxins
5. Nutritional deficiencies
6. Mitochondrial dysfunction
7. Endocrine abnormalities
8. Neurodegenerative disorders
9. Neuropsychiatric disorders
10. Sleep disorders
11. Autonomic nervous system dysfunction
12. Allergies
13. Gastrointestinal disorders
14. Liver dysfunction
15. Pain disorders/addiction
16. Lack of exercise/deconditioning[31]

There is little doubt in my mind that history will ultimately show that chronic Lyme disease is real and prevalent. I have had too many people with classic symptoms improve with treatment for me to believe it is a hoax. The Lyme community has come up with a paradigm that explains very well what is happening to a subgroup of the chronically ill. Thus far, the mainstream medical world has yet to come up with any alternative approach of value. The Horowitz book may influence the debate on chronic Lyme by providing a reference point for medical providers. It may be the support providers need to manage complex patients more deftly with less fear of retribution.

Consider this hypothetical panel discussion with an infectious disease specialist representing the mainstream:

ID Specialist: What about all of the people diagnosed with "chronic Lyme" that are on two or three antibiotics for years and don't get better?

Me: That was my frustration for years as well, but Richard Horowitz provides a framework that explains why some people improve on antibiotics alone and why others need a broader, more sophisticated approach.

ID: Some of the Lyme practitioners are charging exorbitant fees.

Me: Yes. One that I am aware of in particular seems to charge high rates and this issue can undermine good work that's being done. But that doesn't have anything to do with whether or not chronic Lyme disease is real and complex and needs to be managed. Dr. Charles Roy Jones in Connecticut uses most of his income for a legal defense fund so he can continue to practice.

ID: Some of the providers aren't medical doctors but naturopaths and other alternative practitioners.

Me: Experts can be found anywhere. Naturopaths go through rigorous schooling similar to medical doctors and their training is probably more relevant to figuring out complex patients.

ID: Why aren't the blood tests reliable?

Me: There are potentially 100-200 individual species of the borrelia bacteria. Researchers like Raphael Stricker, MD, at Johns Hopkins have described the unique qualities of Borrelia Burgdorferi that help it evade the immune system.[32] Some of these stealth characteristics help minimize the immune response required to have an antibody test be positive. For a summary of the other reasons, read the Horowitz book.

ID: There is no evidence supporting the methods used to manage chronic Lyme patients.

Me: Horowitz.

I am continually searching for better ways to diagnose and manage what I suspect is chronic Lyme disease. The Horowitz book is a revelation, but prior to that I had heard a lot about a Dr. Charles Roy Jones working with pediatric Lyme patients. As part of this endeavor, I spent a day in 2012 tailing the Lyme specialist in Connecticut.

Charles Roy Jones is a major player in the Lyme story. For those with chronic Lyme, he is revered as a pioneer who has saved the lives of thousands of children. The reports I heard about his impact on the health of children were invariably positive. I finally made contact with his office and he agreed to let me sit in with him for a day. I figured I would probably learn a lot about chronic Lyme disease and, at a minimum, it would be an interesting experience. I was not disappointed.

In the spring of 2012, early on a Friday morning, I took the day off from my regular work, drove to New Haven, Connecticut, and found Dr. Jones' office in a building a stone's throw from Yale-New Haven Medical Center. The building was a nondescript gray brick edifice in a row of identical, uninspiring apartment buildings in a low-income section of town. At the end of a long hall on the ground floor, I found his office. There was no one there. I was a bit early, but figured there should be a receptionist or nurse getting ready for the day. I sat down in a chair, picked up a magazine and started browsing.

Fifteen minutes later I heard some activity back in the exam rooms—a bump, then the unmistakable sound of a person slowly walking the hall with one foot dragging behind. Eventually, a heavy man in his 80s appeared, stooped over, wearing thick glasses and a navy blue tracksuit, sporting messy, dark hair. I could tell by the way he was looking down at the floor that he didn't see me or realize I was sitting there.

When I stood up and walked over to him, he was mildly surprised to see me. He had forgotten that I was coming, but then welcomed me and invited me back down the hall to his small office. He said that doctors often came to work with him for a day, a week, or sometimes longer. He said more doctors were needed to take up the cause because he wasn't going to be around much longer.

Dr. Jones told me some of his story. He was working in Connecticut as a pediatric immunologist in the 1960s and 1970s. He and other colleagues, notably Allen Steere, MD, started seeing more and more children with severe joint pain, fatigue and other symptoms. Many of those children were diagnosed with Juvenile Rheumatoid Arthritis (JRA). There was no clear explanation, though, for the dramatic rise in these cases. He said a few of the patients he was seeing got sick with strep throat or a lung infection or some other infection requiring antibiotics. When they were put on oral antibiotics, not only did the acute infection get better, but often their chronic joint pain and other symptoms improved as well. Some physicians, including Dr. Jones, started to suspect that, in many cases, a chronic infection was the root cause of the JRA diagnosis.

Dr. Jones became more and more interested in these cases. He did his best to manage them with antibiotics and, through trial and error, eventually came up with protocols and general approaches for treatment. There were so many of these cases in Connecticut that in the mid-1970s he transitioned his practice solely to helping these kids. It wasn't until Willy Burgdorfer isolated the eponymous bacteria Borrelia Burgdorferi in 1982 that the causative bacteria for Lyme disease was identified.

Up to the time of my visit, Dr. Jones had treated almost 20,000 children for chronic Lyme disease, probably making him the most experienced provider in history. He gave me some additional background on diagnosis and management until the families started arriving. They came from many states, including New York, New Jersey, Pennsylvania and Ohio. Most drove long hours to get to his office.

The cases were varied but shared common themes. Most of the children had had symptoms for many years before they were diagnosed with chronic Lyme. They had seen their primary care providers and multiple specialists before finding their way to Dr. Jones out of desperation. Thankfully, most of them were slowly improving on long-term antibiotics and doing better in school. The families had come to accept that slow progress was better than steady deterioration.

For the whole day, Dr. Jones and I sat in his little room as the children and their mothers were shuttled in one at a time. He drank five or six cups of black coffee. He didn't eat breakfast, lunch or dinner. One time, I saw him sneak a couple of tiny Reese's peanut butter cups, but that was his only sustenance all day. I don't think he ever got up to use the bathroom. He was still seeing people when I left around 6 p.m. The nurses told me on my way out that he usually saw patients six days a week into the evenings. He would then do paperwork until he fell asleep in his chair. When I heard him stumbling around that morning, it was him waking up after sleeping in his office the night before. The idea that somehow he was getting rich and famous from his work was preposterous. It was obvious that he relished his role as a rebel, but he probably drove to work in a Pinto with racing stripes.

Connecting Infection and Neuropsychiatric Disorders

One of the more recent chronic infection developments involves a condition called PANDAS. This stands for Pediatric Autoimmune Neuropsychiatric Disorders Associated with Streptococcal Infections. There are different streptococcus infections, but the most prevalent would be a pharyngitis infection of the throat caused by the Group A streptococcus bacteria. I first heard about PANDAS years ago, but in a vague way that did not stick with me—uncooked spaghetti that bounced off the wall. The issue then came up briefly at the very end of some lecture at a medical conference sponsored by Harvard Medical School. It was mentioned as an oddity with little impact on or relevance to the day-to-day management of primary care doctors.

The classic situation for PANDAS is a child with a new onset tic disorder that is caused by an acute strep infection. There are several different types of tics that a person can develop. Tics are repeated, involuntary muscular movements affecting either limb muscles, facial muscles (e.g. grimacing or eyelid flicking) or vocal muscles (grunting or saying words). There are estimates that suggest a very high percentage of children will have a tic disorder during childhood. This can be up to 20% or higher based on research studies. Most of these children are undiagnosed. The parents, teachers and doctors may not recognize the tic is present or they may recognize it, but feel it is a minor issue not worth investigating or managing. Parents will often keep things to themselves, especially if there are associated behavioral issues.

Many children with tic disorders will also have coexisting behavioral difficulties, including disinhibited speech or conduct, impulsivity, distractibility, hyperactivity and, occasionally, obsessive-compulsive symptoms. There can be an assumption that a poorly behaved child is a reflection of poor parenting. (This "Standard Parenting Model" was discussed in "The Power of the Mind" chapter.) It is possible that by not uncovering the underlying infection causing a tic disorder we are missing an important opportunity to correct a problem that can cause a difficult-to-manage chronic neurologic or psychiatric disorder.

Within a week of hearing about PANDAS at the conference, an eight-year-old little girl named Sally came in with her mother. The complaint was that Sally had developed a facial motor tic over the previous week or two. If I hadn't just recently heard about the PANDAS issue, I probably would have talked to the mom about giving it some time to resolve on its own or getting a consultation with a pediatric neurologist. In primary care, there are issues that providers see often and over time they become extremely comfortable managing them without help. There are other issues, however, so uncommon that most primary care providers do not feel they can keep up with optimal management and choose to seek the help of a specialist. Tic disorders do not come up as chief complaints often enough for most primary care physicians to manage them independently.

For Sally, she had no signs of any recent or ongoing infection—no sore throat or cough or fever or rash. There was no one at home with a sore throat and no close friends were recently diagnosed with strep throat. I did a quick strep test that was negative but, to be safe, I also sent out a 24-hour strep culture. A couple of days later this came back positive for Group A Streptococcus. I called the mom about the positive result and we started the antibiotic amoxicillin for a 10-day course. After a few days, the mom called to say that the tic issue had resolved. I have seen Sally several times since then and the tic has not returned. In retrospect, it was relatively easy to take care of Sally's PANDAS issue because it was an infection of such short duration. With many chronic illnesses related to chronic infections, notably Lyme disease, I tell patients the longer they have had the infection, the harder it is to eradicate. We will see this in another much more complex PANDAS case.

There are precedents for PANDAS. As noted in a review article by Lisa Snider and Susan Swedo, this is not necessarily a new development in medicine. The authors relate: "The first infectious agent shown to cause a post-infectious disorder in the central nervous system was [a different strep bacteria] Streptococcus pyogenes in Sydenham's chorea."[33] Since I have never seen a case of Syndenham's chorea (SD), and probably only heard about it for five minutes while in medical school, I had to read up from another source. The National Institute of Neurological Disorders and Stroke summarized the condition on its website:

SD is characterized by rapid, irregular, and aimless involuntary movements of the arms and legs, trunk, and facial muscles. It affects girls more often than boys and typically occurs between 5 and 15 years of age. Some children will have a sore throat several weeks before the symptoms begin, but the disorder can also strike up to 6 months after the fever or infection has cleared. Symptoms can appear gradually or all at once, and also may include uncoordinated movements, muscular weakness, stumbling and falling, slurred speech, difficulty concentrating and writing, and emotional instability. The symptoms of SD can vary from a halting gait and slight grimacing to involuntary movements that are frequent and severe enough to be incapacitating. The random, writhing movements of chorea are caused by an auto-immune reaction to the bacterium that interferes with the normal function of a part of the brain (the basal ganglia) that controls motor movements.[34]

The article by Snider and Swedo also reviews the principle that only certain individuals are susceptible to the autoimmune inflammatory response caused by various streptococcus species and subtypes. This would explain why most children that get infected with strep do not develop the neurologic symptoms or get severely ill. The paradigm of chronic infection causing chronic illness in the young and old has been around for a long time.

PANS and Courtney

PANS, Pediatric Acute-Onset Neuropsychiatric Syndrome, was proposed as recently as 2012 to describe a subset of acute-onset obsessive-compulsive disorder (OCD) cases. A common element among those with complex pediatric conditions is that many of them have been prescribed multiple courses of antibiotics. Of course, this could be cause or effect. The patient could have a poorly functioning immune system which led to frequent infections that necessitated antibiotics. Or, it is also possible that a young child repeatedly on antibiotics would have their internal flora disrupted, causing a ripple effect.

I've been seeing Courtney in our office for a few years. She is a young woman diagnosed with PANDAS by one of the top specialists in the world in this area. Courtney had ear infections, sinus infections, lung infections and allergy problems starting before the age of two. She saw many specialists in an effort to improve her health. She had her adenoids removed. She had persistent bowel problems and was ultimately diagnosed with irritable bowel syndrome. It was later on that her neurologic and psychiatric manifestations began. She had anxiety, insomnia and severe regular nightmares. Then, the obsessions about food and eating started to pick up momentum. She was ultimately diagnosed with the eating disorder anorexia nervosa.

Courtney was diagnosed with PANS as the explanation for her anorexia nervosa. When I first heard this concept I was dumbstruck. This radical idea will take some time before it is accepted in mainstream medicine but the more I worked it out, the more sense it made. The most typical manifestation of PANDAS and PANS is a tic disorder, and it is well established that tics and obsessive compulsive disorder (OCD) are on the same spectrum. It doesn't take much to put eating disorders in the broad classification of OCD. There is no medical condition I can think of with more profound obsessions and compulsions than anorexia nervosa. This links the field of psychiatry with infectious disease. Who knows how far this link will go and how many psychiatric conditions may ultimately be related to the immune system and chronic infection.

By the time I started seeing Courtney in the office, she was very ill. She was having one sinus infection after another. She had lost a lot of weight. She was having trouble controlling her anxiety. The family was in a state of constant turmoil. The mom described the situation:

What took us to come in is that Courtney is getting tired and just overwhelmed with the OCD, now manifesting with germs (still) and binge eating (although preoccupation on healthy eating, so no significant weight gain and still excessive diarrhea, so not much is sticking to her). She overeats during the day (2600-4600 cals/day) and then feels excessive anxiety at night. That sends her into fear and despair about waking up to the whole nightmare of being out of control the next day. She ramps up and then can't control the anxiety.[35]

We started having conversations about PANS. It was difficult to get her in to see him, but Courtney started working with a specialist in PANDAS/PANS named Denis Bouboulis, MD. The family would drive down to Connecticut to see him on a regular basis. There is an interesting *TODAY* show clip from March 11, 2010, where Dr. Bouboulis describes his success in treating a young girl with PANDAS. This girl had a tic disorder from the streptococcus bacteria causing frequent sneezing and was ultimately cured by his intravenous immune globulin (IVIg) treatments when no one else could help her.

Anorexia nervosa is one of the most difficult-to-manage conditions in medicine. The person has a distorted sense of self and an insatiable desire to be thinner. This leads to disordered eating and, often, excessive exercise because the person will do almost anything to maintain a slender physique and sees themselves as always overweight. For those around them and taking care of them, the mindset behind the obsessions makes no sense.

I remember well a yoga retreat I attended with my wife in Costa Rica. There were about 20 yogis in the group, including a young woman in her early 20s who obviously struggled with anorexia nervosa. During the week, one well-meaning woman after another took her aside, trying to convince her that she was beautiful and should feel better about herself. Each was trying to help but had no understanding of the nature of the disease. These conversations probably made the young woman feel worse because, in her mind, if she really were beautiful and worthwhile, people wouldn't have to work so hard to convince her. She went home at the end of the week more frustrated and alone than ever.

Courtney ultimately ended up working with Dr. Jones as well, because the causative organism for her PANDAS was thought to be Lyme. She went through different antibiotic regimens and had multiple IVIg treatments. We have used a variety of different vitamins, supplements and medications. Sometimes, doctors can have the answer but not the means to correct the condition. In the case of both Courtney and the young yogi, the insights of others, including the savviest medical provider, could not easily resolve the issues. Courtney is steadily improving and each time I see her she is one step closer to recovery. For many complicated people, it is a long, arduous process toward wellness that takes many years and much sacrifice.

Chronic Skin Conditions

There are many chronic skin conditions, including acne, seborrheic dermatitis, eczema and psoriasis that are worse when the person is under stress. This is probably because stress depresses the immune system and disrupts our ability to keep infectious agents in check. The classic example of this is shingles. It is well established that shingles is a reactivation of a chronic infection. If a person is exposed to the chicken pox or varicella virus as a child, most or all will then develop a chronic infection where the virus remains dormant in the root of a nerve somewhere in the body. The virus can be dormant for 50 years or more. When the person is older and their immune system is less effective, they are more vulnerable to a shingles outbreak. If a person at any age is under a tremendous amount of stress, they can get shingles. If I see someone with a painful rash and I'm not sure whether it's shingles, the amount of stress they are under will often help make the call about whether to start antiviral medication.

The herpes virus is a "cousin" to the chicken pox virus. It has a similar modus operandi where it is dormant most of the time but then flares up, producing a painful skin outbreak, if the person is under stress. I suspect we have many chronic infections as yet unidentified. Some of them have more obvious presentations, like a burning rash, but others probably have few symptoms. There is a continuous ebb and flow to our functioning immune system. When we put this all together, it becomes obvious that much of our health is peaceful coexistence with microorganisms. It is essential for us to maintain an appropriate balance internally. All of the elements of a healthy lifestyle help to achieve homeostasis, a well-functioning balance. This creates a strong argument for judicious use of antibiotics and steroids because they can dramatically alter the internal terrain. We have our own internal ecosystems as vast and as complex as any on earth. They are gardens that must be tended. Some are advocating the use of resistant starch (RS) as a way of nourishing our good bacteria. It is possible that by ingesting these forms of starch on a regular basis, we can each enhance the composition of our bowel flora.

Paul

A few years ago, I saw a 52-year-old male with fatigue, joint pain and persistent fevers. Paul had no significant past medical history. He was seen in the ER where they did a battery of tests including blood work, urine studies and a chest x-ray. The only abnormality was mildly elevated liver enzyme levels. The ER started him on doxycycline for possible Lyme disease. This seemed reasonable to me as the blood tests for Lyme disease are often falsely negative and it is crucial to get people on antibiotics as early in the course as possible. I saw him about a week later for a follow-up visit and he was feeling somewhat better. Even so, there was something about his case that didn't sit well with me.

I called an infectious disease specialist to review the case and went over the various symptoms and test results. His fateful words: "You know, acute HIV can present like that." I had only seen the patient in question once before and the subject of sexual activity came up during that initial visit. Paul was divorced, bisexual and engaging in many random, casual sexual encounters via internet "dating" sites. I had warned him about the risks, but I could tell he had shrugged it off.

I called Paul, telling him I had discussed his case with a specialist and asking him to come in for more blood tests, including HIV. By that time, he was feeling better with no symptoms and didn't want to come in. I insisted we do the labs. In the end, Paul turned out to be the first positive HIV test I had had in my practice. If I hadn't trusted my instincts and talked to the infectious disease specialist, he could have spread the virus to many people over the years while asymptomatic.

Once again, the most important factors in preventing and managing acute infections are the most basic. People will do best when they pursue a healthy lifestyle, exercise regularly, get enough sleep, manage their stress and wash their hands. The immune system can take care of the vast majority of infections by itself. Often, the most important thing any provider can do is *not* prescribe antibiotics for an infection that is likely viral. There is mixed evidence for some of the more natural options like Echinacea, andrographis and umcka. Trying those at the onset of a cough/cold is reasonable and may shorten the duration of symptoms.

In summary, there is a growing list of chronic medical issues caused in part or in whole by an underlying chronic infection. The many diverse symptoms include fatigue, headaches, joint pain, and others. It includes all of the organ systems of the body. We know with a high level of certainty that seizures, dementia, peptic ulcer disease, liver cancer, stomach cancer, skin cancer, cervical cancer, oral cancers and tic disorders are often caused by chronic infections. In my Lyme-endemic area, I see many patients with chronic intractable problems that I suspect have tick-borne illnesses as the primary cause. *In over twelve years of practice here, I have yet to see a complicated patient where I suspect chronic Lyme disease successfully diagnosed by a medical specialist.* With PANDAS, we see an entirely new realm of neurologic and psychiatric conditions that may ultimately be treated by eradicating infectious agents and more effectively supporting immune function. But, at this point in our history, we are almost certainly unaware of the role of many other infectious agents that are causing chronic health conditions.

5

Rheumatologyand Chronic Pain

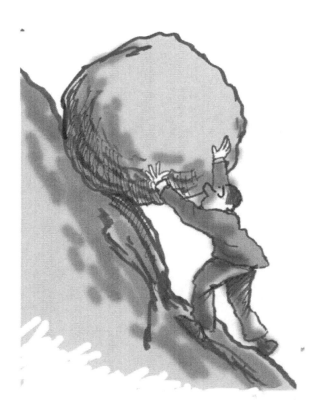

Rheumatology is a very challenging specialty overall with elusive diagnoses and dubious treatment plans. This should be an area where the alternative world has a lot to offer since most of the chronic rheumatologic conditions are complex and difficult to manage. Chronic arthritis and joint issues fall under rheumatology as well as chronic autoimmune conditions.

The most common diagnoses include rheumatoid arthritis, psoriatic arthritis, and fibromyalgia. The rheumatologist will also manage the ill-defined chronic fatigue syndrome and the rare bird lupus. Gout is more often managed by the primary care doctor, but cases can fall into this specialist's lap as well. Not surprisingly, The Royal London Hospital of Integrated Medicine has clinics specifically dedicated to chronic fatigue syndrome, fibromyalgia, irritable bowel syndrome and nutrition.

May's Fibromyalgia

May, now in her late 70s, was diagnosed with fibromyalgia when she was around 50. For over 20 years she had intense, daily muscular pains and could do very little. She had trouble walking up and down stairs, so would often sleep in a recliner on the first floor. She had two side businesses she loved: Tupperware sales and making cards. She would go to people's houses with her supplies and do Tupperware parties for groups of women. Slowly, she had to reduce her involvement with Tupperware because it was so difficult to get around.

I had been seeing her in the office for a couple of years and I was aware of her chronic pain syndrome. Fibromyalgia is a convenient label for a chronic pain syndrome and, originally, a patient has to have 11 out of 18 tender trigger points to officially meet criteria for the diagnosis. There are many other symptoms and problems that often co-exist with fibromyalgia. Most patients will have insomnia and wake up feeling unrefreshed. They will have moderate-to-severe daily fatigue. They often have headaches and unexplained hypersensitivity to touch. The underlying cause or causes of the condition are not well understood. A study published in the August 2013 issue of *Pain*, a journal from researchers at the Massachusetts General Hospital, provides vague insights into the pathophysiology. In the study, about half of a small group of patients diagnosed with fibromyalgia were found to have damage to nerve fibers in their skin and other evidence of a disease called small-fiber polyneuropathy (SFPN). This presents a classic "solution" for our current pharmacologic-based healthcare system where only an intermediate aspect of the process is being targeted. The pharmaceutical industry considers the number of people diagnosed with fibromyalgia, currently two percent of the population, and sees the seductive potential for lifelong treatment. Unfortunately, a new medication option does not get us much closer to understanding the deep underlying cause or causes. In some circles, fibromyalgia is presumed to be caused by a chronic infection of some sort, but that has not been clarified. There is a strong possibility that genetic abnormalities, like a methylene tetra-hydrofolate reductase (MTHFR) enzyme defect, explain the underlying susceptibility of some people to these chronic pain syndromes. Exercise is typically helpful, but someone with pain, fatigue and insomnia may not be up for a three-mile jog.

There are currently three medications being used for fibromyalgia. Cymbalta was developed as an antidepressant and now is touted as a miracle drug for fibromyalgia. Cymbalta itself is a "me-too" medication very similar chemically to another antidepressant, Effexor. There is no evidence that Cymbalta is more effective than Effexor for anything. It is newer, however, and people often assume newer is better. It is name-brand only and, because of this, the profit margin is considerably higher.

Lyrica is another drug being used that can have some benefit(s). The majority of people, however, will probably not do much better than on a placebo. Many will also be unable to tolerate the side effects, notably drowsiness and sluggishness for Lyrica.

The third medication option is the generic medication similar to Lyrica, gabapentin. This medication does seem to have clear benefit for many who have chronic neuropathic pain, like peripheral neuropathy. For fibro-myalgia, however, it probably will not have much real impact in terms of improving patients' quality of life. The patient as consumer needs to always be aware of the medical doctor's strong inclination to do something, even though giving a prescription medication with small chance of benefit and some likelihood of side effects may not be the best course of action. I've been guilty of this in my time so won't judge. It is embedded now in western medical culture to give the patient a prescription under the presumption they will feel better about the visit and the care they received if they go home with something. To "do nothing" often leaves the patient with the sense that the visit was a waste of time and that they aren't getting their money's worth.

Another study, published in the August 21, 2013, issue of *Analyst,* described a new diagnostic tool:

In a pilot study, the scientists used a high-powered and specialized micro-scope to detect the presence of small molecules in blood-spot samples from patients known to have fibromyalgia. By 'training' the equipment to recognize that molecular pattern, the researchers then showed that the microscope could tell the difference between fibromyalgia and two types of arthritis that share some of the same symptoms.[36]

The scientists hypothesized that a reliable diagnostic test could reduce the time to a fibromyalgia diagnosis by five years. This would be a more profound development if we could then cure those people, or even if the pharmaceutical options were better. For many years, fibromyalgia was viewed with skepticism by physicians who thought it was primarily a psy-chosomatic condition. The research that continues to be done has one tremendous benefit at a minimum: it shows more definitively that fibro-myalgia is a real condition.

My patient May was like many people who are extremely sensitive to medications and more prone to side effects. Some people will have a para-doxical reaction, like insomnia from benadryl and drowsiness from sudafed. If I had unlimited time and resources, I would start a massive database to look for common elements of patients who have one or more of the difficult-to-manage conditions. There are many patients with five or six or more medications listed in the section of their chart under medication allergies/adverse reactions. I believe there is some crucial explanation for why some people are unable to tolerate medications, but I am not aware of anyone who has tried to sort this out.

People who are desperate will have a much lower threshold for trying med-ication. To that end, May had tried the lowest doses of Cymbalta, Lyrica and gabapentin. She could not tolerate any of them. It was around this same time that vitamin D[NS] started getting a lot of attention.

There were a couple of studies linking chronic muscle, joint and bone pain to chronic vitamin D deficiency. I reviewed these with May. She was inclined to the alternative side of things, anyway, with regular visits to a chiropractor and an acupuncturist. I checked her level and it came back extremely low, below 10. The goal is generally to have levels over 30. Many in the alternative world advocate for levels at 50 or even higher.

I started May on 50,000 units twice per week with the plan to recheck her level in two months or so. This is a standard approach to building up people's vitamin D blood levels if they are very low. Within 24 hours of taking the first high dose vitamin D supplement, her pain decreased. In less than a week, her pain was completely resolved. It was miraculous. I had hoped for some small benefit and she was cured (or so I thought). She started to walk and then to exercise more vigorously. Things changed so dramatically for her that she went snowmobiling. For six weeks she was virtually pain free. It was, at the time, one of the major developments in my medical life. There have been many others that I will cover in the book where I had little or no expectation the patient would benefit and they dramatically improved or the problem resolved.

After six weeks or so, May's pain started to return. She saw me for a follow-up visit, but I had no answers for her. She was a singularity. Her experience was unique, so I couldn't really explain what had happened on either side of the minor miracle. To this day, she still has muscular pain, but it is significantly improved and she is able to function.

I was so impressed by May's results, even if they weren't sustained, that I had our office manager run a search for all patients in our office carrying a diagnosis of fibromyalgia (FM). I started a database. I called each patient and told them I was doing a study on vitamin D deficiency and fibromyalgia. Unable to control my excitement, I occasionally blurted out what had happened with patient #1 in my study. We certainly couldn't use this "study" to yield rigorous incontrovertible results, but that wasn't really my intention as a community-based family doctor.

I had the group come in so I could check their vitamin D levels. I at least wanted to see if the degree of vitamin D deficiency was higher in the FM population compared to the non-FM populations. In the end, there was a slightly higher percentage of patients with fibromyalgia who had low vitamin D levels. I recommended they all go on vitamin D supplements. Some got better and many did not, so I was unable to draw any firm conclusions.

I did send several emails to a well-known expert on vitamin D, Michael Holick at Boston University. I asked for his opinion on what had happened with May and if he was aware of research linking the two issues. I am a long way from basic science, but I still wonder if some percentage of people with chronic vitamin D deficiency downregulate the vitamin D receptors after a while. Because of this, it can be too late to completely reverse the chronic symptoms of pain. This would potentially explain why the benefit was limited to six weeks.

I never heard back from Dr. Holick. I am convinced that he stole my idea and has been doing intensive fibromyalgia research ever since my emails to clarify the relationship with vitamin D deficiency. I wonder if he will win the Nobel Prize in Medicine for curing fibromyalgia and my name will be left out of his speech.

May is still doing well overall. She loves to travel and made it to China a year later. She may not be able to walk the length of the Great Wall, but she is determined to do as much as she can. Most people have an internal drive that helps them push through such times of adversity. At this stage, I do not expect the majority of patients with fibromyalgia or other forms of chronic pain to be cured by vitamin D supplements, but I feel it can be one of many options that can improve their quality of life. There is likely more value in vitamin D when it is used proactively before a person develops chronic illness.

Another aspect of vitamin D deficiency relates to magnesium. An expert on magnesium, Morley Robbins has described the relationship of vitamin D (which is actually a hormone, so he refers to it as "hormone D") to calcium, magnesium and other electrolytes and minerals. He asserts that those identified with vitamin D deficiency should not be put on megadoses of vitamin D initially but should first have their magnesium levels checked. This would be done more reliably through a blood test called RBC magnesium. The goal would be to raise a person's RBC magnesium level into the 5.0-7.0 range first and follow the vitamin D levels. Many benefit from 1,000 to 2,000 IU of vitamin D daily but will have more long-term success if they also have adequate magnesium levels. A good source of information on the important of magnesium can be found through the Magnesium Advocacy Group at www.gotmag.org.

Slick's Case

Psoriatic arthritis is definitely on the list of underdiagnosed health conditions. Several years ago, I was seeing a young man nicknamed Slick in the office. He had a history of mental health problems and substance abuse. He often complained of joint and back pain at his visits, but I was reluctant to give him any narcotics because of his history. At one of his first visits, he confessed he was borrowing percocets from a friend. Boy, I thought, if he's a drug seeker, he's got some material new to me. I figured he was either the worst drug seeker I had met or the savviest. He might just be playing me, thinking that by being so open about his use of narcotics, I would lower my guard.

He complained of moderate-to-severe pain and, deep down, I suspected he was exaggerating. That is one of the more difficult issues for me. My general tendency is to believe people and trust what they are saying. This can be advantageous and has helped me sort out a number of people's chronic medical problems. This can also, however, lead to overprescribing controlled substances. After being in medicine for a while, I listen to and trust the person in just about every situation…unless pain and narcotics are involved.

We did x-rays and an MRI scan of Slick's back. We tried many different options to control his symptoms with minimal benefit. Then, one visit, Slick reported a dry patch on his left thigh. The light bulb went off in my head. I biopsied part of the lesion and the pathology came back as psoriasis. Even with psoriasis and moderate to severe joint pain, the first rheumatologist disagreed with my diagnosis of psoriatic arthropathy. I sent Slick for a second opinion and that specialist agreed that it was likely.

There are a group of medications called tumor necrosis factor (TNF) inhibitors. The medications in this class include infliximab (Remicade), adalimumab (Humira), etanercept (Enbrel) and certolizumab (Cimzia) and can be used to treat chronic autoimmune conditions like rheumatoid arthritis, ankylosing spondylitis, Crohn's disease, psoriatic arthritis and others. These medications are very expensive and suppress the immune system with increased risk of infection and lymphoma. They can also be incredibly effective for chronic debilitating conditions with no other reasonable mainstream option. I would have preferred that my patient see an alternative provider first to check on other options, but he did not have the money or the inclination to see someone and pay out of pocket. Instead, Slick went on a trial of the medication Remicade and experienced tremendous relief from his chronic pain. Several years later, with ongoing treatment with this TNF inhibitor, his inflammatory joint condition is well-controlled. He is clean from all substances and has improved his diet with a significant amount of weight loss.

Rethinking Chronic Fatigue Syndrome

A cousin to fibromyalgia is the condition Chronic Fatigue Syndrome (CFS). This is characterized by daily, severe, unexplained fatigue, often with sleep disturbances, focus problems and other systemic symptoms. For the person with chronic unrelenting fatigue, doctors will investigate for manageable sources including an underactive thyroid, iron deficiency, B12 deficiency, depression, insomnia, sleep apnea and others. If the work-up is normal, then the label of Chronic Fatigue Syndome could be used. This is the rare diagnosis or, in this case, pseudodiagnosis, that actually has no pharmaceutical treatment. Doctors usually listen patiently serving more of a therapist role before finally telling the person, sorry, we don't understand Chronic Fatigue very well and have nothing to offer you.

The evaluation for thyroid problems is an area where mainstream and alternative providers diverge. For years, I have had patients come in asking questions about the reliability of standard thyroid testing and the use of "natural" options. As with many of the holistic approaches, it took some time for me to see the light. A middle-aged woman, Shirley, came in for an evaluation early in 2014. She had inexplicable fatigue getting progressively worse over several years. She was open to alternative options. She had great success by working with an alternative provider, but not all of her issues had improved. She was reading a book called *Overcoming Thyroid Disorders* by David Brownstein, MD. At one visit, she had the book with her and showed me the areas of interest she had underlined. I was intrigued, so she let me borrow the book over a weekend. She felt that an underactive thyroid was her primary undiagnosed problem. I had ordered a thyroid stimulating hormone (TSH) level for her, the blood test most doctors consider a reliable measure of thyroid function.

For years, I had heard that using the TSH test alone would miss many patients with an underactive thyroid gland. There is an accepted normal range of values for TSH, typically 0.5 to 4.5, but the range can vary depending on the laboratory. TSH is a measure of the feedback loop between the pituitary gland and the thyroid gland. If a person has an *underactive* thyroid gland, the pituitary gland will release more TSH into the bloodstream, so the TSH levels will be elevated. If a person has an *overactive* thyroid gland, the pituitary output is suppressed, so you would see a low TSH level. The first idea contesting the standard approach to thyroid management is that many people with an underactive thyroid will have a TSH level between 2.0 and 4.5. Shirley's TSH level was 2.8. The way most MDs are trained, a TSH level of 2.8 would be considered normal, period, end of story. She would be told that an underactive thyroid could not be the cause for her fatigue.

The next diversion from the mainstream approach to thyroid issues comes in the use of other thyroid blood tests including thyroxine (T4), triido-thyronine (T3) and thyroid antibody levels. The thyroid gland puts out T4 that is converted to the more active form of thyroid hormone, T3. Dr. Brownstein's book advocates for a much broader evaluation of the patient where a thyroid disorder is in question. From his perspective, to truly evaluate a patient for a thyroid problem, the provider needs to check the full panel of thyroid testing. The provider also needs to thoroughly question the patient on signs and symptoms that may reflect a thyroid disorder. The thyroid gland is so important because the thyroid hormones act on most of our cells. It is our thermostat and regulates our metabolism. A person with an underactive thyroid can experience a wide variety of symptoms including focus and memory problems, depression, weight gain, cold intolerance, headaches, fatigue, poor exercise tolerance, dry skin, thinning hair, constipation, menstrual irregularities, infertility and others. Those with an underactive thyroid can also have classic physical exam findings including the loss of hair to the outside half of the eyebrows. They can develop swelling below the eyes. They can have unexplained swelling of their tongues.

Finally, if the diagnosis is in question, the patient can monitor their basal body temperature in the morning. Brownstein asserts that he has reliably diagnosed many patients over the years by finding basal body tempera-tures consistently below the range of 97.8 to 98.2 Fahrenheit. It is only by viewing the issues holistically that the millions of undiagnosed people with thyroid disorders would be appropriately diagnosed.

Dr. Brownstein discusses alternative approaches to the management of a thyroid disorder as well. He feels that iodine deficiency is prevalent in America. I have never heard that from any mainstream provider. He dis-cusses a wide variety of vitamins and supplements that can improve thyroid function. The major deficiency of management in his view, however, is in the use of the synthetic pharmaceutical Synthroid, or the generic equivalent levothyroxine, as the one and only treatment option for an underactive thyroid. Levothyroxine and other similar prescription medications are equivalent to T4. The intention is to give T4 in this derivative form which will then be converted to T3 in the body. The problem with this approach is that many people do not adequately convert T4 to T3. Brownstein lists many causes for poor conversion including chronic illness, smoking, stress, advanced age, vitamin deficiencies and the intake of some other prescription medications including birth control pills.

Brownstein advocates convincingly for the use of "natural" thyroid options like Armour Thyroid, WP Thyroid and Nature-Throid. These options have T4 and T3 so will be more effective in someone who does not convert T4 to T3 very well. I have seen too many patients to remember over the years that did not respond to levothyroxine. Despite taking the medication, they continued to have many of the symptoms of an underactive thyroid. I could never figure out why some patients required such high doses of levothyroxine or were taking levothyroxine yet still had borderline lab results. I suspect the majority of these patients were not adequately converting T4 to T3.

After reading Dr. Browstein's book, I have recalled scattered patients I had seen over the years with complaints of swelling to the face or the tongue. I remembered seeing people with a scalloped appearance to the tongue on physical exam. (It can be scalloped because the tongue is swollen in the mouth, causing indentation from being squashed between the lower teeth.) I had no context or understanding of these findings until I read his book. I wondered about all of the people who came to the office with unexplained fatigue, only to be told by me it wasn't a thyroid issue because they had a normal TSH level. I have seen patients with a wide variety of textbook symptoms of an underactive thyroid only to send them away without answers.

Helen, a woman in her 40s, came to me with a wide variety of symptoms and problems. One of the first areas I investigated was her thyroid. Her T3 level was low and her TSH level was in the high normal range at 2.5. She had many symptoms to suggest an underperforming thyroid gland, so we discussed a trial of armour thyroid. She came back a month later with her husband for a follow-up visit. She was sleeping better and her fatigue was much improved. Her joint pain, muscle pain and frequent palpitations had resolved. There was only one downside: her headaches had actually worsened since starting the thyroid replacement. She had been without a menstrual cycle for some period of time and then, in under a month, started menstruating again. Hormonal shifts around her menses had been a migraine trigger, so reestablishing her normal cycles had contributed to more regular headaches. It is well established that a thyroid disorder can affect hormones, menstrual cycles and fertility. It makes me wonder how many women with infertility and a normal TSH level might have their cycles restored by taking an alternative approach to thyroid management.

Dr. Brownstein estimates that forty percent of Americans have a thyroid disorder. This order of magnitude would be hard to confirm, but the steady rise in autoimmune conditions is well established so it may not be far-fetched. The prevalence of autoimmune conditions will be discussed in more detail in "The Perfect Storm" chapter. Dr. Brownstein also believes that a very high percentage of people diagnosed with fibromyalgia and CFS have an undiagnosed thyroid condition as the primary cause for their issues.

For the person with chronic fatigue, if they have normal testing and a thorough assessment of their thyroid, a focus on the diet should probably be the next line of attack. I would try, through testing or an elimination diet, to find an underlying food sensitivity or intolerance contributing to or causing the fatigue. After this, the SHINE protocol may be the best current treatment approach. SHINE is an acronym for sleep, hormonal support, immunity, nutritional support and exercise. In a study where patients followed the protocol for 99 days, 91 percent experienced an average 90% increased quality of life.[37] The person behind SHINE, Jacob Teitelbaum, did a study in 2012 in 53 different health centers where 250 participants were given the sugar ribose at 5gm three times a day to build up their ATP levels. Patients reported a 61% average increase in quality of life after three weeks, so that may be another option going forward.[38] Teitelbaum suffered from chronic fatigue himself so, once again, we see that it often takes an individual with a personal stake to push beyond normal treatment protocols.

As noted above, magnesium needs to be part of the evaluation of almost every patient with elements of fibromyalgia and chronic fatigue. Some can get their RBC magnesium level above 5.0 through dietary choices that include shellfish, nuts, leafy greens, healthy whole grains (not mass-produced whole wheat products) and cacao. Others would benefit from Epsom salt baths, Anderson's concentrated mineral drops or the Jigsaw magnesium

SRT supplement. The optimal daily dosing is often five times a person's body weight in pounds. A 100 pound female would then take 500mg of magnesium daily. As with all of the other approaches in this book, these interventions should be done in consultation with a knowledgeable health-care professional.

Will's Story

Since early in 2012 I've been seeing a young guy in his 30s. Will came in like a whirlwind. The first visit, he had made a mistake and came in a day earlier than scheduled. He said he only needed a few minutes, so I agreed to shoehorn him into the morning's schedule. Twenty-five minutes later and very behind I had to slip out the door and tell him I'd see him again in a week.

He came back and described severe daily pain to the groin and scrotum area. He said it was like sitting on a fire hydrant. His prior primary care doctor had ordered extensive blood tests, urine tests and a CT scan of the abdomen and pelvis. There was no apparent cause found for his symptoms. He said he really couldn't sit for an extended period of time. The pains would shoot down both medial thighs with numbness. His description certainly sounded like pain from a nerve problem, so I wondered about several things including spinal stenosis. This is a relatively common condition where the spinal canal narrows, pinching the spinal cord. This is much more common in people over 65, but congenital spinal stenosis can be seen in younger adults.

I ordered a lumbar MRI that was normal, ruling out spinal stenosis. We discussed seeing a neurologist, the next logical step. The neurologist really could not come up with a specific diagnosis. Will was having problems urinating as well, so I sent him to a urologist, but that specialist didn't have much to offer him. I tried oral steroids with little or no benefit. We tried other options to control his pain, but none of them worked well. I was prescribing narcotics for him to reduce pain during our work-up, but I didn't sense that he was drug-seeking or abusing the pain medications in any way.

Will saw a colorectal specialist next, but that provider had no explanation for his symptoms. Each time I would see Will in the office, he would tell me he would do whatever it took to find out what was wrong with him. He worked in sales and drove all over the place, which was difficult since his symptoms were worse when sitting. Most visits he would stand leaning against the table. As time went on we talked about his going out on short-term disability, but that would be a last resort.

The next specialist in the loop was a pain specialist. In general, there are two types of pain specialists. The more common version is an anesthesiologist who does focused cortisone shots and other injection procedures to the spine and other areas of the body. The other type takes a more comprehensive approach to pain. The latter type often works with a group of professionals including nurses, occupational therapists, physical therapists, psychologists and acupuncturists, among others. Will ended up seeing the first kind at a hospital in Boston. He was then referred for an EMG test to clarify the source of the problem.

The Electromyogram (EMG) is one of the more painful tests in medicine. Needles are inserted into muscle tissue to check the nerve conduction. This can help clarify a source of nerve impingement. Will was more than willing to have needles inserted into his perineum, the area between the scrotum and the anus. I will tell you that there is no drug seeker on earth that would agree to that test. In my mind, any question of him seeking opioids was over at that point.

The EMG results were inconclusive. The anesthesiologist, however, treated him like a drug-seeker and told him there was no identifiable source for his symptoms. He said that narcotics were inappropriate and implied he would just have to live with the pain. A different medication, tramadol, was offered, but there was really no way that was going to help his situation.

Will was upset when he came back to me for a follow-up. Now, I will say in full disclosure that Will has a strong personality. He can be abrasive and confrontational. With me, there were times when he was difficult and I could tell in reading many of the specialists' notes that he had rubbed them the wrong way. At this follow-up visit, I was very direct with him. I told him he had to change his attitude or he would in effect be blackballed. If he couldn't get a genuine opinion from specialists, it would make our lives more difficult. He understood and, to his credit, took it well. He said he would try to be more diplomatic.

Things went on after that for a while and I really wasn't sure what direction we could go. I told Will repeatedly that narcotics for life would not be an option. Finally, we had a breakthrough. Will came in with a stack of papers. He said he thought he had figured out his problem. He had put his symptoms in the search field on the internet and it came up with pudendal neuralgia.

I read through his materials and pudendal neuralgia did fit perfectly with his symptoms. This gave us something to work with. By this time, however, he had burned many bridges with specialists and it was going to be hard to find someone who would listen to what he had to say. I tried to document my opinion thoroughly in the hopes that the specialists would read my note and respect my impression. Eventually, Will worked his way back around to the same pain specialist. He had procedures to block the pudendal nerve. The symptoms were not completely under control, but he had significant relief. For a while, he was back working and only taking strong pain medications as needed.

Things worsened again after that and we had many extended visits discussing options. He saw several pain specialists and had a number of injections into different areas including his lumbar spine and sacroiliac joint. Sometimes, the injections would reduce his pain for a few weeks, but other times he had minimal benefit. The real breakthrough came when he found the name of a specialist in New Hampshire that did surgery to correct Will's type of problem. It was a hard decision, but Will was desperate to get his life back so would do just about anything. Late in 2013 he went to the operating room. When the surgeon got in, he found that Will's pudendal nerve was trapped within a supporting ligament coming off the sacrum. This is not something that would ever show up on a CT scan or MRI. The surgery took over six hours. Will came to me for follow-up afterwards barely able to walk with six-inch longitudinal incisions to both buttocks. He needed very high doses of narcotics for several months while in recovery, but this finally was the path to long-term improvement. He had a legitimate, although unique and rare, source for severe chronic pain. Doctors would do well to remember that not all patients with chronic unexplained pain are looking for drugs.

Glucosamine and SAMe

There are many alternative options for chronic pain and chronic joint pain. The most commonly used is probably glucosamine[NS], either alone or with chondroitin[NS]. I remember being in residency and first hearing about this option for arthritis. Most doctors who heard about this back then thought the concept was absurd. To ingest one of the constituents of cartilage orally such that it would be absorbed into the bloodstream and then somehow utilized by the body to reduce joint pain either by "growing" new cartilage or by some other novel mechanism made no sense.

Early on, and even now, a lot of the positive reports on glucosamine are anecdotal. When I discuss it as an option with patients, I review that it seems to be safe with no common side effects and no known interactions. Standard thinking is that for a person to get benefit they have to take it every day for at least a month. Of course, this is often a savvy recommendation from vitamin and supplement manufacturers to get people to buy more product. The glucosamine research seems to indicate that it helps about 50% of people in terms of reducing joint pain, with the knees being the most likely joints to be helped. Significant research has been done on glucosamine, as compared with other alternative options. The most compelling result was from a study that showed improvement in knee x-rays suggestive of thicker cartilage in those taking glucosamine vs. placebo.

The following guide from the National Center for Complementary and Integrative Health (formerly the National Center for Alternative and Complementary Medicine) website summarizes the clinical trials comparing SAMe to nonsteroidal anti-inflammatory drugs (NSAIDs) in patients with osteoarthritis of the knee or hip: "In general, trials that compared SAMe with NSAIDs showed that each had similar pain relief and improvement in joint function, with fewer side effects in the patients taking SAMe."[39]

This is a predictable scenario in our current health system. If it is true that SAMe is comparable to NSAIDs for the very common problem of osteoarthritis of the knees and hips, it should be the first line approach. Currently, almost every primary care physician, rheumatologist and orthopedic specialist recommends NSAIDs like ibuprofen (Advil, Motrin), naproxen (Aleve), and others. We know that NSAIDS wear down the stomach lining and can cause bleeding and ulcers. We know that NSAIDs can damage the kidneys and sometimes cause elevated blood pressure.

These side effects and potential problems are even more significant because the population with the most arthritis pain tends to be the elderly. They are more vulnerable, so it is even more important to use a safe, comparable option. What is the MD's solution to the problem? Put the elderly person on a strong acid blocker like Prilosec to minimize the adverse effect of NSAIDs on the stomach. This is absurd on many levels. The elderly tend to have very low levels of stomach acid and we would not generally want to suppress the acid further, which can affect digestion and other functions. Where SAMe might work, the mainstream would instead use NSAIDs and acid blockers, increasing the likelihood for peptic ulcer disease, kidney damage, B12 deficiency and osteoporosis among others.

This is a pharmaceutical approach to health gone mad and is analogous to using Viagra for the sexual side effects of the SSRI medications used for depression and anxiety. It brings to mind the beef industry's solution when they found high levels of E. Coli in cattle. As described in the documentary *Food, Inc.*, rather than change the conditions for the cattle, they realized it would be cheaper to simply treat the beef with a form of bleach during processing. We manage one problem by compounding it with another.

Apple Cider Vinegar

One of the darlings of complementary medicine is apple cider vinegar (ACV), especially the unfiltered version with "mother" floating around. Apple cider vinegar brings an element of nostalgia which probably adds to its appeal: mom's apple pie, Jonny Appleseed, and all of that. This home remedy is purported to help with a wide range of health problems including acne, arthritis, asthma, athlete's foot, nose bleeds, blood pressure, body odor, bones, bruising, burns, cancer prevention, cholesterol reduction, colds, constipation, callus treatment, cramps, dandruff, diabetes, diaper rash, diarrhea, digestion, eczema, fatigue, flatulence, gallbladder flushing, gout, headaches, heartburn, hemorrhoids, hiccups, insect bites, insomnia, jellyfish stings, menstrual problems, hot flashes, poison ivy, shingles, sinusitis, sun burns, ulcers, urinary tract infections, varicose veins, warts, weight loss and yeast infections. I think there are only a few health conditions left after digesting this list and I suspect there is little hard evidence to support all of these claims. The Apple Cider Vinegar Manufacturers of America (the ACVMA if it existed) would probably need a regular stipend from the Bill and Melinda Gates Foundation to fund all of that research. The potential benefits of ACV seem to revolve around two of its properties: alteration of internal pH, its primary mechanism, and a relatively high level of potassium. ACV also contains beta-carotene and phytochemicals that may have health benefits.

The issue of managing a person's internal pH is utterly disregarded by mainstream doctors but widely adopted in the alternative world. There are different recipes for how to consume the ACV but 2-3 teaspoons in eight ounces of water is typical. One rationale for the vinegar and honey regimen is that a person's blood stream tends toward becoming alkaline through a modern diet of fats, starches and de-vitalized processed foods. One of the original proponents, Dr. Jarvis, found that the acidity of cider vinegar, although weak, is enough to correct this excess alkalinity, and that a slightly acidic bloodstream prevents and fights infection.

I found more recommendations for ACV for chronic arthritis than for any of the other conditions above, thus it is discussed in this chapter. There are many books on the use of ACV and my suspicion after reviewing some of the online materials is that there *is* benefit, although again it would be nice to have more definitive proof.

Coenzyme Q10

There is growing evidence that coenzyme Q10 can help reduce chronic pain, specifically the chronic muscle pain associated with fibromyalgia. When statin medications cause myalgias, or muscle pain, it is from depletion of the substance coenzyme Q10. It is plausible, then, that supplementation could reduce pain in those diagnosed with fibromyalgia, and there is some evidence to that end using a dose of 100mg three times a day. A study published in April 2013, comparing CoQ10 to placebo at the dose of 300mg per day, showed a reduction in pain, fatigue and tender points.[40]

Meditation

Perhaps the most effective alternative option for reduction of chronic pain is meditation. A 2011 study showed a "40 percent reduction in pain intensity and a 57 percent reduction in pain unpleasantness"[41] from regular meditation. The meditation produces an analgesic effect greater than morphine and other pain-relieving drugs. The volunteers were trained with four, 20-minute classes, so the approach required minimal resources. The researchers also substantiated the subjective findings by demonstrating changes in the subjects' MRI brain scans. This shows the importance of addressing the mind-body connection in any patient complaining of chronic pain.

To summarize for the areas of rheumatology and chronic pain, there are many options available to providers including magnesium, SAMe for osteoarthritis, and CoQ10 for fibromyalgia. An alternative approach to thyroid dysfunction must be pursued to clarify whether thyroid and other hormones are playing a role. There is enough evidence to support a person trying vitamin D and glucosamine. Almost everyone benefits from exercise and strengthening. Meditation could be used to ameliorate pain more effectively than prescription medications. Mainstream medicine has a very limited understanding of why some people develop autoimmune conditions and other chronic disease processes. The pieces of the puzzle are being put together bit by bit as more and more scientists, researchers and writers are working on it.

The missing piece for many, however, may be the mind-body connection. For those with chronic pain involving multiple systems, true and complete wellness may never be achieved if the psychological aspects of their health are not addressed. We'll consider this further in "The Lost Ones" chapter.

6

Lipitor vs. Guggolipid

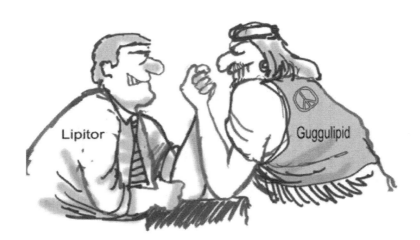

There is one patient of note that I have seen for many years. Aaron is married with children and works as a computer programmer. He has always been focused on wellness and alternative, non-pharmaceutical approaches to health problems. Over 10 years, we watched his blood pressure steadily increase from borderline numbers into the hypertension range. He is active physically with what most would consider an optimal low sodium diet. He has never smoked, drinks 5-6 glasses of red wine or beer per week with no signs of underlying sleep apnea. He meditates and does tai chi almost every day.

For years, I would see Aaron every six months or so for follow-up visits especially to monitor his burgeoning hypertension. He is tall and lean. At visits, he comes across as someone trying to seem at ease, but with an under-lying tension that never softens. He has wanted to do everything possible to avoid prescription medication to lower his blood pressure and I was certainly supportive of his philosophy. He came up with "natural" options such as herbs and other supplements, some of which were familiar to me. Aaron tried hawthorn root, then garlic, then beet root juice for over a year. The beet root juice seemed to work and his blood pressure was consistently lower while he took that natural option, but it caused persistent diarrhea and didn't quite get his numbers into the optimal range.

The natural vs. pharmaceutical question can be philosophical or practical. There isn't always a "free lunch" with the natural options, as we see with Aaron. If something is going to have an action within the body, there is potential for side effects and interactions, although these presumably would be more significant with pharmaceuticals. Many alternative options have less documented evidence (research) as to their effectiveness, a frustration to allopathic doctors as one of the totems of modern medicine. An important development in this regard is the database Natural Standard. Throughout the book most of the alternative and natural options have a superscript *NS* referencing Appendix B at the end of the book. These non-mainstream options are rated from A to F in terms of the level of evidence available. This should not be the last word, however, because there are likely many effective options that have not been studied enough and would get a C rating by Natural Standard.

At one point in the process, Aaron and I resigned ourselves to pharmaceu-ticals since blood pressure control is just too important of a risk factor for stroke, cardiac events and chronic kidney disease. We had taken our shot with natural options, but now needed to bring in the heavy hitters. Aaron, however, had trouble tolerating the prescription medications as well. They all lowered his blood pressure, but I tried several and they all worsened his chronic tendency toward loose stools. In addition to the stool problem, he had fatigue, bloating and progressive inflammation in the rectal area, causing pain during defecation. We were both somewhat frustrated at that point, so I took a step back and we discussed trying to solve his gastrointestinal issue first before managing his hypertension.

I asked him to strip his diet down and avoid caffeine, alcohol, dairy, soy, refined sugar, wheat and gluten. We reviewed his usual diet, and he would still be able to have rice pasta, eggs, goat dairy, cold cuts, tuna fish, chicken, fruits and vegetables. Within a few days of making the changes, the sensitivity to his anal area started to calm down. By a week, his stools had almost completely normalized. There was also some improvement in his blood pressure numbers and they were typically in the borderline range.

After a few weeks, he was remarkably better with no rectal discomfort, less fatigue, and normal bowel movements for the first time in many years. Our plan then was to reintroduce some of the *verboten* foods one at a time to help figure out which were the cause of his chronic symptoms. He was able to tolerate coffee and chocolate. He had some alcohol Thanksgiving evening, one beer and one glass of wine, with a mild return of symptoms. A few days later, feeling ambitious at a holiday party on a Saturday night, he had six Coronas over a few hours. This caused a dramatic return in his symptoms with diarrhea for several days after that. He had some wheat bread and felt fine, so he posited the problem might be with hops. The next week, he reintroduced standard cow's milk dairy and experienced loose stools again. He found overall he could not drink beer or have cow's milk. The blood pressure was improved, so dietary change through an elimination diet seemed at that time to be the most important intervention of all, trumping both herbals and pharmaceuticals.

Later, at another follow-up visit, his blood pressure was very high at 184/102. We talked about his issues with anxiety and stress. For him, the mind-body connection was often working against him. The primary focus needed to be on relieving his underlying tension. We discussed several options for relaxation. We discussed potentially going on a medication, citalopram. I have found this to be very effective for chronic anxiety, as discussed in "The Power of the Mind" chapter. Instead, he wanted to work with a woman who helps clients with relaxation through suggestion and self-hypnosis. She has helped a lot of my patients over the years. Overall, Aaron and I pursued changes to his diet, pharmaceuticals, strategic supplementation and a focus on relaxation to get his blood pressure under control.

The Cardiovascular Landscape

The title of this chapter sounds like the undercard run-up to a championship match between Godzilla and Mothra, but it highlights the dominance of Lipitor, the poster child of mainstream cardiovascular prevention, over alternative options. In the Ambulatory Medical Care Utilization Estimates compiled by the CDC for 2007 [42], the number one reason for a visit to the doctor was to manage hypertension. The management of diabetes, obesity and high cholesterol are also common reasons for visits. In terms of more acute issues, many primary care visits are spent investigating chest pain, leg pain, palpitations and other potentially serious symptoms of cardiovascular disease.

There have been significant advances over the past 100 years in our understanding of the causes of cardiovascular disease, and we now have many pharmaceutical options available to us. There are life-saving procedures done by exceedingly well-trained interventional cardiologists and cardiothoracic surgeons, including angioplasty and bypass procedures. Westernized medicine has made great leaps forward with available technology and advanced surgical techniques.

Many tests can be used in an attempt to clarify the extent of disease and associated risks of heart attack and stroke. These would include standard treadmill stress testing, nuclear perfusion imaging and catheterization. There are also newer tests available such as coronary CT scanning, which may provide better predictive value of those at higher risk of a cardiovascular event.

Like Six-Million-Dollar Man Steve Austin, from my favorite TV show in the 1970s, we have the technology to make us better than we were before. Maybe not "better, stronger [and] faster" like Steve Austin, but embedded in modern culture is the notion that technology is our savior and the best solution to many problems of health and wellness. (For those of you older than 40 who want a stroll down memory lane, the show intro on YouTube is cool.) Will ever-more-powerful CT machines with enhanced imaging fundamentally change our approach? *It is probable that with improved technology and pharmaceuticals, we will still be having the same conversations with our patients.* Almost everyone appreciates that the real focus should be on an optimal diet with regular exercise, weight loss when necessary, smoking cessation and stress reduction.

It is common in our current system to use pharmaceuticals to manage the cardiovascular risk factors of hypertension, hyperlipidemia, diabetes and obesity. The medications are often effective, but we can be too reliant on them and many people are taking medications unnecessarily. In the Pulmonary chapter, "Breathing Room for the Spirit", we will see that millions with high blood pressure have mediocre control with medications because their underlying sleep apnea has not been diagnosed or managed. The benefits of statins to lower cholesterol numbers and reduce cardiovascular risk are greatly exaggerated, and that will be reviewed.

Some people I see with these cardiovascular risks are motivated to change their lifestyle, but many others are not. The best primary care works with people one-to-one to figure out the barriers to change. In the end, however, if we cannot budge people, the risks need to be managed and medication is typically preferred over no management at all. The average person assumes that if they have a good weight with an excellent diet and regular exercise, they can avoid hypertension. It comes as a great frustration, then, when people with excellent lifestyles see their blood pressures rise over time.

In terms of blood pressure, the first thing is to verify whether an elevated number is an isolated, uncommon event or a consistent trend. Optimally, it is better to buy a cuff, verify it as accurate at a doctor's office, and then check it regularly for some period of time. I recommend checking it at different times of day and during work days and weekends. If the numbers are over 140 for the top (or "systolic") number consistently, then the person can be reliably diagnosed with hypertension. There are many people who have been diagnosed with hypertension based on two or three readings in a doctor's office. They can then be overmedicated if their true blood pressure is normal or low outside of the office. In one study, a large group of patients diagnosed with "hypertension" were taken off all of their antihypertensive medications. Twenty percent of those people had normal blood pressure.

Step two for someone with confirmed hypertension is to have a basic set of blood tests, something almost every doctor would recommend. Everyone, thin or heavy, also needs to be evaluated for the possibility of sleep apnea. There is a strong correlation between blood pressure elevation and sleep apnea. One article in the *American Journal of Family Practice* found that about 50 percent of those with hypertension had sleep apnea as a contributor.[43]

After these investigations, the question is: what is the optimal way to keep a person's systolic blood pressure between 120 and 140 consistently in order to lower their risk? The ideal approach involves a focus on life-style first. Lose weight down to somewhere below a BMI of 30. BMI, or body mass index, is simply a person's weight for height. The individual should keep alcohol to two drinks per day maximum. Some minority of people will have elevated blood pressure in part from excessive salt intake. The average American consumes over 3,700 mg of sodium per day, while the daily recommendation is 2,000 mg or less. That is equal to about one teaspoon per day in all of the food a person consumes. Two jiggles of a salt shaker is almost that amount. We typically look at salt as something to be avoided. One of the many revelations from researching this book includes new thinking on salt. Refined salt is generally to be avoided. Unrefined salt like Himalayan sea salt or Celtic sea salt can actually be beneficial because it replenishes essential minerals. One of Dr. David Brownstein's books is dedicated to this topic.

I will often ask people how many meals of 21 during a typical week they make themselves and how many are made by someone else. Take-out food or any meals eaten out will invariably have high levels of the refined, unhealthy version of salt/sodium. If you have a restaurant or work in the food industry, there is a very simple formula for success. Serve sugar, fat and salt in large quantities and the people will beat a path to your door.

Many years ago, researchers developed what they thought was the optimal diet to keep blood pressure normal. It was called DASH after Dietary Alternatives to Stop Hypertension. This is really just a basic, well-balanced diet, but it may not be individualized enough to provide much benefit across the entire population.

Another important contributor to blood pressure elevation is magnesium deficiency. The Magnesium Advocacy Group (MAG) provides excellent resources on this important, underappreciated topic. Each person with a blood pressure issue should at least have an RBC magnesium level checked. The goal level for RBC magnesium is somewhere between 5.0 and 7.0.

Standard magnesium levels that most doctors would order measure the blood serum levels and provide little or no information on whether a person is deficient. Only about one percent of the body's magnesium can be found in the bloodstream.

If weight loss, moderation of alcohol intake, magnesium replacement and dietary change do not control the blood pressure, the person has a fundamental decision to make. Do they have the time and the inclination to alter their lives in such a way that stress will be reduced enough to lower their blood pressure? A crucial, underutilized element of blood pressure control involves ways to relax the cardiovascular system. Meditation, breathing techniques and acupuncture are often effective. The person needs to optimize quantity and quality of sleep to have this area addressed effectively. The typical American is so overworked and overstressed that they live most days in a state of low-level tension. They are so accustomed to this, they don't even realize they are frequently holding their breath and sitting with head, neck and shoulder muscles taut. The person who gets up early, runs out the door while cramming down a Nutri-grain bar, commutes an hour through heavy traffic to a hyper office with deadlines and quotas, survives to make it home by 6:30 p.m. and rushes through dinner before getting the kids to bed probably will not find the time for acupuncture or meditation.

For this person, based on my experience, pharmaceuticals are often the way to go. They are almost always effective with minimal side effects. The choice of medication and dosage would depend on a number of individual factors, and just about any allopathic provider would feel comfortable making that decision. For years, I would say to my patients that Americans are probably overmedicated in every situation except one: hypertension. I would later change that to hypertension and chronic anxiety but continue to search for effective non-pharmacologic solutions.

Alternative Approaches

Lifestyle improvements are the domain of neither traditional primary care nor alternative medicine but the foundation for both. Why? The alternative approaches to cardiovascular risk reduction are not necessarily more effective or less costly. There are many people pursuing vitamins and supplements recommended by holistic providers which can require a significant commitment of time and resources. In my experience, some of those options are excellent with good effect while others have no value.

There are several herbs commonly used to lower blood pressure. These include Coleus forskohlii, the hawthorne (Crateagus oxycantha) which Aaron tried, mistletoe (Viscum album) and Rauwolfia. The last of these is considered the strongest hypotensive botanical, according to the Rienstra Clinic in Washington State. From their website:

Rauwolfia is the name of the plant. Reserpine is the name of the active ingredient in the plant. Reserpine has a soothing effect on excitatory centers in the brain and reduces blood pressure. Rauwolfia lasts for several days in the blood and its effects can last for several weeks, so rauwolfia and reserpine need to be taken just once a day or once every other day, as your physician prescribes.[44]

I attended a naturopathic conference in 2013 and made contact with a group of naturopaths. I asked one of them how he manages hypertension without pharmaceuticals. His response was fascinating to me as it was such a diversion from allopathic medicine. In an email reply, he mentioned the use of acupuncture specifically focusing on the:

BP groove–fold the top of the ear down, there is a groove attaching the cartilage, 1" needle inserted, PC6, H7, SP6, treat twice weekly for 6 to 8 weeks. Cranial electrical stimulation–home units best. Heart Tension [supplement] from Mountain Peak contains rauwolfia reliably standardized... formula contains other cardioprotective herbs hypertine, asparagus extract and vein lite from [Chinese] herbs.[45]

Whoa. I think he was assuming I had a different foundation of knowledge, because I could barely follow half of what he recommended. Over the past 100 years, allopathy and naturopathy have steadily diverged and followed such different paths that we are slowly losing common ground. The farther apart we get, the harder it is for either side to acknowledge the value of the other. It is difficult to avoid a sense of competition. If the heart tension supplement works as well as some pharmaceutical option, is it automatically better because it is more natural? Does a natural option automatically have less potential for side effects and long-term complications because it is not synthetic?

Rauwolfia is a pertinent example in trying to answer these questions. That herb, once used only by naturopaths, was developed into the pharmaceutical drug reserpine as previously noted. There is an interesting history behind the drug. From the Wikipedia entry:

Reserpine was isolated in 1952 from the dried root of *Rauwolfia serpentina* (Indian snakeroot), which had been known as *Sarpagandha* and had been used for centuries in India for the treatment of insanity, as well as fever and snakebites—Mahatma Gandhi used it as a tranquilizer.[46]

In America, reserpine fell into disfavor because of a relatively high frequency of side effects, including nasal congestion, nausea, vomiting, weight gain, gastric intolerance, gastric ulceration, stomach cramps, diarrhea and potentially a blood pressure that drops too low. I learned about reserpine in pharmacology during my second year of medical school, but have never prescribed it and don't know if I've ever seen it on any patient's medication list.

The roots, leaves, and flowers of many plants have been used for centuries to address all kinds of ailments. In the 19th century, researchers began to isolate the powerful constituents of such plants to develop our modern drugs. Although modern medicine has roots in botany and natural science, the process by which specific plant components were isolated actually removed some of the important protective factors hidden within the plants' natural chemistry. Aspirin, for example, also known as acetylsalicylic acid, was derived from the bark of the white willow tree. When ingested, salicylic acid decreases pain, but left alone the acid is too hard on gastrointestinal linings and eventually leads to intestinal bleeding. The bark, however, offers another life-enhancing property. Natural buffers counteract the acidity making the bark safe as well as effective. Unfortunately, the development of aspirin as a powerful analgesic also isolated the salicylic acid from its natural safety check. This reflects a basic question in health and wellness: If you have two identical molecules, one derived from nature and one from a laboratory, would the natural option be in some way preferred?

Diabetes

Diabetes is on the rise in the United States. Its cure is as simple as simple can be—improve lifestyle—but cases continue to mount in correlation with the steady increase in rates of obesity. The majority of people with diabetes are classified as type 2. The number one risk factor for type 2 diabetes is obesity with poor diet, lack of exercise trailing just behind. The type 2 diabetic develops resistance to the insulin his or her body produces. This leads to high levels of glucose in the bloodstream as the mechanisms for maintaining normal sugar levels are disrupted. For this cardiovascular risk factor, we may not need a deeper understanding of the pathophysiology. What we need is more resources dedicated to motivating individuals to improve their way of life. We need to clarify the impact of sugar, wheat, soy, corn and other staples of the modern American diet. Mark Hyman, MD, has said, "Fat doesn't make a person fat; sugar makes a person fat."

A couple of years ago I began seeing John. The labs I did early on revealed type 2 diabetes. The most commonly used blood test for a person with diabetes is the hemoglobin A1C test. Some brilliant person many years ago realized that some of the sugar in the bloodstream sticks to red blood cells. The A1C test measures the percentage of red blood cells with sugar stuck to them. The more sugar in the bloodstream, the higher the percentage and the higher the A1C number. Since red blood cells have about a 90-120 day life span before they are destroyed by the body, the A1C level gives a reliable estimate for a person's sugar levels in the blood over the 2-3 months before the test is drawn. This is incredibly valuable because everyone's sugar levels will fluctuate from day to day depending on many factors, including stress level and diet.

A non-diabetic typically has an A1C below 6.0%. The goal for a diabetic is to keep the A1C number below 7.0% as this correlates with lower risk of microvascular and macrovascular complications over time. John's number was 9.7%. John weighed 360 pounds and complained of chronic daily severe low back pain that he had been experiencing for over five years. I sent him for a lumbar MRI that was normal. He had no interest in narcotics, so that was not an issue.

I sent John to physical therapy. As he did his home exercises, over time, his chronic back pain disappeared. I reinforced the importance of sticking with the plan, as many people in this situation will eventually lapse if they don't have back pain for an extended period of time. In terms of the diabetes, he had seen a nutritionist and was going to the gym every morning. He was following the diet 100% with no junk food. He had lost 20 pounds and we discussed getting him off his medication. He had tried the most commonly prescribed medication for type 2 diabetes first, metformin. When it caused persistent diarrhea, John switched to a different medication, glyburide, which carries with it more risk of having sugars drop too low.

I have found that most people do better with strict, self-imposed guidelines. To have a policy of no junk food keeps it simple with a much higher likelihood of success. If the person instead comes up with some wishy-washy goal of cutting back on junk food or only having it twice a week, they will probably fail. That person will go through frequent internal negotiations, creating convenient rationalizations of why they will allow themselves the cookie at any given moment. They work hard. They deserve it. They are a nice person. Just this one cookie and only today.

At his follow-up visit, John had changed things so drastically that he was well-controlled and able to get off his glyburide. I praised this patient up and down and he was justifiably proud of what he had accomplished. Being optimistic and positive can be very important in the doctor-patient relationship. I sometimes wish for an *It's a Wonderful Life* scenario where I could know the impact of positive statements on people.

There are a number of more natural options that may also reduce blood sugars and improve the health status of those with diabetes. These include cinnamon,[NS] chromium citrate or picolinate[NS] (250 mcg), vanadium ascorbate[NS] (250 mcg), 4% corosolic acid from banaba leaf[NS] (50 mg), French lilac[NS] (150 mg), bitter melon[NS] (150 mg), huckleberry/bilberry[NS] (100 mg) and chaste tree berry[NS] (150 mg). As with many nutraceuticals and herbs, I have little or no experience with patients utilizing these options. I have not seen rigorous placebo controlled studies either. Spending a hundred dollars or more a month for herbs may not be much better than pharmaceuticals, especially if diet, exercise and weight loss would take care of the problem.

In terms of non-pharmaceutical options, we need to bring magnesium once again into the conversation. We have good evidence that many Americans are magnesium deficient. There is also research showing that magnesium deficiency plays a role in cardiac risk through a variety of mechanisms. The magnesium deficient person is at a higher risk of diabetes, elevated triglycerides, hypertension, congestive heart failure, heart attacks, atrial fibrillation and sudden cardiac death.

Consider this office visit from the past, representative of many of the standard issues in allopathic medicine. Debbie was a 55-year-old woman with a history of type 2 diabetes, hypertension and hyperlipidemia with a chief complaint of chest pain. For about one month she had been having left upper back and shoulder pain. To her, these pains felt "muscular." More recently she also experienced pain in her right flank and intense pain in both calves, especially at night. She then mentioned the symptom that brought her in: chest pain. She said there were a few brief episodes over the past week or two where she felt a "pinch" or a "tightness" in the left side of her chest. These chest pain episodes all occurred at rest, which was reassuring to some degree.

Debbie had no family history of coronary disease. She was originally from the Middle East and said she smoked socially for maybe 10 years when she was younger, since it was the thing to do. She exercised regularly, including walking and biking, and had not noticed any symptoms with exertion.

The overall assessment for her chest pain would be that it was "non-anginal" in nature, code for not being related to her heart. As a reflex to cover myself from legal harm, I had the medical assistant do an EKG, though there has not been one time in my medical career where I have seen a worrisome EKG in a clinical setting like this. Most doctors, in fact, would do the EKG to CYA.

As a side note, the CYA model of healthcare is insidious and contributes to a vast amount of over-testing in American medicine. A good friend of mine is an excellent family doctor. When asked what percentage of testing he ordered that he thought was unnecessary, he said 90%! When I first heard him say that, I thought he was exaggerating. But taking a strict view of which tests are absolutely necessary, I realized he may not be so far from the truth.

Consider the predicament of even the most conscientious doctor today. He thinks: Every doctor is ordering unnecessary tests. Why should I go out on a limb and put my medical license at risk if no one else will? Why would I try to cut costs by myself and potentially compromise my career and my family's livelihood? The incentive for any individual provider to do the right thing and not order the CYA tests is relatively small.

I have heard that the average family doctor is sued once in his or her career. A study done by the AMA in 2007 and 2008[47] involving 5,825 physicians found that 95 medical liability claims were filed for every 100 physicians during the course of their careers. To have over 100,000 visits in a career and view every single patient as a potential litigant is sad. It is a shame that doctors are ordering unnecessary tests every day to protect themselves from one or two potential lawsuits.

But let's return to Debbie. I reviewed the high likelihood that her diffuse pains were caused by her cholesterol medication, simvastatin. We also reviewed her diabetes. I looked back through Debbie's A1C numbers and there were none above 6.5 percent and the most recent was 6.1 percent. By almost anyone's standards, these would be excellent results. She was on metformin, however, prescribed by an endocrinologist. When in doubt, specialists tend to order more tests than primary care doctors. When in doubt, specialists also tend to prescribe more medication. Nearly two out of three doctors in America today are specialists, which likely contributes to overreliance on pharmaceutical options.

For Debbie, I could see no clear indication for the metformin. Overall, I tend to avoid micromanaging some other provider's issue. In an effort to be professional and respectful, I will not typically discontinue a medication prescribed by another doctor. There are times, however, when I feel the patient's best interests are more important. I will gently raise the issue to see how the person responds. In this case, she was experiencing some borderline low sugars and working on a healthy lifestyle. She wanted to stop the medication, but did not feel empowered to stop it on her own.

I gave her the green light and diplomatically put in my notes that she was hoping to discontinue the medication and that we would recheck her labs in three months to make sure the A1C level did not increase significantly. The main aspect of our plan involved stopping her simvastatin, as I suspected that was the cause for her muscular pains. In addition, I ordered a treadmill stress test to help rule out any underlying coronary disease. The stress test is a judgment call overall. The argument to do the test is that she had three independent risk factors including diabetes, hypertension and elevated cholesterol. The argument to avoid the test is that her diabetes was well controlled with no worrisome family history and that her pattern of chest pain was not suggestive of a cardiac source.

Questioning the Conventional Wisdom About Cholesterol

Stopping Debbie's statin medication represents a good segway into the murky world of cholesterol and lipids. The general public, in my opinion, tends to overestimate the relevance of cholesterol levels in the blood. They think if they have high cholesterol levels on a blood test their arteries are relentlessly filling up with plaque and they are at high risk for a heart attack.

They also think that if they have normal or low cholesterol levels on the blood test they can relax since their risk of cardiovascular disease must be low.

People tend to fixate on a single goal: total cholesterol below 200. I have told people many times that the total can be misleading and that the individual numbers are what we need to look at. I check the LDL or "bad cholesterol" first, the HDL or "good cholesterol" next, and then the triglyceride number. Overall, though, we should look at the person's cholesterol levels in the larger context of risk. For many years, I used the Framingham Heart study's risk calculator to generate an estimate of the person's 10-year risk of having a cardiac event.

The dubious use of the LDL number alone to decide on use of a statin medication applies in the case of a patient of mine, Greg. Greg has a rare familial tendency to very high LDL numbers. Greg, his father, his brother and his uncle all have LDL numbers over 250 with the fluctuations occasionally drifting up over 300. He is thin with a superb diet and is an endurance athlete getting hours and hours of vigorous physical activity every week. All of the older members of his father's side lived to old age, some over 90, with no heart disease or strokes.

Greg and the other family members with the super high cholesterol levels have probably all been tried on every statin and cholesterol medication at every dosage possible. I tried to put him on a couple of statins and it only caused erectile dysfunction. If having high LDL levels in the blood were so definitively the cause for premature heart attack and stroke, Greg and his family members would be high risk, but they are not.

Another patient is a 60-year-old female I've been seeing for years. Gail is generally healthy with no chronic medical conditions. Her LDL number has been trending upward for years and most recently was in the 240 range. (Current standard of care is a target LDL of under 130 for the general population and under 100 for those with a higher risk of cardiovascular events.) Gail wanted to avoid a statin medication but was spending a lot of her time worrying that untreated cholesterol was putting her at risk. I told her many times that her anxiety over the issue was more of a risk than the elevated serum cholesterol levels.

In the summer of 2014 we found a solution to Gail's predicament. I sent her for a coronary scan that cost $99 out-of-pocket. This would tell us how much plaque had built up in her coronary arteries during her 60 years of life. If there was significant plaque, she would go on simvastatin. The scan gives a score from 0 to 1500 and the higher the number, the more atherio-sclerotic plaque. Her score came back at zero. She is now sleeping soundly, comfortable that a statin would have little or no value for her.

There are national guidelines from the National Cholesterol Education Program (NCEP) called the Adult Treatment Program with the most recent version called ATP III. These are good guidelines overall because they tend to incorporate other risk factors into decision-making. The guidelines say that for any individual with an LDL over 190, medication should be "consid-ered." Thankfully, they did not make a concrete recommendation of a statin for all people with LDL numbers over 190 because then I would be more at odds with the Standard of Care. The Standard of Care for any medical issue incorporates the most up-to-date information from research with expert opinion. It is an unwritten standard by which doctors in practice would be judged, especially in a court of law.

The relevance of cholesterol in diet to levels measured on standard blood testing is much more complex than was once thought. When I started in medicine back in the 1990s, conventional wisdom said that the most important thing a person could do to lower cholesterol was to decrease fat intake in the body. Eggs were a prime target, as it seemed to be common sense that a food high in cholesterol would raise blood cholesterol. Not so.

The next development was the good fat/bad fat approach that still seems to make more sense. Nuts, avocados, olive oil and some other fats are good for health while salami, hamburgers and deep fried Oreos, sadly, are not. This still is not the last word on dietary items and their effect on cholesterol numbers.

There is a significant difference between "good" fats and "bad" fats. Harvard School of Public Health explains that trans and saturated fats, not mono-unsaturated and polyunsaturated fats, increase the risk of certain diseases. They point to the increase in easily digestible carbohydrates such as white bread and sugar in the effort to decrease fat.

In the 1960s, fats and oils supplied Americans with about 45 percent of calories; about 13 percent of adults were obese and under 1 percent had type 2 diabetes, a serious weight-related condition. Today, Americans take in less fat, getting about 33 percent of calories from fats and oils; yet 34 percent of adults are obese and 11 percent have diabetes, most with type 2 diabetes.[48]

Dietary changes can also help lower bad cholesterol, notably increasing soluble fiber, soybeans or soy protein, phytosterols and Omega-3 fatty acids. Phytosterols interfere with intestinal absorption of cholesterol and can be found in plant sterol and sterol esters in whole grains, fruits, vegetables, and vegetable oils. Omega-3 fatty acids decrease the rate of LDL production by the liver, decrease growth of arterial plaques, thin the blood and have an anti-inflammatory effect. Omegas can be found in fish, flax seed and walnuts. Furthermore, hydrogenated and partially hydrogenated oils should be avoided because they increase LDL (bad) cholesterol and decrease the heart-protecting HDL (good) cholesterol, while increasing the body's inflammatory response.

I have found over the years that most people's bad cholesterol numbers (LDL and triglycerides) will rise and fall as their weight changes. That is often the primary driver. More weight equals more adipose tissue. I have said many times that waist size and fitness level are better indicators of how a person is doing with lifestyle. Weight alone, and thus the BMI number, can be misleading. If we only went by the BMI, then a six-foot one-inch, 225-pound NFL cornerback with 10% body fat who can run a 4.45-second 40-yard dash through a brick wall would be classified as obese.

In terms of the lipid numbers in the blood, the degree of exercise may be the second determinant and diet the third, but there is significant variation. Some people can do everything right and still have poor numbers. Less often, people will be overweight with terrible lifestyles and have excellent numbers. It would seem that for the HDL (good cholesterol number), people have a genetically-determined range. The HDL number will go up and down somewhat but will seldom rise significantly. Exercise is the number one way to raise it, but I remember a cardiologist saying it usually takes the equivalent of running 25 miles per week to really push it up.

Overall, I tend to prescribe statins less than most doctors. There are two scenarios where they are prescribed in medicine: primary prevention and secondary prevention. Primary prevention means that we are working to prevent a person's first cardiovascular event, typically a heart attack or stroke. Currently, it is estimated that 80 percent of people taking statins are taking them for primary prevention. The other 20 percent take statins for secondary prevention, already having had some cardiovascular event.

A few years ago, I read a scathing article about statins and a new version of a blood test, c-reactive protein (CRP). The CRP blood test is a measure of inflammation in the body. The writer described the lengths to which the developer of the CRP-hs test went in order to manipulate data to make the newer version of CRP seem like a major development in preventative medicine. She also revealed that, up to that point, there had been 13 studies done by the pharmaceutical industry that tried to show risk reduction for statins in the setting of primary prevention. Of these 13 studies, not one showed significant risk reduction. Yet statins are still touted as miracle drugs. These studies were, of course, buried because drug companies really don't need hard evidence to get doctors to prescribe medications.

An excellent book that successfully analyzes and reinterprets pharmaceutical data is *Overdosed America* by John Abramson, MD.[49] He prodigiously researched the studies typically cited in support of many of the most commonly prescribed medications in America. In his chapter "A Smoking Gun: The 2001 Cholesterol Guidelines," he spends much time going over the statin studies. I will hit a few of the high points, but anyone who wants to grind it out and review the statistics in detail should get this book. In a study with those at "moderately elevated risk" for coronary artery disease, 100 people would have to be treated with a statin for 25 years to prevent one death from a cardiac event. In the highest risk category, men with known coronary artery disease, a different study showed that you would have to treat 166 people for one year to prevent one heart attack.

When discussing statins, I usually raise my right hand and make a series of elaborate movements in the air with an imaginary magic wand. I say that, in my opinion, a spell has been cast over the medical community and the general public. For someone with an LDL above 190, however, I will often say that if they saw 100 cardiologists, all 100 would probably recommend a statin. This is the Standard of Care at its most profound. I want the patient to have all of the information at their disposal so they can make an informed choice.

For years, I have imagined a scenario where I do not prescribe a statin for one of my patients with an LDL over 190 and they have a cardiac event. This, fortunately, has not happened. (A related situation did occur in 2013; see "The Power of the Mind" chapter.) In this nightmare, the person is convinced to sue me. I get called into court and the lawyer for the prosecution puts me on the stand. It might go something like this:

"So, Dr. Lenhardt," the lawyer starts his questioning, "you are aware that your patient, Mr. Smith, had a heart attack recently?"

Quietly, I reply, "Yes. I'm glad he's ok."

"You were also aware that Mr. Smith had high cholesterol?"

"Yes, by the standard definition."

"Do you remember his last LDL number?" Here he glances over at the jury, which is made up of 12 lobbyists for the drug companies. "I think doctors refer to that as the 'bad cholesterol.'" Shudder.

"Yes." I cough. "It was 210." There's a collective gasp from the gallery. An older woman in the back row faints and has to be taken out the side door as her granddaughter fans her face with a playbill from Annie.

"Well," the lawyer continues, "we have sworn affidavits from the Chiefs of Cardiology at Massachusetts General Hospital, Johns Hopkins, the Cleveland Clinic and 20 other major institutions in the United States and Guam. We asked them if they would have prescribed a statin for Mr. Smith. Can you guess what they said, Dr. Lenhardt?"

I shrug my shoulders and give a blank look like Ralphie in *A Christmas Story* when the class is asked if anyone knows where Flick is. Flick? Flick who? Their friend Flick is outside in the cold with his tongue stuck to a metal pole after getting the double dog dare.

"Well, each of these eminent cardiologists responded that they would use a statin medication for a patient like Mr. Smith. You decided not to, so are you saying that you know more about cardiology and preventing a heart attack than these titans of medicine?"

I don't know what I would say to that. Conventional wisdom and expert opinions do not always add up to the best advice. In the end, physicians should be doing what is best for their individual patients.

When I first read the article highlighting statins' lack of risk reduction, I was surprised at the magnitude of the studies, but not completely stunned that this information is largely unknown in the medical community. Shortly after reading it, I sent an article to a cardiologist I know and respect asking him if he was aware of any evidence for statins and primary prevention. I didn't hear back for a few weeks, so I emailed him again.

He emailed that he had been searching around trying to find a study that supported the reason why 80% of people were taking these blockbuster drugs. In the end, he said he was going to make contact with his mentor, a cardiologist at the Cleveland Clinic. I did get a reply from the second cardiologist who was aware that the studies did not show benefit. His explanation was that it was only because the incidence of events was so low in the younger populations that they didn't have enough of a sample size in each study to show statistical benefit. *That's the best you've got for why we're bombing people with these medications?*

[Since I wrote this section, I have come across a study that shows risk reduction benefit from a statin in the setting of primary prevention. The WOSCOPS (West of Scotland Coronary Prevention Study) showed that after 20 years the participants on 40mg of pravastatin had a 27% lower coronary heart disease mortality rate compared to placebo controls. New information is coming in all the time reinforcing that no piece of information and no study result should ever be considered the last word. For statins, the possible benefit for primary prevention still needs to be put in context of the pros and cons of therapy for each individual.]

The statins themselves may be their own worst enemy. It is incontrovertible that statins often cause muscle pain. It is relatively clear that statins raise the risk of diabetes. I have seen a number of people with high cholesterol improve their lifestyle only to have their blood sugars go into the prediabetes range when taking a statin. People taking statins may have an increased risk of developing cataracts. There is evidence that statins may cause memory problems and cognitive deficits. This may be relevant only for patients over 65 years old, however, because a study published in *Family Practice News* in September of 2013 showed that in 58,000 Taiwanese patients on statins there were significantly lower rates of dementia.[50]

For those with low overall cardiovascular risk, the statins will lower cholesterol numbers but probably have only a small benefit for risk reduction. Of course, I tell them that being on a statin is the Standard of Care to reduce their risk of heart attack and stroke. I tell them that just about every cardiologist would recommend it and I document all of that in the medical record.

A 68-year-old patient of mine, Bill, sees a cardiologist in Boston. Bill is on several cholesterol medications, including a statin, and his numbers are still not at goal. A couple of years ago, he paid out-of-pocket for a special CT scan to look at the degree of calcification in his coronary arteries. The scan suggested some degree of coronary disease, not necessarily a surprise in a 68-year-old male, and also not a surprise given Bill's lifestyle. He is now exercising after getting the CT results but is still significantly overweight and tends to overindulge. He also continues to work vigorously at his insurance business. He is high-strung and worries quite a bit.

At one point, I saw Bill for an unrelated visit and he told me his cardiologist was adding back yet another cholesterol medication, his fourth, called Zetia. Zetia came out a number of years ago and the research showed that it did indeed lower cholesterol by 10-15 percent, but it didn't lower heart attack or stroke risk. What is the point of lowering his cholesterol numbers if it doesn't affect his risk? I almost never interact with pharmaceutical reps, but after the Zetia study came out, I couldn't help myself. The Zetia rep showed me the data where total cholesterol was lowered by Zetia. I asked the rep if he had any research showing a reduction in risk. He said, "Well, no. We found that the doctors we spoke to wanted to know more about how well it reduced cholesterol levels." Yeah, right.

I have told Bill multiple times that he would lower his risk more by eating well, exercising, reducing stress in his life, and losing weight—this as opposed to taking multiple cholesterol-lowering pills. But he's a believer in the expert opinion. Is he really going to listen to the family doctor from the suburbs instead of the prominent cardiologist from a major teaching hospital? No, not usually.

Statins often cause the side effect of muscle pains or myalgias. People can have leg pain for months or years and not realize that the cholesterol medication is the cause. Because of these pains, some on statins will avoid exercise. The irony, of course, is that the medication purported to reduce the person's risk is probably increasing it because the person decreases physical activity. Another insidious effect I often see is the person on a statin eating poorly because they think the cholesterol medication is protecting them.

Alternative Options for High Cholesterol

Garlic[NS] has been used for thousands of years as a spice and as a medicine for high cholesterol, heart disease and high blood pressure. Its positive effects tend to last only in the short term (1-3 months). Guggolipid/gugulipid[NS] from the gum resin of the mukul myrrh tree showed reduced LDL and total cholesterol levels in clinical studies in India[51]; however, clinical trials in the U.S. produced negative results,[52] requiring further research. Other non-pharmaceutical alternatives include artichoke, barley, psyllium found in seed husk, oat bran found in oatmeal and whole oats, and some oral supplements and cholesterol lowering products such as the OTC fiber supplement Metamucil. These more natural options should, of course, be scrutinized with the same vigor as the pharmaceutical options. Some or all of them may reduce cholesterol levels in the blood, but that is of no real consequence if it doesn't lower risk.

Question the Conventional Wisdom Further

Most people would have smoking as the number one risk factor for cardiovascular disease. A March 2002[53] study featured in the *The New England Journal of Medicine* evaluated risk factors for cardiovascular disease. The study population was 6,213 men referred for exercise testing. In the end, the testers formulated a list of factors with the lowest age-adjusted risk of death. The variable associated with the lowest risk was peak exercise capacity. This reflected a person's degree of conditioning from regular exercise. Coming in at number two was the number of pack years of smoking. (A pack year represents a person smoking one pack per day for the whole year. If someone smokes two packs per day for 20 years, they would then have smoked for 40 pack years.) The rest of the list included hypertension at number three, diabetes at number four and total cholesterol level at number five. There were several limitations of the study. The study only had male participants, so results cannot always be extrapolated to the general population. The testers also did not assess for some difficult-to-quantify factors like stress and strength of a person's relationships. In my experience, these issues are often as important as, or more important than, the traditional risk factors like cholesterol.

The simplest way to reduce the risk of heart attack may be to increase hydration. The *American Journal of Epidemiology* published a study in 2002,[54] that followed more than 20,000 men and women over six years, comparing those who hydrated well (drinking five or more cups of water per day) to those with poor water intake (two or fewer cups of water per day). With the better-hydrated group, the relative risk of fatal coronary heart disease events was reduced by 54 percent for men and by 41 percent for women, other risks being equal. The risk reduction likely relates to water diluting the blood and lowering viscosity.

An Unappreciated Cardiovascular Risk Factor

Not everyone I see is interested in a collaborative therapeutic relationship. I see Peter about every two to three years. He is burly, in his late 50s, and not much for conversation. He usually wears wool shirts and is a successful entrepreneur with a security business. Peter has several chronic medical issues including borderline diabetes. I have tried to convince him to come in for regular visits, but he won't have it. We seem to go through the same routine once or twice a year: He calls for some issue to be managed over the phone and I will tell the nurses he needs to come in for a visit, blood pressure check and lab tests. Typically, he refuses to come in, but every so often he makes a cameo appearance.

One time Peter had a visit for severe knee pain. His blood pressure was elevated, which at that time was a new issue for him. He was taking non-steroidal anti-inflammatory drugs (or NSAIDs) like advil and aleve for his knee, but it wasn't getting better, so I arranged for him to get physical therapy. He called a few times in the next six months for one thing or another. He was seen a couple of times and at each visit his blood pressure was elevated. It wasn't clear to me whether pain was contributing, but during one of the visits where the blood pressure was elevated, his pain was significantly improved, so we discussed medication to lower his blood pressure. He declined. Even with consistently high numbers, he wanted to get his knee fixed first. Many months went by after this and I got a few notes from his orthopedic specialist in Boston. Then, in August of that year, Peter finally had his knee replacement. Miracle of miracles, he showed up about a month after the surgery. It may have been the first time he scheduled a visit spontaneously. In retrospect, I think he just came in to give me the business.

When I walk into an exam room, I usually study the patient. I do it automatically now without thinking. I want to get some sense of their mood and whether they're in pain. People will often notice that I'm scrutinizing them and comment on it. "What?" they say. "What's wrong? Do I look sick or something? Is something coming out of my nose? What?" I then reassure them that I'm just trying to take them all in.

I walked in to the visit with Peter and I could tell he was upset. Before I even sat in my little chair that spins around, he was all over me. "Listen," he started, "I'm not sure you're running too good of an office here." I was startled, as I don't often get verbally attacked by patients.

"I don't think your nurses even know how to take a blood pressure," he continued, as I looked at the chart to see what his blood pressure was that day.

"Oh, no, I wouldn't let them check it." He jabbed his finger at me. "I want *you* to check it."

I could feel the warmth rising in my chest and neck. A phrase I cannot abide is: The patient is always right. They are not always right and have no business being rude to me or my staff. I have asked a few people to leave our practice over the years for consistent rudeness.

I settled myself down, curious as to where this was going. "Why do you think the nurses don't know how to check a blood pressure?" I asked. He was quite definitive on a subject he knew nothing about.

"Every time I come here, your nurses check my blood pressure and get a high number. Then I go to my ortho's office and it's normal. I go into the hospital for my knee surgery and all they're getting is normal numbers." He finished with a smug look on his face.

In an effort to figure things out, I asked a series of follow-up questions. I wondered if he had sleep apnea and had lost weight before the surgery causing his blood pressure to normalize. No, that wasn't it. I asked him if maybe his pain was high when he saw us, but better at the orthopedic visits. No, he claimed. If anything, it was getting worse. In fact, the specialist put him on vicodin a few weeks before the surgery. Eureka!

"How many ibuprofen were you taking before they switched you to vicodin?" I asked, hoping for the right answer.

"Geez, I don't know. I was popping 5 or 6 at a time at least a few times per day," he said.

"That's probably the reason why your blood pressure was elevated. High doses of anti-inflammatories can raise some people's blood pressure. It sounds like your blood pressure got better right after they put you on the vicodin to replace the high doses of ibuprofen."

He gave that idea a few seconds, then said, "Nah, I don't think that was it," rejecting what was almost certainly the explanation for the blood pressure discrepancy. He much preferred the idea that our nurses were incompetent. He relished the experience of putting us in our place.

Peter illustrates some elusive but key elements of wellness: attitude and positive connections with other people in the world. His weight, blood pressure, diet and stress may not be his primary risk factors for serious health problems. *Schadenfreude* could top his list. This German word is defined by Merriam-Webster's online dictionary as "a feeling of enjoyment that comes from seeing or hearing about the troubles of other people."[55]

There was a study done as an offshoot of the Framingham Heart Study which evaluated the degree of happiness among subjects as correlated with people they were connected to, including family members, friends and co-workers. The conclusion was: "Clusters of happy and unhappy people are visible in the network, and the relationship between people's happiness extends up to three degrees of separation (for example, to the friends of one's friends' friends)."[56] So, if I'm happy, then a friend of mine is more likely to be happy. If my friend is happy, then a friend of his or hers and a friend of their friend is also more likely to be happy. With each step outward from the core individual, the effect was smaller, but my emotional state could influence someone far away whom I will never meet. (Perhaps this represents a feature of the quantum physics principle of entanglement.[57] It is only recently that quantum mechanics has been shown to act on a macroscopic scale.)

Given the importance of cardiovascular health to our long-term well being, our approach must be proactive and focus on *lifestyle*. Medications have their place, especially in the management of hypertension, but high cholesterol is almost certainly overmedicated, leading to a false reliance on statins. Type 2 diabetes can almost always be managed through weight loss, diet and exercise. Good hydration with water is a simple way to help reduce the risk of coronary events. Magnesium supplementation should play a bigger role in risk management and prevention.

Pharmaceuticals and alternative options like herbs should be evaluated on whether they reduce end points like the risk of heart attack and stroke. We have seen many pharmaceuticals lower cholesterol but have little or no impact on risk reduction. I suspect many of the alternative options would produce similar results. Natural is not always better, especially in a for-profit world where manufacturers of vitamins and supplements are hoping for a good income as well. In the end, a minimalist approach, with only essential additions, should form the basis for long-term health for most people in most situations.

7

Breathing Room for the Spirit

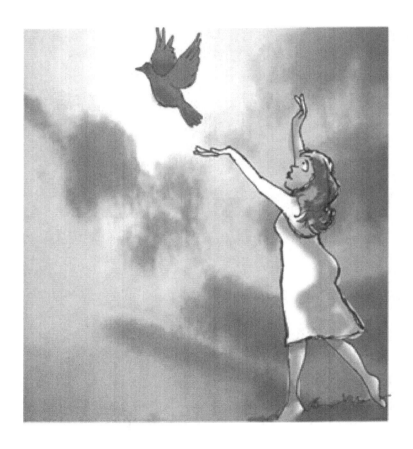

"What art offers is space–a certain breathing room for the spirit."[58]

—John Updike

The prolific American writer John Updike was a member of my community until he died from lung cancer, which brings us to the field of pulmonary medicine, a field which has not changed much in the past 25 years. There are several common diagnoses that cover most pulmonary visits to primary care providers and specialists: bronchitis, asthma, pneumonia, obstructive sleep apnea (OSA), and chronic obstructive pulmonary disease (COPD). There are others that are important but much less common, including a pulmonary embolism (the medical term for a blood clot to the lung) and lung cancer. Mainstream medicine has done well, overall, but again the system would be better off with more resources dedicated to smoking cessation and a more complete understanding of allergies and asthma.

Albert Can Finally Smell and Breathe

In my current position, I have seen one person who, by his account, had his allergy and asthma issues resolve after pursuing regular acupuncture sessions over a couple of months. Albert has told me anecdotally that he has not needed an antihistamine, nasal spray, inhaler or steroid since he started working with the acupuncturist many years ago. This could be an anomaly of sorts or it could represent an opportunity for some significant percentage of people with chronic allergies and asthma to be cured. It is difficult to clarify this question because of a lack of research in the area and because acupuncture is not typically covered by health insurance companies. Most people are reluctant to spend money out-of-pocket if I cannot predict a high likelihood of success. A more rational, unbiased medical system truly dedicated to patients would probably invest a couple hundred thousand dollars to see if acupuncture could cure allergies and asthma for a significant percentage of patients. Even if it cured five percent, it would almost certainly be cost effective.

Most physicians and scientists will discount the singularity, ignoring a unique event or outcome because they feel that "evidence" or truth can only come from the double-blind, placebo-controlled trial. I think this is a mistake. Albert's experience should, in my opinion, be the basis for further inquiry. As the following events all took place before I became his primary physician, I can take none of the blame for mismanagement or praise for his turnaround.

In the winter of 1981, I returned from being stationed in the desert Southwest for four years. I was home for about a month, when early one evening I had trouble breathing. I went to the emergency room (ER) and was given an injection of epinephrine. I was told I had asthma and needed to see a respiratory care physician. The respiratory doctor started me on albuterol. For the next 15 years, I was treated for asthma. During that time, I developed other allergies, experienced a constant runny nose, watery eyes, inflamed sinuses and constant sinus infections. For the allergies I was given several drugs, including claritin, allegra, allegra-D, clarinex, dimetapp, benadryl, flonase, nasalcrom, etc., etc.... Every time I got a cold or the flu, I developed either a chest infection or sinus infection. In these cases, I was always prescribed prednisone [an oral steroid] with antibiotics, sometimes three times a year. In 1999, I started seeing a new GP, and he added some additional drugs to my regimen: flovent and singulair. While some of these drugs seemed to provide some relief, they never seemed to 'fix the problem.'

One day, after three rounds of antibiotics for a sinus infection and a serious headache that would not go away, I was sent for an MRI (to check for a tumor). The doctor also sent me to the pharmacy with a prescription for a double dose of claritin. The pharmacist did not want to fill the script until he spoke to the physician. I returned the next day to pick up my prescription and asked the pharmacist 'why' He told me, 'There is nothing in the literature to explain why the physician wants to prescribe a double dose, but after speaking with him, I understand what he's trying to do.' At that point, I told him, 'No, thank you.'

For years, I walked around with a constant running nose, my jackets, pants and coats were all filled with Kleenex. I couldn't sit down to a meal, go for a walk, watch TV or anything else without a chapped, running nose. Sometimes foods and wines set off my asthma, and there was no way I could visit a friend who owned a cat. In 2001, a friend of mine started school to become an acupuncturist. She told me I should 'give it a try.' To be perfectly honest, I wrote this off as voodoo, and thought 'no way,' but after more time and more sinus infections, I heard from a friend that his daughter, Joyce, had just finished up acupuncture school, so I decided to take a chance and made an appointment.

At the first appointment, Joyce spent an hour talking to me, asking me questions and assessing my lifestyle. She asked me about everything from diet to home environment, and then explained the treatment. As she treated me, she placed pins at various points on my body—some at the top of my forehead, one on the right side of my nose, and even a few in my foot. She also burned moxa in the background. I can only explain the physical and mental experience as by far the most relaxing and euphoric feeling you can imagine. I felt as though I had had a massage when I left.

Ten minutes later, I went to the coffee shop next to my work. All of the sudden it hit me: I could smell everything, …the coffee flavors mocha, cinnamon and hazelnut, …all baked goods, the breads and the pastries. I had not realized until that moment that I had had no real sense of smell for many years. I also realized that the swelling in my sinuses was gone. I was able to take a deep breath with no phlegm at the bottom of my lungs. I spent the next half hour sampling all of the muffins and breads. I never realized my sense of taste, as well as my sense of smell, had been so diminished. The best part was, unlike with the allergy drugs, I had no strange side effects. I made an appointment with my doctor and told him about my experience. He told me he tried acupuncture in China, but it made the problem worse, and that I should keep using the flovent, albuterol and claritin. I took his advice and finished all three prescriptions, but never took a one [again after that]. This was December 10, 2001. Since that time, I have continued to see Joyce on a quarterly basis, and although I have had two or three ear infections and a sinus infection, they have resolved quickly and I have not experienced any asthma or allergies. I continue to enjoy the smell and taste of food. I have no idea why acupuncture works, or why it feels so good, but it does.[59]

Albert's experience highlights the difference between mainstream and alternative approaches. The primary care doctor and the specialists gave him one prescription after another in an effort to control the symptoms—the standard mainstream approach. Especially in the early part of my medical career, I managed patients similarly. I wanted to help people feel better and I was trained to recommend antihistamines, nasal sprays and inhalers.

Doctors can respond to the success Albert had with acupuncture in several ways. They can dismiss it as an outlier with no application to the treatment of allergies and asthma or to the broader world of health and wellness. They might be intrigued and potentially utilize alternative options more often. They also could start to question the entire system in which they were trained. They could step back and take a hard look at how our current medical system has evolved. I am, of course, in the third camp. It's analogous to someone who learns how a magic trick is performed. Once you see the world as it truly is, there is no going back.

Questioning the Conventional Wisdom

It is crucial for the long-term wellness of a population to minimize the overuse of antibiotics, yet antibiotics have been overprescribed for many years. Most acute middle ear infections (acute otitis media), pharyngitis, sinusitis and bronchitis will resolve without antibiotics. It takes a disciplined provider and a reasonable patient to not give in to the easy solution of bombing away with antibacterials. The use of these antibiotics has major implications for the health of our internal flora, especially as it pertains to the more vulnerable younger children whose micro biome is still developing.

A major dividing line, when it comes to providers, is how much value they give to the color of the phlegm when someone is sick. The conventional wisdom for many years was that clear phlegm was viral (or allergy related) but yellow and green phlegm were a sign of a bacterial infection. There was a physician that would hold up a paint stick and have the person indicate the particular shade of green of their phlegm. He chose a stronger antibiotic if the phlegm matched the Torrey Pine color on the spectrum.

It is clear now that the color of the phlegm has no predictive value in determining viral vs. bacterial infection and who will respond to an antibiotic. One of the studies that shot down this idea came from the *Scandinavian Journal of Primary Health Care* in 2009[60] and another was reported in the *European Respiratory Journal* in 2011.[61] The problem isn't that conventional wisdom exists, because it will always exist. The problem is when people are unable or unwilling to accept that the conventional wisdom is wrong. The incorrect notion often will hang around for many years after it has been debunked. Every week, a patient will diligently try to describe to me the color of their phlegm.

There's an old maxim for the card game bridge: "The hardest bid in bridge is pass" (which means to do nothing). Likewise, in medicine, often the hardest thing to do is nothing when someone comes to you for help, sick for a couple of weeks with a spouse at home expecting relief and a $30 co-pay for the visit. During my residency training, I remember a preceptor's idea that would help reduce the use of unnecessary antibiotics for viral infections. She recommended giving patients prescriptions for cough and cold medications. The prescribed medication would be roughly equivalent to what the person could get over the counter. She reasoned that this would make the person more content that they had not wasted their time coming in when they were sick. That didn't work for me. It is worse to reinforce the idea that the person needed to come in to the doctor's office for their cold. It maintains a sense of dependence on the all-knowing doctor who will take care of everything.

Finding the Triggers

There are many people that are prone to bronchitis and they come to the office expecting an antibiotic. Instead, I try to give them my impression of the episode in the big picture. The asthma spiel is definitely one of my more commonly invoked mini speeches which has been modified and crafted over the years. When people with an asthma history come in with acute bronchitis, I explain that the two issues are related and need to be viewed as a spectrum. To quote myself: "Anyone can get bronchitis, but the more susceptible a person is, the more likely they have a mild case of asthma. If someone gets bronchitis every 10 years, they probably don't have asthma. But if someone gets it every winter, I would argue they do have a mild version of asthma. There is some underlying reason why a person gets bronchitis every year. It is not a random occurrence for that person."

For the person with underlying asthma, the mainstream world has a wide array of medications used to treat symptoms, including cough syrups, bronchodilators like albuterol, steroid inhalers, and oral steroids like prednisone. The more severe a person's wheezing and breathing difficulty, the more important it would be to use strong medications like steroids. Prednisone has many negative associations for people, but short courses are very safe and incredibly effective. These treatments represent the standard reactive approach of allopathy, however.

There is a medication—singulair—that can be taken every day. It has been around for over 15 years and there are no known long-term problems and very few side effects. In my experience, it is often incredibly effective at preventing both allergy symptoms and asthma flare-ups. I have had a number of people use singulair to replace an antihistamine, a nasal steroid, albuterol for as-needed use, and an inhaled steroid like flovent. Believe it or not, the mainstream can be proactive with pharmaceuticals.

The best approach, however, is to try and identify the environmental factors that trigger symptoms for the individual. The most common cause of a flare-up is a respiratory virus, so preventing viral illnesses can be as simple as handwashing and maintaining a healthy lifestyle to maximize the effectiveness of the immune system. Pollen, mold, dust, pets, perfume, and smoke will often cause symptoms. Allergy testing can help to focus efforts within the home. One person may do well with dust mite covers for pillows and mattresses. Another needs an air purifier. The next will have symptoms improve with a dehumidifier in the basement to reduce mold counts. If we were using our resources in a better way, we would have environmental specialists go into the home of every person with allergies and asthma to make changes that minimize allergen exposure.

There is solid research that honey is more effective in suppressing a cough than all of the OTC cough medications. In one study,[62] a small amount (10gm) of any of three different varieties of honey was more effective than placebo for nocturnal cough in kids with upper respiratory infections. I would say in full disclosure that some of the OTC medications seem to be effective as decongestants and that, overall, the majority of OTC medications have some value—but the cough syrups, probably not.

"No, You Didn't Have Croup."

The person who is prone to bronchitis is much more likely to have a personal history of both allergies and eczema or family history of allergies, eczema or asthma. So many times, I see a bronchitis-susceptible person who tells me they had "croup" eight or ten times as a child. In my head, I think, "No, you didn't have croup. You had bronchitis and probably mild, intermittent asthma."

I've also heard many times that a person has had "pneumonia" five or six times and I think the same thing. I'll tell them that being prone to bronchitis is very common, but being prone to pneumonia is very uncommon. I often go on to say that the only individuals who are typically prone to bacterial lung infections are those with immune deficiency or a condition called bronchiectasis. Out of 3,000 patients, I have two with bronchiectasis and one with an actively deficient immune system who requires monthly immunoglobulin therapy. I probably have a few hundred patients, however, who are prone to bronchitis.

There is almost no doubt in the medical and scientific communities that the rates of allergies and asthma have been on the rise over the past 30 years or so, and there is an abundance of articles supporting this. The rise in allergies is somewhere in the range of two to five times in 30 years, depending on the source. The most prevalent hypothesis for this rise is the hygiene hypothesis.[63] British researcher David Strachan first proposed this back in 1989. The idea is that children are less exposed to dirt and microorganisms from a very young age and the under-stimulated immune system does not develop in such a way that it can readily distinguish between pathogens and benign articles in our environment like dust and pollen. Research has shown that children in daycare centers exposed to other sniffly kids have fewer allergies. In a Finnish study, the authors found that subjects living on farms or near forests had more diverse bacteria on their skin and lower allergen sensitivity than individuals living in areas with less environmental biodiversity, such as in urban areas or near bodies of water.

It has always been assumed by mainstream medicine that asthma is fundamentally an allergic or atopic condition. This may not be the case. In a review in 1999,[64] Neil Pearce found that half of the people with an asthma pattern have an allergic component triggering their symptoms, but the other half had no discernible allergic cause. Perhaps this distinction is relevant in deciding who would respond to acupuncture. Some of our assumptions can be incorrect and many chronic processes are more diverse and complicated than we realize.

There are many other ideas about why allergies and asthma are on the rise. Some research links the rise to climate change, questioning whether earlier flowering of plants with higher pollen counts is contributing. There is research to suggest that air pollution and chemical exposure in the environment are playing a major role, especially in the steady increases in the rates of asthma. This would potentially explain why inner-city children have much higher rates of asthma than children in suburban and rural areas.

There have also been links made to overuse of antibiotics that could alter a young child's internal flora irrevocably. One research group focused on the increasing use of tylenol in young children. Another posited that increasing rates of obesity cause higher levels of inflammation that play a role internally. Yet another researcher suggested that we are just diagnosing allergic conditions more often, as the "dry skin" of the past is now classified as "eczema" by today's physicians.

To figure all of this out is to figure out much of what is fundamentally wrong with our health. This represents a convergence of the worlds of allergy, immunology, pulmonology, gastrointestinal health, microbiology and infectious disease.

Breathing Like a Yogi

In July of 2013, I attended the International Congress of Naturopathic Medicine. It was an enlightening conference in many ways, and I will reference much of the information from the conference later in the book in various chapters. As a starting point, though, there was a lecture on something called the Buteyko method of breathing, including its benefits for people with asthma.

Back in the hotel room, I talked to my wife about the Buteyko method and its alleged successes. I reviewed the details and demonstrated some of the techniques. My wife said they were all based on Ujjayi breathing developed in yoga and first described maybe two thousand years ago—just a wee bit before Buteyko presented them to the world in the 1960s.

Ujjayi is a diaphragmatic breath which first fills the lower belly (activating the first and second chakras), rises to the lower rib cage (the third and fourth chakras), and finally moves into the upper chest and throat. The technique is very similar to the three-part Tu-Na breathing found in Taoist Qigong practice. Inhalation and exhalation are both done through the nose. The "ocean sound" is created by moving the glottis as air passes in and out. As the throat passage is narrowed so, too, is the airway, the passage of air creating a "rushing" sound. The length and speed of the breath is controlled by the diaphragm, the strengthening of which is, in part, the purpose of ujjayi. The inhalations and exhalations are equal in duration, and are controlled in a manner that causes no distress to the practitioner.

There is a condition called "chronic hyperventilation" that potentially links pulmonary symptoms to various chronic medical conditions. Chronic hyperventilation typically would cause dry mouth and bad breath. (Or, the person needs to brush and floss their teeth more often.)

The thinking is that stress causes "overbreathing," and because of a relatively high respiratory rate, the airways become dry and irritated. This leads to lower carbon dioxide (CO_2) levels in the blood because the exhaling is out of proportion to the normal physiologic exchange. With lower CO_2, the oxygen (O_2) in the blood stream is more tightly bound to the hemoglobin in red blood cells, causing decreased O_2 to the tissues. If there is less oxygen, then the person can experience headaches, poor sleep, numbness and tingling to the extremities (also called paresthesias), dizziness, poor focus and other symptoms. It can theoretically affect any part of the body with smooth muscle, like blood vessels, airway and bowel. The signs of this effect can include recurrent unexplained chest pain, indigestion, shortness of breath, cold extremities and excessively uncomfortable menstrual cycles, also referred to by doctors as dysmennorhea. I see many people in the office who have these symptoms with no obvious cause. They typically will have a work-up and ultimately normal tests. They are given various medications like non-steroidal anti-inflammatories, muscle relaxers, acid blockers and pharmaceuticals for anxiety and stress.

The Buzz Saw in the Bed

A major underdiagnosed and undermanaged condition related to breathing is obstructive sleep apnea (OSA). This condition is important in terms of its effect on health and productivity. It has been estimated that 90 percent of sleep apnea cases are undiagnosed. There are many scenarios where sleep apnea should be considered, the most obvious being the middle-aged obese male with the thick neck who sleeps at the other end of the house because the snoring is so loud his wife gave him the boot.

Most presentations of sleep apnea are more subtle, though, and most patients underrepresent, underreport and "underunderstand" what is going on. Patients typically confuse insomnia with sleep apnea, so it's good for a practitioner to be aware of that misunderstanding and address it early in the conversation. "Oh, no, I sleep fine, Doc," they will say, or "Yeah, I do have problems sleeping and often wake up around 3 a.m."

Snoring is embarrassing, so people tend to minimize the issue. I remember a classic patient. He had not been seen in our office yet but called frantic because his blood pressure had been checked at work and was 190/100. We said we could squeeze him in that afternoon, but he retorted he was too busy to come in. Reluctantly, I started 10mg lisinopril over the phone, with a visit the next day.

Brian came in, pleasant and large, about six feet tall and 280 pounds. Right there, I'm thinking sleep apnea. I asked him if he snored and he said occasionally, but nothing on a regular basis. In an effort to avoid jargon, I asked him if his wife had ever commented on any irregular breathing at night or gasping for air. He said no, but why don't we just ask her since she was out in the waiting area.

The nurses brought his wife, Allie, into the room. I asked her if Brian snores. Oh, sure, she said—every night like a buzz saw. I asked about breathing and she said every night he's gasping and sputtering and seems to almost stop breathing. The patient and I were both incredulous, but I did a better job of hiding it. After Brian closed his gaping mouth, he asked her why she hadn't brought it up. He had no idea what was going on. Patients with obstructive sleep apnea can stop breathing 80 or 90 or 100 times per hour for many years and have no idea.

Any person with elevated body mass index (BMI) should be questioned about sleep apnea. Any person with hypertension should be questioned, especially someone with variable blood pressure numbers. Many times I've seen a patient showing 128/84 one visit and then 154/100 the next, with numbers all over the place. "White coat hypertension" will come up as a possible explanation. The person will say they're under stress or had too much coffee that morning. They rushed to the office and got stuck behind a school bus and continue to grumble about the rotten kids interfering yet again with our timeliness and productivity.

The person with erratic numbers, especially with an elevated diastolic component, often has sleep apnea. The person with sleep apnea can also have relatively normal blood pressure but unexplained fatigue. For a couple of years, I was seeing a 75-year-old thin woman, Anne, with severe unexplained fatigue, memory loss and focus problems. She had an extensive workup and saw several specialists. She did not have undiagnosed thyroid disease, which was my first thought. I remember the thought popping into my head about sleep apnea, although she seemed to be the opposite demographic.

One visit I told her the only test I could think of that we hadn't done was a sleep study. Anne was motivated because she felt so terrible every day.

The sleep study showed severe obstructive sleep apnea. That diagnosis was made years ago and, to my frustration, she still does not acknowledge the sleep apnea as the probable cause for her severe fatigue. I see her every 3-6 months desperate for some explanation for why she feels so terrible every day. At those moments, I often look around the room for the hidden camera. Someone must be playing a prank on me, having this patient come in so often so we can have the same exact conversation. Deja vu all over again. Groundhog Day. Strike up the polka, the band has begun.

I saw a younger woman—Lisa, in her 40s—for visit after visit for fatigue with no apparent cause. She worked in a private practice as a psychotherapist. She was mildly overweight but slept alone, which made it more difficult to get information on any commotion she might be making at night. Many years before coming to see me, Lisa had been diagnosed with chronic fatigue syndrome (CFS). She was so intent on improving her quality of life, she was considering taking atripla (a medication used to treat the Human Immunodeficiency Virus or HIV) when it looked like a retrovirus might be the cause for chronic fatigue syndrome. A sleep study showed moderate sleep apnea. Since then, Lisa has had some improvement with Continuous Positive Airway Pressure (CPAP) therapy. She still has fatigue overall, and investigations are still ongoing, but it was still important to uncover her sleep apnea.

Detecting sleep apnea is crucial for many reasons, one being it can prevent overtreatment of blood pressure. Many people with OSA have grown accustomed to fatigue, drowsiness and trouble concentrating. If better managed across the United States, the benefit in terms of health, quality of life, and work productivity would be incalculable. Chronic Fatigue Syndrome has been discussed in the Rheumatology section.

At the International Congress on Naturopathic Medicine conference, there was also a lecture on pulmonary issues where the speaker brought up sleep apnea. She said that sleep apnea was "invented" in the 1960s. Most of the speakers were reasonable, but some, including this one, were hostile toward mainstream medicine. She implied that somehow sleep apnea was a concocted diagnosis, perhaps invented by a group of MDs trying to keep people sick and make a lot of money. This would be a difficult conspiracy to pull off. If I send an obese snorer with uncontrolled hypertension for a sleep study and the results show that he stopped breathing 50 or 60 times per hour in the sleep lab, I'm thinking there is something real going on. I don't think sleep apnea was invented in the 1960s, I just believe the incidence has gone up steadily as Americans have become more obese.

"Doc, I Don't Understand Why I Feel So Good."

Chronic Obstructive Pulmonary Disease (COPD) incorporates a high percentage of patients seen in any medical office for respiratory symptoms. Obviously, helping people with smoking cessation is the best proactive option. For smokers, I try to bring up the issue at every visit, no matter why they have come in, searching for the right angle to help stoke their motivation. I have seen an older gentleman, Milton, in my office for many years. He starts each visit by asking how my family and I are doing. He was a long-term smoker and we talked often about quitting. For some time, it didn't seem like he was ready to cut back, but then one visit we had a longer discussion than usual and he told me the time had come. Smoking for him was over, done, kaput. We left the room together and I stopped at our nurse's station. Milton kept going, walking out toward the front desk. I started talking to one of our nurses about how great the visit had been and how optimistic I was that he was going to finally stop smoking. In the middle of my monologue, I looked out the window only to see Milton, cigarette in hand, ready to spark up. Eventually, he did quit and we still joke about that incident.

For the person who has already smoked for many years with permanent damage to the lungs, inhalers are the mainstay of treatment. Some patients with more advanced disease need supplemental oxygen. The mainstream medications typically improve a person's quality of life. I'm not sure if any alternative options would be comparably effective.

In pulmonary medicine, as with all medical subspecialties, it is important to individualize care. There is a 78-year-old male I have seen in the office for several years named Fred. He is retired and lives alone. Over a period of time he was showing signs of slow, unexplained weight loss. He had a long history of smoking, over 50 pack years, but had quit several years prior to seeing me. He went out of his way at each six-month follow-up visit to tell me, "Doc, I don't understand why I feel so good." He had no aches or pains and was remarkably stable. He spent a good deal of his free time volunteering at an animal shelter and loved it there.

Unexplained weight loss, to a doctor, is often cancer until proven otherwise, especially in a smoker or an elderly person. At one visit, he mentioned that, for the past year or so, he was going down by a few pounds each month. I reviewed his diet in detail and it turned out he really wasn't getting much in the way of calories—I estimated around 1,000 calories per day. I ordered some lab tests including electrolytes, glucose level, kidney function tests, liver panel, complete blood count, thyroid test and CRP. CRP or C-reactive protein is a non-specific measure of inflammation in the body. You can see elevated CRP levels if a person has an active infection. You can also see elevated CRP levels in someone with underlying cancer.

For this 78-year-old, there were no concerning results. His CRP was mildly elevated, which is uninterpretable. If it were low, it would be mildly reassuring that cancer is not present. If it were high, it would be another red flag that cancer is more possible. I arranged for him to come in for close follow-up one month later.

To my partial relief, he had gained four pounds. I reviewed his diet and he had increased his calorie intake by having a full bowl of raisin bran for breakfast and by having two Snickers ice cream bars every evening. I started to talk with him about doing a lung CT. In my mind we would be trying to rule out lung cancer. There are many reasons to finesse that discussion. In the past, I assumed that deep down, when I recommended a CT scan in this context, people understood that I was investigating for a potential malignancy. I have found, however, that people generally don't put these things together. I have learned to assume nothing about what a person knows or does not know.

After I brought up doing the lung scan, Fred said he really didn't want to do a lot of tests. He confessed that every time he came to see me, he was worried I would find something seriously wrong with him. For all of my well-intentioned listening, I had missed that one. When Fred was saying how he couldn't understand why he felt so good, he was really indicating that he expected to have some serious medical problem (i.e. cancer) diagnosed by now. With his head down, looking at the floor, he said that he really didn't expect to be alive for more than a few more years.

I said we didn't need to do the lung scan if he didn't want to and we also didn't need to have more visits if he would rather just come in every six months. I told him I worked for him and we would always do as much or as little as he wanted. I worried that on some level he had picked up on my fears. The cat was out of the bag now and I couldn't take back that visit.

Within a few months of that encounter, Fred's COPD grew worse and he went to the ER. They did a lung CT scan that showed fluid in the lungs, also known as a pleural effusion. Fred saw a pulmonologist, who drained the fluid and sent it off for analysis. The results showed that he had advanced lung cancer. This diagnosis, which he had feared for many years, was now official. The illusion of his good health was now altered and he became a sick person with steady deterioration in his status.

Physicians are trained to run tests and make diagnoses. We are motivated to find problems and treat aggressively in almost all situations so, in many ways, it goes against the grain to respect a person's decision to let things be. Looking back, it is impossible to say whether my conversation with Fred had any influence on his symptoms or made a difference in the sequence of events that led to a diagnosis of lung cancer.

To summarize pulmonary issues, we should do whatever we can as a society to continue to encourage smoking cessation. COPD and lung cancer would plummet. Once again, we should work hard on improving lifestyle and maintaining healthy weight, as this would cure most cases of sleep apnea. It would be worth researching the benefits of alternative options, especially acupuncture, for allergies and asthma. Curing those conditions would be preferable to bombing away with pills and inhalers year after year after year. Figuring out the triggers in our diet and environment is a crucial piece to the puzzle. This point will come up over and over in the subsequent chapters.

8

The Others

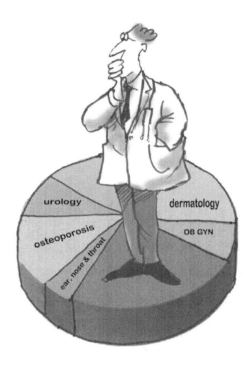

So far, there have been chapters for each of the primary medical subspecialties. This chapter is a hodge podge encompassing most of the other areas of medicine. Many of these are surgical subspecialties, but much of a surgeon's work is done outside of the operating room. The goal is still to review some of the best of what the mainstream and alternative worlds have to offer.

The Head and Neck

I will often see people in the primary care office with sinus symptoms. If the symptoms are improving, we will pursue supportive care in some form, avoiding antibiotics whenever possible. One hypothetical patient comes in with two weeks of progressive symptoms including focal sinus pressure to her left cheek with intermittent low-grade fevers. This would be considered more likely bacterial and, for most providers, she would meet criteria for antibiotics. Basic primary care would include a brief physical exam and some first line oral antibiotic. Her overall history shows that she is prone to sinus issues and comes in once or twice per year for similar episodes. She doesn't typically come in after four or five days of symptoms and understands, to some degree, the viral vs. bacterial distinction.

A better primary care visit would not only address the acute issue but also discuss (1) ways to reduce the incidence of the primary viral infection and (2) ways to minimize any progression to a secondary bacterial infection. I try to reinforce the importance of adequate handwashing and avoiding touching the mouth, nose and eyes if possible. It may be a boring topic to discuss, but the simplest solution is often the best solution. I may also review the importance of adequate sleep, stress management and regular exercise to maximize the functioning of the immune system.

Repetition is valuable and people often need to hear the same information over and over before it sticks. One study revealed that a person needs to hear something three times to remember it. Another suggested the range is more like seven to ten times. Hearing you won the lottery probably takes one time. Someone badgering you about cutting back on weekly beer intake may take 20 or more reminders.

Several things can be effective in reducing the progression of acute sinusitis. The first is a nasal steroid such as fluticasone. For those prone to sinusitis, starting the nasal spray early on in the course of the URI (upper respiratory infection) probably cuts back on progression by at least 50 percent. I couldn't find a study that supports this degree of success, but there may never be a "double-blind, placebo-controlled, multicenter trial with a low p value" constructed in such a way that it will definitively answer my clinical question.

The other common option is nasal irrigation with a neti pot or some similar device with a saline and baking soda concoction. This is typically preferred by the "holistic" person and can be helpful, especially if done on a regular basis. It has been interesting to see the little neti pot rise to prominence in American medicine. Remember ABC, in the 1980s, copying successful original shows developed by the other networks? Health is no different. Companies started copycat sinus rinse devices relatively quickly after the neti pot from aryuveda became popular. Surgery to improve sinus drainage is an option for the small percentage of people with nasal polyps or some other anatomical issue.

An interesting alternative treatment for excessive ear wax is candling or coning. A candle is used to supposedly generate negative pressure that draws wax from a person's ear canal. Over the years, I have repeatedly heard people say it worked for them. Studies seem to refute this, saying the material alleged to be earwax is actually residue from the candle itself. It may have value for those with blocked Eustachian tubes but I don't have enough anecdotal experience to know.

The debate reminds me of the ionic foot bath that is purported to draw toxins from the body. My wife and I had this done where you put your feet in the little tub and the device is turned on. Gradually, with both of us, the water became darker and darker. After 30 to 40 minutes, the water was a reddish brown with thick sludge floating around. The effect is so dramatic it is easy to see why a person would believe the junk was extracted from their toxic body. *Theguardian.com*, an online British newspaper, sent a doctor to have an ionic detox footbath.[65] He took water samples before and after and sent them to a lab for analysis. Neither sample contained any toxins. And when a reporter for the publication suspected that the discolored water might be due to rust, he tried an experiment: he rigged up a bowl of salt water with two metal nails attached to a car battery (to simulate the metal electrodes used in the ionic detox footbaths). That water also turned brown with some sludge on top. Analysis of the "after" sample of water from the detox footbath showed that the change in water color was a result of increased iron content from the nails.

There are so many "alternative" and "natural" options out there, including innumerable vitamins and supplements and potions, that we will always need to weigh the available evidence to make the best possible judgment. The goal is to find a cozy place in the middle of the gullibility/cynicism spectrum.

Orthopedics

Many medical issues and patient visits are related to the field of Orthopedics which focuses on the musculoskeletal system. I see numerous people with chronic joint pain, especially of the weight-bearing joints, the hip and knee. I actually think it's stunning that the joints of the body can take so much abuse for so long. The cartilage in joints is tough and maintains adequate cushioning year after year.

John

A patient I've seen for years, John, is in construction. He works mostly in a supervisory role, but he sometimes has to get out from behind the clipboard and do physical work. He has the standard middle-aged American male belly. He came in one day complaining that he had experienced knee pain for about six months but had also begun to experience hip pain in the past few weeks. The most common cause of hip pain isn't really hip pain at all, but trochanteric bursitis. True hip pain typically involves the crease of the hip not the sides. The majority of people come in with pain localizing to the side. At the angle of the femur as it turns into the hip joint there is a prominence called the greater trochanter where there is a bursa sac. Repetitive friction and stress can cause inflammation to the bursa sac referred to as "bursitis."

The relatively simple approach to any short-term musculoskeletal problem is rest, ice and *consistent* NSAIDs for up to seven days or so. Most people take an Advil here and two Advil there, but don't take them with a dosage or regularity that will resolve, rather than just reduce, the inflammation. A naturopathic provider would typically view acute inflammation as a normal process of the body and not something to be suppressed. For more chronic inflammatory musculoskeletal issues, they prefer natural or homeopathic options like arnica in a topical application.

(There is a book called The Calcium Lie and a follow-up book called The Calcium Lie II by Robert Thompson, MD, that blow the lid off many issues of health and wellness. It is an incredible resource and as important as anything I've read but by the time I read The Calcium Lie II, it was too late to incorporate the ideas from that book into this book. One of the most important principles described is that most Americans have too much calcium in their system and that this plays a major role in the development of chronic arthritis. Almost 100% of Americans have other mineral deficiencies and imbalances implicated in a variety of chronic health problems.)

If John were merely experiencing bursitis, the simple approach would likely be enough. However, he had more chronic knee pain and, on review of symptoms, some intermittent low back pain as well. Optimal primary care in this or any case involves looking for the underlying causes of symptoms rather than just bombing away with medication.

There are several common reasons why a person has multiple musculo-skeletal problems. The person could be obese, which causes stress to the joints. The person could have a physical job leading to wear and tear. The person could also have some chronic medical condition like rheumatoid arthritis, though this is relatively uncommon. Psoriatic arthritis tends to be underdiagnosed, since the person and doctor seldom relate the person's dry skin with chronic diffuse arthralgias, but this is also not seen very often.

The most common causes of multiple musculoskeletal problems are muscle weakness/deconditioning, repetitive activity and alignment problems. The stronger a person's core muscles, the fewer back problems they have because the spine is more stable. The stronger a person's quadriceps muscles, the less knee pain they tend to have because the knee is more stable. Chiropractors catch a lot of grief in mainstream medicine, but over my time in medicine I have come full circle. Now, I will often do a poor man's assessment of a person's alignment: I have them stand facing away from me and I look for asymmetry. One of my more commonly used spiels involves asymmetry. "All people have asymmetry," I start. "People have a dominant side and a weak side; a more flexible side and a less flexible side. Over time, this asymmetry often gets more pronounced and affects the alignment of the spine and joints. This causes areas of mechanical stress which lead to pain and inflammation."

I have been stunned by how many people have one hip higher than the other or one scapula more protracted that the other. People will have shoulders at a grossly rotated angle with their cervical spine. Physical therapists and chiropractors are both valuable in addressing these underlying issues. The home exercise program is the most important element long-term if a person wants to prevent these diverse musculoskeletal problems.

The Mind-Body Connection

Several books have been written about the psychological aspect of chronic pain. Many people with chronic pain likely have the mind-body connection working to their detriment. This element probably explains why some have a bad-looking MRI of the spine and seem to manage well without the need for strong prescription pain medications, while others complain of severe, disabling pain with a relatively normal MRI. One of the main proponents of this idea is John Sarno. He has written three books: *Mind Over Back Pain*, *Healing Back Pain: The Mind-Body Connection*, and *The Divided Mind: The Epidemic of Mindbody Disorders*.

Sarno defines "psychosomatic" as physical disorders generated by the mind. He explains that these symptoms appear to be purely physical but are either directly induced or contributed to by unconscious emotions that may have arisen due to childhood trauma, feelings of inadequacy, or inappropriate desires long suppressed. Sarno believes physical symptoms are present "not to protect you from foreign substances, but to keep your conscious attention focused on your body."[66] In short, Sarno implies that these deep, dark thoughts are worse than bodily pain and that the mind decides to inflict physical pain to distract from mental anguish.

Sarno defines "psychogenic" disorders as any physical disorder that is either induced or modified by the brain for psychological reasons. For example, he explains that blushing and "butterflies" in the stomach are harmless and short-lived but are, nevertheless, examples of the mind inducing specific reactions from the body due to emotional elation or stress. Blushing and "butterflies" show that emotions lead to seemingly unrelated reactions in the body, implying that deeper and more complex emotions could give rise to even more intricate and confusing physical symptoms.

Another psychogenic disorder Sarno identifies is increasing pain of a physical disorder when the mind is anxious or overly emotional. If someone has a headache because they forgot their morning coffee, it will only get worse when they walk into the office and they realize they also forgot to bring the prepared morning presentation, that their child is waiting for pick-up in the principal's office, or their mother's doctor calls with bad news from the recent PET scan. Conversely, take an injured soldier, perhaps an amputee, and bring him to the countryside, wheel him along the beach (therefore removing him from the stressful scenario of wartime hospitals), and you will improve his state of mind and accelerate his physical progress. Whether one agrees with Sarno or not, he gives a foundation for the mind-body relationship, especially in the context of chronic pain.

Larry came to me as a new patient in early 2014. He described a long history of low back pain. He had seen many healthcare professionals including physical therapists, occupational therapists, pain specialists and several neurosurgeons. He did prolotherapy (injection therapy intended to stimulate the body's ability to repair injured areas). He learned hypnotherapy so he could try and cope with the pain. He eventually became so frustrated that he flew out to California to see another back specialist. The specialist was performing a unique surgery with claims of great success. There were countless people with videotaped testimonials describing how well they had done. Larry had to change his health insurance and finagle an out-of-network approval to see the physician.

He had the surgery in California and was discharged to his hotel on strong pain medication. He was seen for a follow-up visit a few days later. The nurse brought him to a separate room with a movie camera and they started to film him. He felt drugged from the medication and had difficulty answering the questions. They wanted him to say that the surgery had been a great success. It hadn't worked, however, so he walked out. He went back to the hotel, recuperated on his own for a few days and then flew back home.

His primary care physician recommended another consultation with a specialist in Boston. Larry agreed and, to his surprise, the back surgeon did not recommend surgery or more physical therapy. He didn't recommend cortisone shots. He recommended a book by Dr. Sarno.

Larry read the Sarno book and it helped him to start putting the pieces together. At that first visit with me, he descreibed some of his relevant experiences. When he was five years old, his mother died in a tragic accident. When he was eight years old, his father died suddenly. He was an orphan, forced to live with his grandparents that didn't want him. For the rest of his childhood, he had to endure physical and emotional abuse by his grandfather. He finally escaped to college and it was sometime in early adulthood that his back pain started. By the time we met, Larry had already started intensive psychotherapy and was optimistic that it would be his true path to recovery.

It is often challenging for physicians to sort out those with "legitimate" chronic pain, those with a psychosomatic component, and those that are knowingly seeking narcotic pain medication. Most physicians would acknowledge that a high percentage of those with chronic pain from any source have related psychological issues, but teasing out the chicken/egg aspect is difficult. Either way, the pain needs to be addressed and managed for the person to attain true long-term relief. There is an interesting parallel with addiction management. Many groups that specialize in addiction recovery have higher rates of success if they incorporate an understanding of the individual's psychological make-up and background.

I am also wondering more and more about whether a person's genetic background is relevant to how a person experiences pain. Those people who have not experienced severe chronic pain may assume the "hurting" person is exaggerating their symptoms. They could think the person is looking for a convenient way to get out of work or avoid the challenges of life. In private conversations, there can be talk reflecting some inherent weakness or flaw in the character of those with chronic pain. We may find that people with genetic anomalies, like an MTHFR defect, are more prone to chronic severe pain with less of a response to treatment. MTHFR represents an enzyme called methylene tetrahydrofolate reductase and has been brought up earlier in the book but in other contexts. This enzyme is important for a wide variety of cellular processes, but one action in particular may be relevant to chronic pain.

Normal MTHFR enzyme activity is essential for production of a powerful, naturally produced antioxidant called glutathione. We all have glutathione produced on a daily basis. Glutathione helps us to detoxify our tissues and it reduces inflammation. Genetic MTHFR anomalies are very common: about 40% of people have moderately reduced activity of the enzyme and about 10% of people have severely reduced activity. Research may show that the tendency toward intractable chronic pain correlates with MTHFR.

My Wife the Healer

My wife Mary is a yoga teacher. She has had extensive training and is certified in more areas than anyone I know. She has been trained in yoga, pilates, aesthetics, massage, reiki, aromatherapy, spinning, dance, barre, horticulture, holistic nutrition, lymphatic drainage and other modalities.

From 2012 to 2013 I had problems with my left shoulder. If I was doing anything over my head there was discomfort and, sometimes, severe pain. What I could do physically was limited and for six months I felt some degree of achiness every day. This would be classified as "impingement" by just about any orthopedic specialist. As far as I could tell, the shoulder problem was caused by intensive Rip Trainer sessions at the club down the street. I think I was trying to show the suburban housewives who was boss.

I tend to be a bad patient and don't always follow my own advice. If I saw someone like me, I would recommend about a week of consistent high dose anti-inflammatories. Of course, I never followed through with that simple option. If that didn't work, physical therapy would probably be my next recommendation. This would typically involve one or two hourly sessions a week for 4-8 weeks and then a home exercise program. If regular anti-inflammatories didn't work, the PT program would probably work. But I'm too impatient for all of that.

In the winter of 2013, my wife grew tired of my grousing and told me to get on the floor. She had me on my stomach and started walking on my back. It was uncomfortable and, at first, I thought it was all a ruse because she didn't like my anniversary gift last year. She worked me over pretty well with her feet, then had me flip over on my back and she continued an intensive massage to my shoulders, neck and upper back. "You're a mess," she kept saying. I could feel her working out knots of muscle.

After about 45 minutes of this, she let me up. My shoulder felt better. I could lift it over my head with no discomfort. Within a week, it was 90% better. Within two weeks, it had resolved completely. At that time I had been in medicine for 15 years and had seen hundreds of people with similar shoulder problems. She did for me in under an hour what would probably have taken 20 hours of therapy and 20 hours of a home exercise program. Yet massage is still considered by many to be an "alternative" therapy.

Here's another personal experience with what would broadly be considered alternative medicine. For more than five years I had had problems with my right knee. It got progressively worse, causing more limitations in terms of regular exercise. It got to the point where I could barely run a mile on the treadmill before having to quit. Around this time I was looking for a single supplement to take for general health. There was a lot of focus on vitamin D deficiency and omega-3 fatty acids and resveratrol, one of the active substances found in high quantities in red wine. I found a single supplement, Omegaberry, and started taking it every day.

I kept trying to exercise and found that my knee was getting better. I was able to run farther and harder with less pain and swelling. Things improved with the knee and, for a few weeks, I really couldn't come up with any good explanation. It then dawned on me that the only thing that was different in my life was the Omegaberry. I stayed on it and my chronic knee pain essentially resolved.

Since then, there have been several times where I stopped taking the supplement because I was on vacation. The knee pain returned within a week. I restarted when I got home and the knee pain resolved. More recently, the knee pain got much more intense and I resigned myself to needing an MRI and possible surgery. I then realized that, once again, I had forgotten to take the Omegaberry for over a week. I don't know what in the supplement is helping my knee, but I'm probably on it for life. Research shows that omega-3 fatty acids reduce inflammation, so that is the ingredient most likely reducing the knee pain.

Possibly the most effective solution to chronic neck or back pain is again non-medical: a new mattress. There is no telling how many people with chronic neck pain, chronic back pain, chronic fatigue and other medical issues would get dramatically better in a relatively short period of time if they purchased a new, high-end mattress like Tempurpedic or Sleep Number. I have seen this happen over and over again. Most people are reluctant to spend $1,500-$2,000 or more on a mattress. It seems like a waste of money. But we spend almost a third of our lives in bed. If you get 10 years out of it, the cost is relatively small, especially if your productivity is higher and you're saving on heating pads, ibuprofen, Tylenol and all the other items people purchase to get through a day more comfortably.

Urology

Some of the more common problems affecting the genitourinary system include urinary tract infections (or UTIs), kidney stones, prostate enlargement and incontinence. There are also issues that come up with prostate, bladder or kidney cancer. As in other systems, prevention and a more proactive approach are preferable to procedures and other interventions.

Urinary Tract Infections

Women are much more prone to UTIs, mostly because they have a short urethra so there is a shorter distance between the hostile bacteria in the outside world and their bladders. One of the quickest, most straightforward visits to any primary care doctor is a patient coming in with urinary frequency, urgency and burning. Bing, bang, boom! Check a urine dip, send the sample for culture and start an oral antibiotic. Naturopaths will often use D-mannose for UTIs. It is the active ingredient in cranberry juice and is thought to interfere with the bacteria's ability to adhere to the bladder wall. There are reports that D-mannose can be 90% effective in curing UTIs. Once again, if we were truly dedicated to an integrated health system, there would be resources for a study comparing the efficacy of D-mannose with standard antibiotics for UTIs.

I had two elderly patients over 85 years old, a man and a woman, both prone to UTIs. For the male, the D-mannose supplement taken every day worked well for him. He went from a multi-drug-resistant UTI every two or three months with several admissions to the hospital for urosepsis (where the infection progresses from the bladder up into the kidney and then into the bloodstream) to no UTIs for over a year. The female patient, however, took the D-mannose faithfully every day and continued to have UTIs on a regular basis. I have also tried D-mannose a few times to treat acute UTI episodes with no success. It does not make sense to me to dogmatically reject the use of all antibiotics. As with many issues, there is wide variation of underlying causes and the simple solutions do not always work.

If a woman presents with acute urinary changes, it is not always a straightforward UTI. There is a chronic poorly-understood condition seen in younger women with flare-ups that mimic a urinary tract infection. This bladder problem is called interstitial cystitis (IC). I have often called this the

Irritable Bowel Syndrome of the urinary system.

The classic scenario for making the diagnosis is a young woman who comes in with acute or sometimes sub-acute urinary changes. I have found that the symptoms are usually similar but not textbook for a UTI. A woman with burning during urination, frequency and urgency for two days probably does have a UTI. The woman with vague discomfort, with unclear timing relative to urination and possible other dubious symptoms for a week, may or may not have a UTI.

For the patient with underlying interstitial cystitis, there are typically some mild abnormalities on a urine dip test, but not the 3+ leukocytes, 1+ protein and moderate blood typically seen with UTIs. Standard practice in these situations is to start an antibiotic and send the urine sample for a culture. If the urine culture comes back negative and the provider finds a history of multiple other negative cultures, the patient probably has interstitial cystitis.

There is a good treatment regimen to use during flare-ups—doxepin at bedtime and piroxicam, a prescription anti-inflammatory, twice a day, although the majority of women can control flare-ups and symptoms through lifestyle changes like cutting back on/eliminating coffee, alcohol, acidic foods and vinegar-based foods like salad dressing. At least half of the women I've told of these instigating lifestyle factors, will say, "You just described my whole diet!" This is almost as high as the percentage of males over 50 who will say "What?" when you ask them whether they have any hearing problems.

Overactive Bladder

There is a chronic urologic condition that is representative of many of the failings of modern medicine. If a person goes to a physician complaining of frequent urination with an intermittent urgency to go, a work-up will be done to rule out diabetes, kidney disease, bladder cancer and other potential causes. If the work-up is negative, a diagnosis of Overactive Bladder (OAB) will often be made. The primary care doctor or urologist will often prescribe a medication like oxybutynin for the problem and consider it a victory. The medications for OAB however, generally have side effects like drowsiness and dry mouth. Making the diagnosis also is not much of a victory because the provider and the patient still have no idea of the underlying cause and there is not typically any effort made to cure the problem.

If we studied the issue more, it would likely be shown that a significant percentage of patients with OAB, have hyperactivity of their bladder muscle because of chronic magnesium deficiency. I have never seen a study done to clarify this relationship, which reflects poorly on our pharmaceutical-focused healthcare system. Anyone with OAB should, as part of their work-up, have an RBC magnesium level checked. Diet and supplements should then be used to get that person's RBC magnesium level at least over 5.0, if not above 6.0, to see if the symptoms improve or resolve.

Blood in the Urine

Joe, a 55-year-old high tech consultant and long-term smoker, came in and was found to have microscopic hematuria. This means that the blood in the urine was not grossly evident and only picked up by a urine dip or urine analysis. I sent him to urology for prostatitis and for the hematuria. He said the urologist wanted him to have a CT scan and that they wanted to put a scope in his bladder. I could tell by the way he was talking that he had no idea the specialist was working him up to rule out kidney and bladder cancer.

I often have to decide how specific and direct I need to be with a person for a particular issue. I try to avoid alarming patients unnecessarily and typically won't tell them the important potential problem I'm trying to rule out as long as they are going for the test. If they ask me directly what I am doing the test for, I can usually finesse that one, too. For example, for a long-term smoker with a subtle abnormality on a chest x-ray, I'll say we're doing the lung CT ("lung scan") to get a more thorough picture of their lungs. Occasionally, but not often, a person will ask if I'm worried about cancer. I will minimize the likelihood but acknowledge that, yes, that is a possibility.

Joe started by saying, "No way am I going to let them put anything up my pecker." At that point, I had to be specific about the potential for bladder cancer. People, especially males, will often minimize these issues. He tried to say that bladder cancer didn't run in his family. He didn't understand why he would get bladder cancer at such a young age. I pointed out that the majority of people with bladder cancer don't have a positive family history and that smoking is the number one risk factor. Deflated, he now understood what was at stake.

At this point, it was not clear to me whether he would agree to the cystoscopy or not. My prediction is that the issue will simmer with him and he will probably agree to the procedure after he's had time to think about it. The main reason I was direct with him was to encourage him to get a full evaluation—because bladder cancer is generally very treatable early on. Another reason, though, is to cover myself legally. I know this patient well and have a very good relationship with him. There is almost no situation I can imagine where he would sue me. But the inclination to protect myself is embedded in just about every visit.

Kidney Stones

Kidney stones are a common issue in the field of urology. The most common type of kidney stone is a calcium oxalate stone. For many years people were told to avoid calcium to reduce their risk of getting another stone. One of the great lessons in life and in clinical medicine is: Even if something seems like common sense, that doesn't make it true. It turns out that oxalate is the real problem. Oxalate can be found in different types of foods, but the big three are probably colas, teas and dark green leafy vegetables. Not only does dietary calcium not increase the risk of developing a calcium oxalate stone, it seems to actually have some protective benefit because calcium will bind the oxalate, helping to remove it from the system.

Bedwetting

One of the most compelling cases I have seen in my time in medicine involves a 9-year-old boy, Jake. I have seen Jake since he was a baby. His family is generally focused on health and wellness. The dad is a personal trainer and the mom is a pharmacist. When I see anyone in the family for a visit, our conversations tend to be collaborative. Jake is a patient that I usually only see once a year for well visits. He has the odd sore throat and sprained ankle, but even those seem less common relative to other children. Every year Jake and his mom would come in for physicals and the only complaint was his nocturnal enuresis, the medical term for bedwetting. The problem is more common that most people realize. It affects boys at the rate of about ten percent at five years old, five percent at ten years old, and one percent at fifteen years old.

Jake had some basic testing to rule out diabetes, kidney disease and other underlying conditions that could cause frequent or difficult-to-control urination. We discussed the use of alarms that can be used to try and train a child to wake when they are starting to urinate. We discussed the variety of pharmaceuticals that American doctors have at their disposal. The parents were hoping to avoid drugs and decided to wait it out since it almost always resolves on its own. By the time Jake was nine, both he and his family were frustrated with waiting. They had adopted a plan where one parent would wake him at 11:00 p.m. and shepherd him to the toilet. The other parent would set the alarm for 2:00 a.m. and do the same. Even with this burdensome schedule, Jake would still often wet the bed.

At his well visit I discussed with the mom the potential that something in Jake's diet could be contributing. As with many great ideas, it just popped into my head. It wasn't an original idea, but I remembered reading it somewhere in some context. I had already had some success resolving chronic bowel issues in kids by their doing an elimination diet (see the chapter "The Gut is the Center of Our Universe"), so I brought it up. Mom was open-minded and interested.

I saw Jake just over a month later and his mom said he was cured! She took various food types out of his diet for a week or so to see what the effect would be. She eventually went almost Paleo (avoiding cow's milk, gluten, wheat, soy and corn) and then reintroduced foods. It turned out that if Jake had any gluten during the day, he would wet the bed that night. If he had any cow's milk, he would also wet the bed. If he didn't have either during the day, he would be completely dry all night. At one point, Jake started wetting the bed again. Mom was perplexed until she talked with him and found out he was having one of those small cartons of milk at school with his lunch. The only problem with the success was that Jake was a relatively picky eater and by eliminating gluten and dairy he started to lose weight.

Low Testosterone

When I was going through medical school and residency, almost no thought was given to the issue of low testosterone, yet I have been seeing more and more of it. the issue came up, it was reflected as being part of "male menopause," where men over 50 have had a decline in their testosterone level as part of normal aging. Now, I am seeing low testosterone in all ages. It is more common in obese males and those on opioids, but I am seeing many thin, fit males in their 20s with sexual dysfunction caused by idiopathic low testosterone levels. I checked with a specialist in the area about whether low testosterone, a.k.a. hypogonadism, is increasing in frequency or if we are just more aware of the issue in medicine and checking levels more often. His opinion was the latter. He didn't think the incidence of males with low testosterone was increasing.

My instinct was that something else was going on. I thought the issue might be part of the larger autoimmune, food, allergy maelstrom we find ourselves in. I couldn't substantiate this until I came across an article on obesity in the Winter 2013 edition of *Holistic Primary Care*. The article first discussed how the obesity epidemic is more prominent in males. At the time of the article, 72 percent of males in America were overweight. The article focused on a "worldwide testosterone decline" with corresponding drops in average sperm counts by 50 percent over 50 years of research. This was linked potentially to "46% more men getting testicular cancer and 76% more getting prostate cancer."[67] The central problem causing declining levels of testosterone, increased insulin resistance and weight gain was the "deposition of visceral fat." This type of fat, classically represented by the large belly, is an "estrogen factory," converting testosterone to estrogen. The question is then: Is it primarily fat causing low testosterone, low testosterone (with a lower corresponding metabolism) contributing to obesity, or more likely both?

The primary expert cited in the article, John La Puma, MD, thinks that environmental toxins, pesticide residues and drug metabolites are also playing a major role in the estrogenization of men. There is reference to 75 million pounds of the herbicide atrazine pumped into the earth every year to help corn production. Atrazine is a male hormone antagonist (androgen blocker). Pthalates, founds in paints and plastics, and BPA, in plastic bottles and containers, both have hormonal effects on estrogen and testosterone and may contribute as well.

These chemical exposures may be playing a primary or a secondary role in the problem. The *Wheatbelly* book gives its own compelling argument that the current wheat strain that dominates the American diet is the primary cause for obesity. The author, William Davis, MD, would almost certainly link low testosterone to wheat intake, but both may be important causes.

I have a theory that chronic iodine deficiency is playing a role in low testosterone levels. David Brownstein, MD, has written a number of books on holistic health including *Io*ine: Why You Nee* It, Why You Can't Live Without It.* [68] He asserts that 96.4% of his patients have tested positive for iodine deficiency. He describes in his book how crucial iodine is for proper functioning of all of the hormonal and glandular tissue in the body including thyroid, adrenals, breast, ovary, uterus and testicles. His opinion is that iodine deficiency is a major risk factor for prostate cancer. I wonder if it is also playing a role in the low testosterone epidemic. I have started using iodine supplements to try and raise testosterone levels, but that is a long-term approach and the success or failure of iodine for this issue will have to come in my next book.

The current mainstream approach to low testosterone, assuming no signs of any serious cause, is replacement with gels, patches, intramuscular injections or an implanted pellet. Sometimes replacement works incredibly well and the male patient has significant improvement in his quality of life. More often, the benefit is meager and the patient is not really sure if it is worth continuing the treatment. I had one patient who used the gel for a month but stopped when he found his female dog repeatedly making love to his dirty clothes. He was worried about the gel coming in contact with his wife and children.

I contacted my mole in the Naturopathic world and asked for his take on the issue. He summarized a variety of options including a chinese herb, myomin, which he would use if there were signs of excessive estrogen. Or he might use something called Orchex for "those stressed out types." He listed other options like wheat germ oil[NS], tribulius[NS], maca[NS] and deer antler[NS] for those with impaired sex drive. This already is potentially a better approach, compared to what MDs offer, as it is more individualized. The naturopath also said he sometimes uses Symplex M from Standard Process for overall endocrine support. It has protomorphogen nucleic acid extracts (whatever those are) for pituitary, thyroid, adrenal and testicular action.

Sadly, we may never see any trials comparing standard allopathic and naturopathic options. It would be relatively easy. We could have medical Olympics—giving medals to the providers that most successfully increase a male patient's testosterone level and improve symptoms. I would simply start with wheat avoidance and a weight loss program.

Benign Prostate Enlargement

In this area, I would actually make a case for more minimally invasive prostate procedures to improve urinary flow. All males develop prostate enlargement if they live beyond 50 or 60 years old. Saw palmetto, an herb, can be helpful at improving the symptoms of benign prostatic hypertrophy (BPH), but only in the early stages. There are Pharmaceuticals like tamsulosin (Flomax) typically help as well. The older a male gets and the worse the symptoms, the more the impact on their quality of life. If an older male has dribbling and overflow incontinence and is sleep deprived because he is up three or four times every night, that is not optimal living. Overwhelmingly, the person who has a Transurethral Resection of the Prostate (TURP) or Transurethral Needle Ablation (TUNA) or similar surgery almost always enjoys dramatic, long-lasting relief. I don't think there is a natural option that can come anywhere close.

Dermatology

Dermatology is an area that leads to a relatively high number of office visits in primary care. Some of the most common chronic skin conditions include eczema, acne, psoriasis, and seborrheic dermatitis. The underlying causes for these chronic skin conditions are not well understood. My management plan these days uses topicals only for symptom relief as my goal is to cure the problem or at least improve the situation enough that creams and lotions are hardly ever needed.

The skin is not an isolated organ. It often provides a window to internal problems. I have seen some people improve with dietary changes and others improve with a high quality probiotic. Stress often causes a flare-up of these chronic conditions. I suspect, like in many chronic disease processes, the immune system and the gastrointestinal system play a crucial role. There are probably multiple triggers and each plays a variable role for any given individual. That would explain why some people do not respond to diet changes.

Causes of Dry Skin

Seborrheic dermatitis is a more widespread version of common dandruff, ·

also known as seborrhea. A person with seborrheic dermatitis will often get dry, itchy, mildly inflamed areas around the nose, into the eyebrows, behind the ears and other areas. I am slowly coming to find that some percentage of people with this chronic condition have a sensitivity to cow's milk as the underlying cause.

A representative 40-year-old male came in wondering what could be done about this frustrating condition he had endured for many years. The standard approach from a primary care physician or dermatologist, ninety-nine percent of the time, would be to prescribe a low- to medium-potency steroid cream or ointment. This usually calms things down and seems to work well but, of course, is not a real solution. For this 40-year-old, I recommended he stop all dairy. Within three or four days, his skin cleared up and did not flare up again for about six months. Then, when he was under a lot of stress, the dry, flaky patches returned. He limited his diet and the condition improved, but the flare-up did not resolve for a few weeks.

I see many people in the office with eczema. Often, the person will have a flare up of severe eczema mostly involving the hands, with the non-dominant hand slightly worse. Once again, the quickest approach is to give a medium-potency steroid ointment and coax them out the door. Better than that would be to review the many contributors to worsening eczema, including stress, excessive hand washing and chemical exposures. Identifying and helping to manage a person's stress may be the most important long-term aspect of managing eczema. It is worth a question or two to rule out an obsessive compulsive disorder (OCD) as the cause. It also helps to get detailed information regarding the patient's occupation as it may pertain to the severity of the skin changes.

Dry skin is a common issue, especially in the winter. It often causes itch. Yet again, the simplest solution is often the best. One new patient was a pleasant 82-year-old man. We discussed several issues and then he brought up an ongoing frustration. For many years he had itchy skin all over. His scalp was particularly bothersome. He had seen a couple of dermatologists. He had tried many different lotions and creams. A discussion of his bathroom habits revealed that he was using soap excessively and shampooing his hair every day. On a primitive level, people often associate itching with being unclean or having some infestation. A person sometimes gets into a cycle of soap drying out the skin, which causes the skin to itch, which in turn leads to using more soap. I recommended this gentleman use soap sparingly and only shampoo twice per week. In a short time he was cured.

Acne

Acne is caused by a buildup of natural oils, dead skin cells, and bacteria in the pores or hair follicles of the skin. The mainstream approach to acne is relatively simplistic. As is typical, it does not treat the underlying causes but aggressively manages the end result. There are two strategies employed by primary care physicians and dermatologists: dry out the skin and kill off bacteria. The topical creams and gels and the oral antibiotics used serve these purposes. They can gradually improve the cosmetic aspect but do not fundamentally correct the problem. It is obvious to most that bombing away with oral antibiotics month after month can have unintended negative systemic consequences. Oral contraceptive pills can be used for their anti-androgenic effect.

The pendulum has swung back and forth several times in my career regarding the question of whether dietary change can help acne. Nutritional approaches to controlling acne involve avoiding foods such as refined carbs (sugars), saturated fats, chocolate and/or cow's milk. Whole grains, raw or steamed vegetables, fruits and beans, on the other hand, can help to promote healthy skin. For patients that are dedicated to changes in diet, I more often see benefit to the acne.

From the alternative world's perspective, supplementation with selenium, vitamin A, and vitamin E can have a therapeutic effect. Vitamin B6, in particular, can help normalize hormone levels in women, and zinc has an anti-inflammatory effect. In a two-month-long French trial comparing daily doses of zinc to placebo, the subjects who took zinc had significantly fewer and less severe blemishes. Cleansers help to eliminate oil buildup, nutrients help to normalize hormone levels, and avoiding certain foods can help to lower oil production.

There are certain herbs that seek to eliminate bacteria *inside* the body and clear the skin by a different mechanism. Tea tree oil was shown to be just as effective as benzoyl peroxide lotion and, although the herb took longer to do the job, it was less harsh on the skin than the 5% benzoyle peroxide lotion commonly used. Calendula (marigold) tea, when steeped and cooled, can be an effective facial wash. Detoxification through fasting and colon therapy can rid the body of toxins which would otherwise be released through the sebaceous glands and lead to breakouts.

Homeopathy and hydrotherapy may be used to eliminate toxins and soothe the inflammation of breakouts. Meditation can also help as acne is caused by stress or nervous tension. Facials and masks may help to lower inflammation, clean and minimize pores, and remove bacteria. A number of natural remedies suggested by health enthusiasts to quiet acne breakouts include: baking soda and water paste as a mask; apple cider vinegar diluted and applied to skin; coconut oil to moisturize without clogging pores; tea tree oil with equal parts water as anti-inflammatory and antibacterial; egg whites as a mask to decrease oil and draw out impurities; lemon juice as an astringent and antibacterial; garlic, sliced and applied topically in addition to being a natural antibacterial when ingested; ice cubes to decrease inflammation and help close pores while forcing bacteria out; and aloe vera to reduce inflammation and redness. I have not used many of these options in my practice so it is difficult for me to make any comments on efficacy. These alternative approaches generally require more commitment, so adherence rates would likely be on the low side.

Adult acne is a curious development. With the teenager and adolescent, it seems straightforward that increases in male hormone cause a sequence of events ultimately leading to comedones and inflammation. Recently, I have seen adults with unexplained severe acne experience complete resolution within a few weeks by eliminating wheat and/or dairy from their diet. This is a positive development, especially relative to some of the other options that include a daily suppressive antibiotic.

Poison Ivy

In terms of mainstream vs. alternative options, I think of a case from the summer of 2013. Poison ivy is a common acute scenario. The person is working in the yard, gets some of the plant resin on their skin, and within a day or two breaks out in a raised, red, itchy rash. For mainstream providers this is a straightforward problem to manage. If waiting it out is not an option, you can use a steroid cream or a steroid pill, typically prednisone. I try to use steroids less often these days, but they can be incredibly effective and, if used sparingly, I doubt they have any long-term repercussions. I have found that the most effective option, by far, for acute nerve impingement is five days of prednisone. If a person is having a severe asthma attack with difficulty breathing from airway inflammation, prednisone is typically the most effective outpatient option. Likewise, prednisone is usually the most effective mainstream option for poison ivy.

A mom and her young daughter came in together because the daughter had a fairly severe case of poison ivy. This family, relatively new to me, was oriented to more natural options and preferred avoiding pharmaceuticals. With the poison ivy, the daughter was clearly struggling with severe itching that was keeping her up at night. I reviewed the options and the mom declined steroids in any form.

A week later they came back and things were about the same. They had tried some natural topicals and some oral homeopathic remedy. The mom told me she thought the homeopathic option seemed to be helping. She was doing all of the talking, but with this statement the daughter was shaking her head. By my exam, the rash looked worse if anything from all of the scratching. There is a condition called lichen simplex chronicus where the skin becomes thicker and thicker from excessive scratching. The more lichenification (thickening) of the skin, the harder it is to reverse. The daughter desperately wanted relief, but even at that follow-up visit, the mom was reluctant to use steroids. It wasn't clear to me why they returned for a second visit if only to reject the steroids another time.

During visits like this we have to ask ourselves this question: Is natural always better? Some would seem to think so, but I don't know if a rigid, dogmatic approach on that side of the equation is any better than the opposite. People will usually try to shoehorn things so they fit into their world view. This mom had trouble accepting that the homeopathic option was inadequate. If the daughter took the course of prednisone, is there reason to believe this would somehow compromise her long-term health? After 15 years of practice, there really is no evidence, or even a reasonable assertion based on the facts, that says that a short course of oral steroids used infrequently has deleterious effects on the individual.

Molluscum Contagiosum

Molluscum contagiosum is a relatively common skin condition in children caused by a skin infection from the molluscum contagiosum virus or MCV. The child will develop pale bumps on an area of the body. The bumps classically have a small dimple or umbilication in the middle that can help clinch the diagnosis. Typically, not much is done to manage the condition as it resolves eventually over time, but many parents will come to the office repeatedly, frustrated that there isn't some option to clear the unsightly bumps. For years, I really had no option. I then heard about using H2-blockers like Zantac or Pepcid, which sometimes works.

In early 2014 I saw a family in the office. They had lived in India for several years and two of the boys had developed molluscum contagiosum. The mom said they went to an Aryuvedic practitioner and the treatments worked in less than a week. The treatment consisted of topical thuja with canthan ointment plus ½ tsp of dried ginger powder mixed with ½ tsp of honey applied to the lesions twice a day. They were also told to drink ½ tsp of turmeric in a cup of boiled milk once a day. I am often skeptical of the shotgun approach to treatment. It goes against my nature to use five things to solve one problem, but that may be a strength of Aryuveda. It would be interesting to know if successful treatment required all of the components or if less was more.

Osteoporosis

Another relatively important medical condition is osteoporosis, or low bone density. As people age their bone density declines. This is almost a universal process among men and women. Because men have relatively high bone density as young adults, they are at much lower risk of developing osteoporosis over time, so the issue is predominantly relevant to women's health. There are many risk factors for osteoporosis in addition to age: low body mass index (BMI), smoking, excessive alcohol intake, hyperthyroidism, vitamin D deficiency, some seizure medications, and a long list of others.

The standard approach to osteoporosis prevention involves regular weight bearing exercise, like walking, or anything that builds muscle. If a person strengthens their muscles, there will typically be a corresponding increase in bone density. It is also recommended that women maintain good levels of vitamin D, which often requires supplementation. The use of calcium and magnesium supplements is standard as well.

If a woman has a bone density study that shows a result consistent with osteoporosis, she would typically be started on a weekly medication like Fosamax or, more often, its generic, alendronate. Firstly, a study done in

2012 showed that roughly half of the generic alendronate were of such poor quality that they did not have an equivalent benefit for risk reduction compared to the name brand. Even more compelling is the relatively small benefit. A study printed in the *Journal of the American Medical Association* (JAMA) in 2006[69] showed that those who took Fosamax for four years had a 56% reduction in hip fractures. But the *Overdosed America* book points to this as another case where statistics can be misleading. A cleaner look at the numbers shows that for those women who did not take medication, 99.5% did not have a fracture over the period of a year. This was compared to 99.8% on Fosamax who did not have a fracture. There was benefit, but 81 women would have to take the medication for 4.2 years to prevent one hip fracture.

One Thanksgiving dinner I found myself talking with an erudite white-haired gentleman in a tweed jacket about issues in healthcare. He was a professor of medicine at one of the most prestigious medical schools in the country (the University of California, San Francisco) specializing in the area of nephrology. It was clear to me after a short time that he was a brilliant individual with a sophisticated understanding of the inner workings of the body that comes with an academic focus on research.

He referred to a recently published study on the use of an inexpensive supplement, potassium citrate, in an elderly population demonstrating improvement in bone density.[70] He talked about how humans have had an alkaline diet for most of history. Modern diets tend to be more acidic affecting many systems in the body, including the kidneys and bones. In a review article, an author noted: "The modern Western diet imposes, for the first time in human evolution, a chronic acid load on the human bone. Shorter-term studies on the neutralization of a dietary-induced acid load in humans have shown promising results in providing calcium retention and inhibiting bone resorption."[71]

This potassium citrate supplement, at a dose of 60 meq (milliequivalent) per day, could potentially be used as a safe, inexpensive option for the prevention and treatment of osteoporosis. The professor said it may not ever be adopted into widespread clinical use, however, because the pharmaceutical industry would never get involved. The National Institutes of Health, in his opinion, would not get on board because of their cozy relationship with pharmaceutical companies as mediated by lobbyists. On a positive note, he said there was a small chance that the Swiss government would start using the medication because they did not seem to be influenced as much as the United States government and the other European governments.

My brief contribution to the discussion was a comment that the alternative world has been addressing the issue of pH and excessive acidity for many years. I asked if he had heard of the book *The pH Miracle*. His monologue interrupted, he responded with four words: "They have no data." I still don't know who "they" are and how he knows so quickly that "they" do not have any data, i.e. hard evidence or research. Even if non-MDs had worked out much of pH management—with solid recommendations on how to correct underlying issues that helped a wide variety of chronic medical issues—it would be dismissed because it did not come from an institution within the establishment.

Cancer

I will only briefly talk about cancer, as this is too ambitious of a topic to be covered in this book. It is hard to argue that mainstream physicians have not had success in the management of many cancers after diagnosis. Most of our resources are currently dedicated to managing the problem after it has been diagnosed, but some prevention programs like pap smears and colonoscopies have clearly been beneficial. Pap smears are a relatively simple procedure of obtaining cells from the cervix to check for cancerous and precancerous change. We could assume that with newer options and better technology our screening approaches would improve. The development of the 3-dimensional CT scan shows us this is not necessarily the case.

For someone to have a 3D CT scan for colon cancer screening, they still have to do the full preparatory routine ("prep") to clean out the colon. The majority of people who have a colonoscopy say that the prep the day before is the miserable part and the colonoscopy itself is relatively quick and easy. If someone has a 3D CT scan and polyps are seen, they then have to do the prep a second time and have a colonoscopy to remove the polyp(s). The number one reason, however, that the 3D CT scan is rarely used is cost. The national average cost for the procedure was calculated at $2,400, but procedure costs, which vary with geographical location, range from $1,550 to $10,700.

Mainstream Medicine Success Story?

Consider also the following excerpt from an article by Laura J. Martin, MD, that got a lot of press in *WebMD* "Health News":

Jan. 17, 2013—Cancer death rates have fallen by 20% from their peak about 20 years ago, according to the latest statistics from the American Cancer Society. This means that from 1991 to 2009, 1.2 million lives were spared, including 152,900 lives in 2009 alone. "The big picture is that progress is steady, and for the four major cancer sites, progress is even more rapid," says researcher Rebecca Siegel, MPH. She is the director of surveillance information at the American Cancer Society in Atlanta. The four major cancer sites are breast, prostate, colorectal, and lung. "Cancer death rates peaked in the 1990s, and we have seen a 1% decline per year, but we are seeing much larger declines for the most common cancers."

Specifically, death rates have dropped by more than 30% for colorectal cancer, breast cancer in women, and lung cancer in men, and by more than 40% for prostate cancer.

There are several factors that may be driving these drops. It's less smoking for lung cancer, and earlier detection and better treatments for colorectal, breast, and prostate cancers.

Still, not all the news is good. One in four deaths in the U.S. is due to cancer, and rates of certain cancers, including liver, thyroid, and pancreatic cancers, are on the rise."[72]

There has been a steady improvement in survival of the most common form of leukemia in children, Acute Lymphocytic Leukemia or ALL. From the website *www.cancer.org*: "Researchers from the University of Colorado Cancer Center found that the 5-year survival rate for children and adolescents with ALL improved from 83.7% for those diagnosed between 1990 and 1994, to 90.4% for those diagnosed between 2000 and 2005. In the 1960s, the 5-year survival rate was less than 10%."[73]

Would alternative providers like naturopaths have had similar success rates? If they were the predominant health provider in North America, would we see cancer rates in decline? Maybe we would have seen lower rates of cancer in the first place. In this scenario, there would probably have been more of a focus on prevention and maximizing the body's innate capacity to deal with aberrant cancer cells. The human body has a wide range of mechanisms to identify precancerous cells and wipe them out before they progress. In an optimal system, the majority of research would be dedicated to this approach. In our current, reactive system, though, not many question the development of newer chemotherapeutic agents as the fundamental approach to cancer treatment. These drugs are generally toxic to healthy cells and often cause intense side effects. They are incredibly expensive and burdensome to individuals, families and society.

We assume that mammography is a worthwhile pursuit. In a review on breast cancer screening, "Effect of Three Decades of Screening Mammography on Breast-Cancer Incidence," published in the *New England Journal of Medicine* in 2012[74], the researchers found that mammography had a relatively small overall benefit and that more than a million women have been falsely diagnosed with breast cancer over that time. The statistical analysis showed that these early stage cancers would not have progressed, thus the combination of surgery, chemotherapy and radiation that most of these women underwent was unnecessary. Worse than that, however, is the psychosocial fallout. We potentially have had one million women and their families, friends and co-workers dealing with the diagnosis of breast cancer over the past 30 years with all of the collateral damage that comes with it. These women likely live every day of their lives in some fear that the cancer will return. Their psyches have been disrupted and permanently altered in complex ways we could never calculate statistically.

Technology's place in modern medicine is not going away any time soon. If only we could use the best technology at the right time for the right people, then it would more often be to our benefit. Deborah Rhodes is an internist who led a team that developed an improved breast cancer screening method. The new technology uses gamma rays and is better at detecting breast cancers in women with dense breast tissue. A study published by her group in the January 2001 issue of *Radiology* showed that, out of 936 participants, 11 had cancer (one identified with mammography only, seven with gamma imaging only, two with both combined, and one with neither).[75]

Rhodes' TED talk reviews the clear advantage of their machine but then hits upon what is probably the most important issue at hand: overcoming the establishment. In a fantasy world, the best would rise to the top and be adopted into practice. She makes the distinction that the gamma technology makes it incredibly simple to spot suspicious lesions in breast tissue. Mammography, in contrast, is exquisitely challenging, especially in women with dense breast tissue. Currently, there are many with a high financial stake in maintaining the status quo, including the mammogram manufacturers and the radiologists that read the images. They will push back against any new technology that reduces their income.

There may be an even better way to diagnose breast cancer and other cancers: dogs. Because of their strong connections with people and their exquisite sense of smell, it has been shown that dogs can detect cancers at an early stage. They apparently can pick up chemicals released from our bodies. There is a compelling video on the BBC earth website where an English woman describes how her dog, Max, diagnosed her breast cancer. Over a short time, his personality changed from outgoing and frisky to quiet and subdued. He would occasionally touch his nose to her right breast and then back off seeming very discontented. There was a lump there, but the mammograms were read as normal. Eventually, she had a procedure to remove the lump and it was found to be cancerous. After it was removed, the woman says that Max almost immediately returned to his normal energetic self.

9

A Perfect Storm

"Let me tell you why you're here. You're here because you know something. What you know you can't explain, but you feel it. You've felt it your entire life, that there's something wrong with the world. You don't know what it is, but it's there, like a splinter in your mind, driving you mad. It is this feeling that has brought you to me. Do you know what I'm talking about?"

—Morpheus talking to Neo in *The Matrix*

Our minds deceive us. We rely on our senses to interpret the physical world, yet the hyperevolved human eye can only see about 1/10,000[th] of the light spectrum. In many ways, we live in ignorance of how things truly are. It is like *The Matrix* trilogy where the human race is churning along mindlessly until a small group of people come to appreciate the truth of their reality. We are not simply human beings. We are complex symbionts living in an entity that, at least by cell count, is more microbial than mammal. We have hundreds, maybe thousands, of foreign substances flowing through our bloodstreams and trapped in our tissues. We cannot see or smell or feel these substances, but they are affecting us every day. Things have changed radically over recent decades. We are seeing increasing rates of allergies, asthma, eczema, autism and a variety of autoimmune conditions, including more type 1 diabetes in adults.

The paradigm of many triggers adding up and pushing someone over a threshold toward systemic health problems is gaining recognition. There is an excellent resource, prodigiously researched, that reviews much of the most current information—*The Autoimmune Epidemic* by Donna Nazakawa. In this book, the author describes what she calls the "The Barrel Effect,"[76] the idea that at some point the body cannot process the foreign material bombarding it and the barrel overflows. These instigators of symptoms and chronic illness silently accumulate for months and years, according to Nazakawa.

This concept is relevant for many chronic medical conditions including chronic migraine headaches. The best headache book I've read is *Heal Your Headache*[77] by David Buchholz, MD. His scenario is that each person has a genetically determined threshold for having headaches. Some have a threshold that is so high they never experience even a mild headache. Others have a threshold that is relatively low and will get several mild headaches a week and, occasionally, a full, severe, pounding, unilateral migraine with vomiting and light and sound sensitivity. This paradigm explains very well the ebb and flow of someone with chronic headaches. They will experience some stretches with few headaches and then other stretches where the headaches are frequent and debilitating. If a woman with a headache tendency comes in to see me confused because one Saturday night she had three glasses of red wine with no headaches and the next Saturday night she had one glass of the same red wine and got a blinding migraine, we will review the many other potential triggers. On the migraine day, she may have been dehydrated and had coffee with Splenda in the morning and then Chinese food with MSG for dinner.

I suspect that many chronic conditions, like irritable bowel syndrome and interstitial cystitis, also follow this paradigm. It would explain the rollercoaster most patients go through. It is challenging to try and sort out which of the many potential triggers are in play. Some of those triggers are major and, by themselves, can set off symptoms; other triggers are minor with multiple needed to generate symptoms. Some of the triggers are processed through the body and so have relatively short durations of action. Others accumulate in the fat tissue and stay there for years or perhaps even a lifetime.

The perfect storm often starts with a genetically susceptible individual influenced by elements in their environment. This is not a new concept. The start for many chronic health problems may be in utero. The book *Why Don't Zebras Get Ulcers?* by Stanford biologist and stress expert Robert M. Sapolsky was a compilation of most of the research on the impact of stress on human beings.[78] There is clear evidence that a pregnant woman under stress is more likely to have a child with anxiety and other mental health problems. This effect was independent of other factors including whether or not there was a family history of anxiety. A pregnant woman's diet and use of psychoactive substances will likely have a profound influence on the child's development as well.

For the individual to have the best chance at long-term health, they would probably do best to be born by vaginal delivery rather than Cesarean section. The process of exiting via the vaginal canal provides newborns with a bolus of good bacteria, the full impact of which is not yet clear. More important may be the distinction of breastfeeding vs. bottlefeeding. Breastfeeding rates have increased over the past 10-20 years, following the dark times when the formula companies pushed the idea that formula was a comparable alternative to breastmilk. (Formula company representatives would visit Labor & Delivery units providing free cases of Enfamil and Similac to influence the moms into starting the easier option.) Breastmilk, though, is clearly superior to formula in many ways the most significant difference between the two likely having to do with the transference of antibodies to the newborn which stockpiles their immature immune system. The breastmilk also gives the newborn abundant microflora along with the nutrition the microflora require to thrive in the GI tract of the baby. Breastfed babies have lower rates of ear infections, lung infections, allergies, eczema and asthma.

We apparently have to be reminded over and over to respect nature and what it has provided. Complex systems have evolved over millions of years and are not so easily ignored or reproduced. We need to inhale oxygen and exhale carbon dioxide. Plants thrive on carbon dioxide and, in turn, provide us with oxygen. Migrating animals trim down the grasses, dump manure as fertilizer and then circle back around the next year to do it all over again. A plant releases a seed that an animal eats. The animal travels elsewhere, poops it out to provide natural fertilizer, extends the plant's territory and spreads its DNA. A wife cares too much and a husband too little and a balanced child is raised.

Environmental Chemicals, Toxins and Pollutants

To anyone who has read a credible source on chemical exposures in our environment, this is likely the smoking gun for why so many health conditions are on the rise. We are exposed every day to a wide variety of toxic substances. The list is too long to cover fully here, but some include: airborne pollution, chlorofluorocarbons (CFCs), insecticides and weed killers used on lawns, teflon pans, chemical fireproof coating of mattresses, dry cleaning chemicals, hair dyes, car exhaust, food dyes and artificial flavors, plastics with phthalates, cleaning agents and chemicals sprayed around the house for ants, termites and other insects. From *The Autoimmune Epidemic*:

In 2005, the National Institutes of Health (NIH) released a report called *Progress in Autoimmune Disease Research* in which the director of NIH pronounced that nearly one hundred known autoimmune disease—such as multiple sclerosis, type 1 diabetes, rheumatoid arthritis, myositis, lupus, scleroderma, thyroiditis, Graves' disease, ulcerative colitis, Crohn's disease, myasthenia gravis and eighty-some other—now afflict 23.5 million people in the U.S., or one in twelve Americans, and these diseases are now on the rise worldwide—for reasons unknown…. Rates are rising dramatically among children, as are other related syndromes in which the immune system becomes hypersensitive, such as food allergies and asthma. Over the past decade, labs around the globe have proven definitive links between a list of commonly used industrial-age chemicals, heavy metals, and toxins and the development of numerous autoimmune diseases. As hundreds of industrial byproducts interact with the immune cells of our bodies, they are sabotaging an extraordinarily complex and fine-tuned blueprint for healthy cellular communication.[79]

Our immune systems, starting while in utero, are now bombarded with so many exogenous chemicals that our bodies cannot possibly process them all. A useful analogy is seen in a mountain lake. There is a flow of water into the lake and there is a flow out of the lake. If either the inflow or the outflow is corrupted and compromised, the lake will stagnate. The clear water will become murky and thick. The inflow for humans is represented by our water, air, food and all of the other things unseen that are taken into our bodies. If the intake of deleterious material is too great, it can overwhelm our liver, kidneys and bowels, the primary organs for processing and elimination. Many alternative providers will focus efforts on detoxification. This usually involves liver enhancement and an effort to improve bowel health. These simple yet crucial principles get no attention from MDs, other than the maverick who recommends better hydration.

In *The Autoimmune Epidemic*, Nazakawa references a 2003 study by the Mount Sinai School of Medicine in New York City in collaboration with the Environmental Working Group (EWG), an advocacy organization in Washington, D.C. Their findings reveal the "body burden" of environmental chemicals and heavy metals carried by the average American.

After testing the blood and urine of nine representative Americans from around the country for 210 substances, these scientists discovered that each volunteer carried an average of 91 industrial compounds, pollutants and other chemicals—including PCBs, commonly used insecticides, dioxin, mercury, cadmium and benzene, to name just a few. Then in 2005, researchers working through two major laboratories found an alarming cocktail of 287 industrial chemicals and pollutants in the fetal cord blood of ten newborn infants from around the country. These chemicals included pesticides, phthalates, dioxins, flame retardants and breakdown chemicals of Teflon, among other chemicals known to damage the immune system.[80]

The presence of heavy metals, such as mercury and lead, from occupational and other environmental exposure may be important and gets a lot of attention in *The Autoimmune Epidemic*. Mercury is said to be a primary player in autoimmune conditions including autism. In addition to our levels of exposure, under-regulation may be part of the problem. For many years the

Occupational Safety and Health Administration (OSHA) permitted blood lead levels between 40 and 60 mcg/dL. In 2012, a scientific review from the U.S. National Toxicology Program linked concentrations between 5 and 10 mcg/dL with elevations in blood pressure. Lead can also have cognitive effects, causing behavioral changes and hyperactivity among other things, though it is not fully clear whether lead plays a role in the growing number of kids with these problems today. It is standard to check a lead level at 12 months and at two years of age, but perhaps, as above, the current acceptable blood level is not strict enough, especially for children that are presumably more vulnerable to the toxic effects.

Immunizations

There is some evidence that immunizations can be one of the wide range of triggers. It would be just one small addition to the stew, thus explaining why many studies have not demonstrated any risk. Any whiff of a suggestion hinting that immunizations may play a role in chronic disease, autoimmune conditions and autism typically leads to an immediate strong push back from scientists and doctors. For most of my career, I did not want to hear anything negative about immunizations either. That was until I read *The Autoimmune Epidemic*. Nazakawa reviews several well-done scientific studies linking immunizations like diphtheria, tetanus, and oral polio (now replaced with an injection) with an increased risk of the autoimmune conditions like Guillian-Barre syndrome. There are correlations between two vaccines—hepatitis B and measles, mumps, rubella (MMR)—and multiple sclerosis. There is also evidence linking MMR to rheumatoid arthritis.[81]

Putting it all together, Nazakawa summarizes that the benefits of immunizations far outweigh the potential for harm. I also still feel that immunizations remain an important part of prevention. But the controversy around immunizations is growing in scope. More and more parents are coming in with concerns. I have found that their concerns are often varied and difficult to predict. I can assume nothing about why they are worried. Some parents want all the immunizations without question. Some want to pick and choose which ones are appropriate for their child. Some want to delay immunizations. Some parents have very clear information from a good source, but more often they have vague ideas from a dubious source.

I tell parents that I don't believe the medical community has ignored concerns. On the contrary, I think medical researchers have gone to extraordinary lengths to verify the safety of vaccinations.[82,83,84,85] It seems that the well-being of children has prompted a relatively large scale evaluation. The researchers probably are looking out for their children and grandchildren as well as the children in the world at large. There have been many studies done in the U.S., Great Britain, Denmark and other countries involving tens of thousands of children with none so far showing any link between vaccines and autism.

People generally have no idea that these studies were done. They have no background in medicine or science. They would rely on loose anecdotal information rather than medical research. They all too easily assume that there is some conspiracy in play and that all mainstream doctors are just going along with it.

The trepidation with immunizing children has now spilled over to adults. There is a nurse I see often in the office who works with some of the group home patients. I asked her one day if she had gotten the flu shot. She said she hadn't. I played the devil's advocate and asked her why she didn't get the flu shot. In my mind, as with most doctors and public health personnel, it was very important for her to get the flu shot because she was taking care of vulnerable individuals and could potentially give them the flu.

Her first answer was that she had never had the flu. She said she had a very good immune system. Not a bad first salvo but, in my mind, still a weak rationale since anyone could get the flu in any given year. She continued to say that the body should be able to build up immunity on its own rather than have immunity come from a vaccine. Since viruses typically mutate and different strains prevail from year to year, this did not hold water.

I pressed her further and this educated healthcare professional went through a series of reasons for not getting the flu shot that really made no sense. She said if she got the flu shot, she would probably get sick. That is generally not the case. She said if she got the flu, no problem, she would just stay home from work so as not to infect anyone else. People who get the influenza virus, as with many viruses, will have an incubation period of up to a few days where they are contagious without having symptoms, so that reasoning didn't make sense either. She then said she got shots when she was younger, so it shouldn't be as important. This was irrelevant. Getting a polio shot when you are six months old doesn't help protect you from the flu when you're 40.

I didn't let it go, so she kept rattling off reasons. She said she didn't want to get the flu shot because it might take a shot away from an elderly person who really needed it. The altruistic angle would have been more convincing if she had used it as her one and only reason for declining the flu shot. Finally, she may have given the real reason. She said she didn't like being forced to do something.

This laundry list of reasons, some reasonable, but most misguided, is part of the frustration around this controversy. If I probe people as to why they don't want immunizations for themselves or their children, they typically have no clearly stated concerns. I usually can't get out of the person where they got their information. It's often that they heard from some of their friends that there may be some problems. It's not scientific. It's not based on a credible source of information.

I'm an open-minded person. I remember watching the *Frontline* special "The Vaccine War"[86] from 2010. I was not begging for the producers to put these anti-immunization zealots in their place; I was hoping that they would give me some insights into why people are worried and whether there is any basis in fact for these concerns. I do think the producers did an excellent job of being fair and balanced. If I am going to have continued discussions with parents on the subject, I will often recommend they watch the PBS episode.

After I watched it I understood better why some parents are worried. Many of them said their child was fine with normal development, then went to their pediatricians for a well visit and immunizations. Some short time after those immunizations, most often ones that included the Measles, Mumps and Rubella (MMR) vaccine, their child changed dramatically. The interviewed parents said their children declined and were never the same again. If my child was walking and talking normally and got shots and then a week later started showing signs of autism, I would wonder about a link as well.

There are several potential explanations for this phenomenon. The numerous studies to date have not found any link between immunizations (including MMR) and autism. It is possible that the vaccine did contribute to the development of autism, but these episodes are so uncommon that they did not show up statistically in the retrospective analyses. The next option often hypothesized by mainstream doctors is that autism is often picked up for the first time around the same time as the MMR, so it was only a coincidence. The last option is that the parents are somehow misrepresenting what happened for some secondary gain. This seems unlikely.

Based on all of my research, what I now feel is probable is that the MMR vaccine was not technically of harm to this small group of children. By that point the child's immune system had become so compromised by exogenous substances that the vaccine pushed the system beyond the tipping point. The incidence of side effects from MMR tends to be higher than from other vaccines. In about 5 to 15 percent of children given MMR, a fever and flu-like symptoms may occur—usually beginning about 7 to 12 days after the vaccine has been administered. It would not be a coincidence, then, that MMR would overstimulate an already bombarded and overburdened immune system leading to the physical manifestations of the autoimmune process autism for the first time. Since the other factors had already been damaging the vulnerable central nervous system, the patients did not regress but only became sicker over time. There is research suggesting that acetaminophen, or Tylenol, may also be one of the triggers for autism.[87] If that turns out to be true, then perhaps it's the Tylenol given before or after shots by the conscientious parent that causes or contributes to the first signs of autism shortly after a visit for immunizations. These explanations of the autism/vaccination link, to me, are the only way to reconcile the opposing sides of the controversy. It would explain the changes some parents noticed after immunizations and why so many studies have found no statistically increased risk of autism in immunized children.

I will often say to parents at a follow-up visit that it is possible that there is some small risk associated with immunizations that the researchers could not uncover. Even if that is true, though, it is my opinion that the benefits of the immunizations would far outweigh those risks. I believe we should individualize our approach to shots in the same way we do every other aspect of health and wellness. If a child is believed to have an increased risk of autism, it is reasonable to delay immunizations or pursue some alternative schedule. If the immunizations are spaced out, as is recommended by some including Dr. Robert Sears in *The Vaccine Book*, that would decrease any potential exposure. Potential risk factors include a sibling with autism, a strong family history of autoimmune conditions or children showing signs of allergies or an abnormal tendency to infections. Sears explains:

- By only giving two vaccines at a time (instead of as many as 6), I decrease the chance of chemical overload from grouping so many vaccines' chemicals all together at once. This allows a baby's body to better detoxify the chemicals one or two at a time.

- I give only 1 aluminum-containing vaccine at a time (instead of the recommended 4). Overloading on this metal can be particularly toxic to the brain.
- I give only one live-virus vaccine component at a time to allow the body's immune system to better handle the live viruses in these vaccines.
- Giving fewer shots at a time may decrease the side effects, in my experience.
- Giving fewer shots at a time also makes it easier to figure out which vaccine a child is reacting to if a severe reaction occurs.[88]

In doing my research for this book, I found many excellent sources regarding the safety of immunizations. The Center for Disease Control website in particular was well organized and easy to understand. They reviewed many of the concerns that I have heard from people over the years and also addressed many issues of which I was unaware. I really could not find any compelling evidence saying that the risks of immunizations outweigh the benefits.

We can evaluate immunizations in a simplistic all-or-nothing way or we could go through them individually assessing each for their relative merit. I'll go through a few of them as they are each different in terms of their importance.

A hepatitis A infection, for example, is relatively rare and does not pose much risk for the individual infected with the virus. It has a broader importance in terms of public health, as an unimmunized person could spread the virus to many other people if they worked in food service, for example. In over 15 years of clinical practice, I've only managed a few cases of acute hepatitis A and they all recovered uneventfully.

The chicken pox, or varicella, vaccine is actually more important now that there is a vaccine because the potential for someone to develop natural immunity is much lower. As most know, if a person gets a primary varicella infection as an adult, they tend to be much sicker than if they had had their first exposure as a child.

It is hard to argue that the Hib vaccine hasn't been a major public health success. In the past, the Hemophilus influenza type B (Hib) bacteria was the leading cause of meningitis, pneumonia and a severe infection called epi-glottitis that often caused swelling of the upper airway with compromised breathing. There were about 20,000 cases per year in the United States, pri-marily in children under five years old. Early on in my training, I remember seeing cases of meningitis in the Emergency Department. Within a few years of the introduction of the vaccine in the early 1980s, the rate of Hib infections began to steadily decline. Today, the number of cases has overall decreased by over 99 percent.

I recently saw a new 15-month-old. The parents had declined immuniza-tions, so the prior pediatrician had told them he would no longer see the child as a patient. I started the conversation and one of the first things the mom said was that they wanted to wait because their daughter's immune system was immature. I countered by reviewing the success of the Hib vaccine. The father sat in the corner wearing sunglasses and quickly shot down anything I had to say. The success of some of the immunizations can actually work against them. Because these illnesses are now rare, people become complacent and feel the vaccines are unnecessary.

But some of these vaccines offer benefits even beyond their original purpose. One of the newer immunizations, Prevnar, has been available since 2000 and has been shown to reduce the incidence of ear infections, sinus infec-tions and pneumonia in young children. Because of the impact on "herd immunity," it was found unexpectedly that the rates of pneumonia in the elderly declined over a timeframe that corresponded to the introduction of Prevnar.

The flu shot was found to reduce risk beyond getting influenza. A study showed people who got an influenza vaccine were fifty percent less likely to experience a major cardiac event, such as a heart attack, stroke or cardiac death, compared with those who had a placebo vaccine. Study author Dr. Jacob Udell, a cardiologist at Women's College Hospital and the University of Toronto says "the use of the [influenza] vaccine is still much too low, less than 50 percent of the general population; it's even poorly used among health care workers," Imagine if this vaccine could also be a proven way to prevent heart disease."[89] The study he speaks of involved 3,227 patients, half of whom had established heart disease and were part of earlier studies dating back to the 1960s. Half of participants were randomly assigned to receive the flu shot. Besides reducing cardiovascular risk, the study found those who had a flu shot also were 40 percent less likely to die from any cause compared with those who had a placebo.

The Food Supply

In addition to chemical toxins, the other major shift in the last century that has adversely affected our health is the food supply. Any number of journalists, researchers, scientists and doctors have been trying to get our attention, but it seems they are unable to penetrate Americans' insatiable appetite for low quality food high in sugar, fat and salt. It is the Walmart factor, but applied to what we consume.

One of the best sources on the horrendous state of our food supply is *The Omnivore's Dilemma* by Michael Pollan. He describes the feedlot process[90] where most of the cattle in America get their sustenance. Cattle evolved to eat grass but, because corn is so cheap and available in such massive quantities, the corporations that manage the cattle shifted a long time ago to corn as the primary source for calories. When Pollan's book was published in 2006, there were four companies (Tyson, Cargill, Swift & Company and National) bringing eighty percent of cattle from birth to table. The goal for them is quick turnover and today's cattle gain enough weight by 14-16 months to be slaughtered. In the past, before the current system was adopted, cattle were typically 4-5 years old at slaughter.

These cattle are fed three times a day with a rush of corn mixed with liquefied fat, protein, liquid vitamins, roughage, antibiotics and synthetic estrogen. The liquefied fat is often beef tallow trucked in from a slaughterhouse. The protein is typically molasses and urea. Urea is a form of synthetic nitrogen made from natural gas, similar to fertilizer. The process overall is brutal in its simplicity. The cattle are essentially machines that transform the cheap, corn-based calories into protein for mass consumption. If MacDonalds can sell a hamburger for 89 cents and make a profit, it doesn't take a genius to understand the beef is of poor quality.

The feedlot environment is detrimental to the cattle's health and they can only survive there for a certain amount of time, estimated at 150 days in *The Omnivore's Dilemma*. The author quotes a veterinarian who notes that even with the steady use of antibiotics, an average of 15-30 percent of cattle have abscesses in their liver at time of slaughter. It is distinctly possible, and maybe even probable, that this industrial use of antibiotics is one of the primary reasons behind antibiotic-resistant bacteria and the slow, steady evolution of "superbugs" that cause life-threatening, difficult-to-treat infections in people.

The overall estimate is that the average American consumes—in one form or another, directly or as processed by livestock—a ton of corn every year. Low quality corn is *the* staple of America. This corn can be in the form of beef, chicken, pork, soft drinks, soda, breakfast cereal, snacks or even occasionally corn. Two thousand pounds of a cheap, nutrient-poor pseudo-vegetable down the gullet of every man, woman and child. In effect, we are cattle ourselves only with slightly more physical activity, bigger brains and less manure.

So, what can a person eat? Mass-produced, hormone-rich, antibiotic-rich, corn-fed, manure-soaked beef? Um, no. Chicken raised in a similar environment, substituting chicken poop for manure? No again. Whole grains... those have to be good for you. Right? I have come to believe in the *Wheatbelly* literature, so yet another check in the no column. Avoiding wheat, often crucial for improving a person's health, may be more difficult than people realize. I took a field trip to the grocery store and checked different breads. The number one ingredient in wheat bread was, of course, wheat flour. The number one ingredient for white bread was...wheat flour. Oat bread? Wheat flour. Whole grain and multigrain breads? Wheat. What about rye bread, pumpernickel bread, potato bread, banana bread and pound cake? Wheat flour was the main ingredient in all of them. The American public is being bamboozled. Is wheat flour the predominant flour in all of these breads because it is the healthiest option? No. It is almost certainly because it is the least expensive option. Rice crackers and rice pasta are better for most people but have low nutrient-density. Fish can be tricky because farm-raised fish living in pens gobbling up low-quality corn are not ideal, and many forms of fish—especially tuna and swordfish—have high levels of mercury, which is likely a major player in today's autoimmunity issues.

Fruits and vegetables are a no-brainer, right? Yes and no. They often have high levels of pesticides and need to be scrupulously rinsed before consumption. Many fruits and vegetables are also sprayed with bromine as a preservative. Bromine is a toxic agent that contributes to a wide variety of endocrinological problems involving the hormonal and glandular tissue of the body, including the thyroid and adrenals. Also, some fruits and vegetables can be triggers for headaches, including bananas, peas, onions and citrus fruits. Nightshade vegetables—like tomatoes, potatoes, eggplant, peppers and different spices like paprika, cayenne and the main ingredient in Tabasco—potentially contribute to arthritis pain. Doctors and patients need to be very savvy to uncover those foods that may be contributing to their individual acute and chronic health issues.

We come back full circle to what is probably the optimal diet: Paleo. A Paleo diet of foods grown locally and lean, grass-fed meat is great, but it's still relatively expensive for most people and a lot more work. The Paleo diet, for the record, does not match how cavemen ate. Anthropologists and scientists have picked that one apart. But it still is an excellent diet for most people nonetheless.

The decision makers in the food industry are no fools. They follow the trends in American culture and are sophisticated in their understanding of consumer behavior. The modern American is harried with a short attention span. TV, movies and video games had better get the viewer's attention in about five seconds, and keep it, or the viewer will move on. The mom wandering down the food aisle of the local grocery store, trying desperately to keep her children healthy, may just pick up a few words strategically positioned on the box. "Whole grains" and "protein" and "fiber" are all over the place, but have little or no predictive value for the quality of that item.

Even the term organic has been corrupted and abused in recent years. There are chapters in *The Omnivore's Dilemma* about what the term organic should mean and what it means today. The FDA has really not developed specific guidelines for how and when the term can be used. According to FDA policy:

"Natural" means the product does not contain synthetic or artificial ingredients. "Healthy," which is defined by regulation, means the product must meet certain criteria that limit the amounts of fat, saturated fat, cholesterol, and sodium, and require specific minimum amounts of vitamins, minerals, or other beneficial nutrients. Food labeled "organic" must meet the standards set by the Department of Agriculture (USDA). Organic food differs from conventionally produced food in the way it is grown or produced. But the USDA makes no claims that organically produced food is safer or more nutritious than conventionally produced food.[91]

Genetically Modified Foods

When I started writing this book, I was not aware of any concrete evidence showing that immunizations can have serious negative effects. I also had a negative view of genetically modified (GM or GMO) foods. This was based mostly on my frustration that these foods, with unknown long-term consequences, were slipped into our food supply without much public debate. In researching both of these topics, I have had to modify my opinion.

GM foods may not be the villain for all people in all situations. If we take a step back, we can consider the issue from either a first world or a third world perspective. Genetic modifications have increased the productivity and yield of food crops. This tends to keep the costs down and can enable poor families more access to fruits and vegetables. Some modifications have been introduced to reduce the need for chemicals and pesticides. Others are designed to increase the nutrient density in the food.

There is no better example of this than the crop Golden Rice. Unknown to most people in the industrialized world, vitamin A deficiency is a significant cause of disease in poorer countries. This genetically modified rice could save a million lives and 500,000 cases of blindness every year.[92]

In 1991 the World Health Organization challenged scientists to look for a way to make vaccines accessible to everyone. This would mean that children in impoverished areas of the world wouldn't have to travel for hours to a nearby village to get a shot. The scientists succeeded faster than expected, creating a cholera vaccine-like component by injecting a series of genes into a potato. These genes prompt the human immune system to produce its own cholera antibodies or "vaccine."

The GM salmon known as AquAdvantage is meant to be grown in fish farms. According to proponents of the modification, this would reduce fishing of wild salmon, in turn protecting both the wild population of fish and the environment from human intrusion.

At the Naturopath Conference I attended, one lecturer spoke of the perfect storm of foods, chemicals and toxins and how they affect our immune systems causing illness. He referenced studies showing that GMO foods had been found to cause inflammation in people. He thought GMO foods had contributed to the rise in the rates of autism. Toward the end of his lecture, he said that GMO foods were a "crime against humanity," and that led to a vigorous burst of applause from the audience.

I would like to see the research to know if the cited studies evaluated a wide range of GMO foods. We need to be careful about cherry picking. Everyone is guilty of picking and choosing the information that supports their position and selectively ignoring the rest. The entrenched, rigid position on either side may not be for the best. Some GMO foods may be safe, while others may cause harm. For the estimated billion people in our world who are hungry every day, genetic modification may ultimately be one of the greatest developments in human history. We need a clear head, ongoing research and a broad perspective.

There is a strong parallel between GM food and immunizations. The mainstream scientific opinion supports both, and any physician or scientist that questions their safety is an outlier. In a *Scientific American* article:

More scientists would speak up against genetic modifications if doing so did not invariably lead to being excoriated in journals and the media. These attacks are motivated by the fear that airing doubts could lead to less funding for the field…Scientists say that after publishing comments in respected journals questioning the safety of GM foods, they became the victims of coordinated attacks on their reputations.[93]

We see the same issue with the primary wheat crop in America, a dwarf species developed in the 1950s by a man named Norman Borlaug. His successes in increasing the yield of an acre of wheat helped to feed many of the poor around the world, especially in Mexico, China and India. He was ultimately called "The man who saved a billion lives." He is one of seven people to have won the Nobel Peace Prize, the Presidential Medal of Freedom and the Congressional Gold Medal. He bred wheat to favor shorter, stronger stalks that could better support larger seed heads and improve yield per acre. In describing the majority of environmental lobbyists, he said:

They've never experienced the physical sensation of hunger. They do their lobbying from comfortable office suites in Washington or Brussels. If they lived just one month amid the misery of the developing world, as I have for fifty years, they'd be crying out for tractors and fertilizer and irrigation canals and be outraged that fashionable elitists back home were trying to deny them these things.[94]

American wheat is feeding millions of people at a relatively low price, but a food supply dominated by the staples of corn, wheat, soy, beef, pork and chicken is undoubtably one of the major contributors to our chronic health problems. We can see the effects of poor food and environmental exposures on our gastrointestinal systems. More and more people are going to doctors' offices with complaints of bloating, abdominal pain, loose stools and constipation.

The "leaky gut syndrome" is one most doctors have never heard of and, if it does come up, they have no foundation to think it is a real phenomenon. This situation results from a perfect storm as well, analogous to many of the processes described above. The intestine is the means by which we absorb vitamins, minerals and nutrients from our food. If working optimally, it also is an effective barrier keeping chemicals and toxins and pathogenic organisms from getting into our systems. The hypothesis behind leaky gut is that, in our current environment with our current food supply, the intestinal barrier is subjected to a battery of exogenous substances and becomes more permeable. The chemicals, toxins, bacteria and other microorganisms meant to stay in the intestine get into the blood stream, causing adverse systemic effects.

Five hundred food additives, two hundred chemicals in the bloodstream, plus antibiotics, hormones, and stress equals a rising incidence of chronic medical problems. With this chaos, most Americans are unknowingly deficient in magnesium, iodine, vitamin D, B-vitamins and other essential nutrients. In some ways, it's stunning that we are not sicker. This speaks to the incredible capacity of the human body to maintain health.

10

Toward Integration

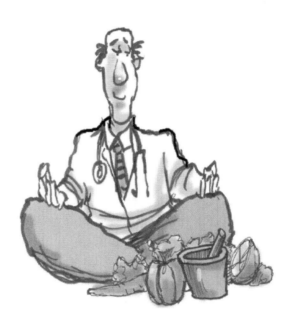

The trend in medicine today is toward more and more specialization. Orthopedic specialists, as an example, used to work on all joints of the body including the spine. Now in orthopedics, we have the shoulder specialist, the hand and wrist specialist (who will battle with the shoulder guy over who gets the elbow), the hip specialist, the knee specialist and the foot and ankle specialist.

The other medical specialties are following the same general trend. There is obviously a huge advantage to this methodology. In this superspecialized system, if you have a knee problem and you see an orthopedic specialist that only works with the knee joint, then you're getting someone supremely expert in that area who will see mostly knee problems day after day until retirement.

There is, however, a major disadvantage to this trend. We are becoming more fragmented in our care. The only medical professional who is looking at the big picture and pulling it all together tends to be the primary care provider. The primary care provider—physician, physician's assistant or nurse practitioner—ideally will look at the person holistically and try to explain a wide variety of symptoms with some unifying underlying explanation. This is not typically the case, however, because that is not how primary care doctors and other allopathic healthcare professionals are trained. Instead, they are trained in a way that mimics the disjointed world of the specialists.

A central tenet in primary care, though, is in the area of prevention. Being proactive is embedded in how PCPs do their work, and this is a great advantage if we are to move forward in American healthcare.

Naturopath vs. MD

It would serve us well, at this point, to contrast the approach of naturopaths to the now more mainstream approach of the allopathic MD. Naturopathy is rooted in thousands of years of health and wellness. In its current form, it encompasses many disciplines of alternative health, including herbs, acupuncture, homeopathy, and a focus on lifestyle, particularly nutrition and diet. There has been a resurgence of naturopathy over the past 30-40 years, with the epicenter for North America found in the Pacific Northwest. A Doctor of Naturopathic Medicine (ND) can be licensed to practice medicine now in 17 states. The current ratio is about 900,000 MDs and DOs to somewhere between 1,000 and 2,000 NDs.

At the International Congress of Naturopathic Medicine meeting in July of 2013, one of the major activists for Naturopathy, Dr. Jared Zeff, outlined the basic principles of Naturopathy. These include:

1. *Vis Medicatrix Naturae*: This reflects the concept that the body has an innate capacity to heal itself and be well. I naively assumed that most practitioners would agree with this idea. I read a "scientific" website, however, with the mission of debunking false health claims, and the blogger ripped this idea as being simplistic and unscientific.

2. *Tolle Causam*: Search for the cause. The current system is often set up to treat the symptoms with no understanding of the underlying cause for a person's presentation. There often seems to be no inclination for doctors and researchers to uncover the deeper causes that could potentially lead to a more robust, long-term cure. The approach of treating symptoms and conditions superficially and piecemeal is so entrenched in America, it is often pursued without question.

3. *Docere*: The doctor serves in the role of teacher and mentor. Naturopathic physicians educate their patients and encourage self-responsibility for health. This can be in contrast to the paternalistic approach of MDs. Historically, doctors instructed the patient on what to do and the person accepted the recommendation without question. This has been steadily changing over the past 50 years or so as the modern patient is more likely to be empowered and work collaboratively with physicians.

4. *Primum Non Nocere*: This translates to 'first do no harm.' This is also a tenet of allopathy, but the application of this principle is different for the naturopath. For the naturopath, this often means avoiding pharmaceuticals with their side effects. It also means avoiding unnecessary surgeries.

5. *Toll Etotum*: Treat the whole person. This speaks to the importance of understanding all aspects of a person including their physical, emotional and spiritual domains. The person I see in the office at a moment in time has a long, complex history, and I am well served to incorporate their beliefs and values. Evaluating a person's genetic background will also have more relevance going forward.

6. *Prevention*: It is more effective to prevent illness than it is to treat health problems after they develop. Our healthcare system needs to adopt this in ways that go well beyond pap smears, mammograms and

colonoscopies.[95]

As I mentioned in the introduction, the majority of Americans want the best for their health, no matter where it comes from. The use of alternative options has become more and more prevalent in America over the past 10-20 years. There are different estimates for the percentage of adults in America using some form of complementary or alternative medicine (CAM). The range is from 40-60 percent, depending on what you include in CAM.

A study done by the National Institutes of Health (NIH) way back in 2002 quantified the extent by which Americans pursued an alternative approach to health matters. The list of the most common forms was as follows:

1. prayer (43%)
2. natural products (18.9%)
3. deep breathing exercises (11.6%)
4. meditation (7.6%)
5. chiropractic (7.5%)
6. yoga (5.1%)
7. massage (5.0%)[96]

If you included prayer, at that time 62% of people had participated in at least one form of alternative health in the 12 months prior to the survey, with many participating in more than one. Even if you took prayer out of it, 43% had used some alternative option. I can safely assume that the numbers are higher these days. With the internet and word of mouth, people are taking more control over their health than ever before. This is a positive development in many ways. There is a fundamental shift that comes with the increased use of untraditional options. What is considered "alternative" is also slowly changing as people's knowledge and awareness expands. Many would not consider vitamins or yoga or massage alternative these days.

Changing a Doctor's Mind

One of the great teachers in my life is an older man I saw for many years. Antonio, a devout Jehovah's Witness, was married to the love of his life and had children and grandchildren. He had curly gray hair and was quick to laugh. He had his priorities in order, dedicated to his family and his faith. He was also one of the most intellectually curious people I've ever met, a voracious reader consuming just about any book on health and wellness he could find. His primary medical problem involved prostate cancer that would eventually spread to his brain. He saw mainstream and alternative providers and often struggled, unsure of which path to follow in his efforts to get well. At many visits he would make biblical references. He was completely and utterly sure that everything the Bible had to say was the truth, the whole truth and the only truth in this world. During patient visits I'm generally respectful and try to avoid disagreements.

One day, many years ago, Antonio and I were chatting amicably at a follow-up visit. He started asking me questions about my belief system. I went into some of the common arguments against organized religion. I said that if there were three people raised in different parts of the world born into three different religions and each of them assumed that what they believed was the absolute and incontrovertible truth, how could we know which one it would be? Organized religions have such a high degree of specificity that only one can be right. Or maybe they all are tapping into the same central truth and the details are less significant. When I was in my younger, more ignorant days, I would use a rhetorical statement like, "Aren't we lucky to have been born into a culture that teaches the only correct view of the world?"

When I started talking like this to Antonio, he did not get upset. He sat in the chair quietly listening to what I had to say. He replied calmly that it was very simple to differentiate which religion was the one and only path to truth. "You see," he started, "in Leviticus page 3-16...." I don't remember exactly what Bible passage he quoted, but that was his source for all answers, so it was logical to use it as the answer to the question I had posed. I felt bad about arguing with him and I knew at once it had been a mistake. It was the last time I ever haggled with him about religion and his views of spirituality. But thanks in part to him, my growth as a physician and as a person has included more of a focus on the spiritual aspects of wellness.

At many of the early visits with me, Antonio would bring up alternative approaches to health and wellness. In the beginning, I mostly shut out what he had to say because it seemed like nonsense. I figured that since the concepts he was bringing up had never been mentioned in all of my medical training, they must be quackery and without value. I was generally polite, so he kept talking to me about leaky gut syndrome and chakras and all kinds of things I knew nothing about. A recurring theme from him was the importance of the gastrointestinal system for overall health. This relatively simple notion is, in some ways, the poster child for how far apart practitioners on either side can be. Allopathic providers think of the gut as important for certain specific functions but do not see much connection between bowel health and general health. Providers can refer to the mind-body connection and the integration of various parts into a whole being, but this is parlor talk if it isn't part of their daily practice.

Over time, as I was seeing the deficiencies of mainstream medicine, I started to listen to Antonio. He gave me a book by Brenda Watson called *Renew Your Life: Improve* Digestion an* Detoxification.*[97] I read a lot of the book and it didn't seem crazy or half-baked. The book was well-written and Ms. Watson clearly had a wealth of knowledge and experience in the area of bowel health and how it potentially affected general health. This was really a turning point for me. I had to be ready, though, to hear what Antonio had to say. The shift in my awareness was gradual and incremental. Even with our fundamentally different views of the world, Antonio became a very important person in my growth as a physician.

In my life, I have obviously learned a lot from my parents and teachers in school. I have learned much from my wife. I have learned much from my co-workers. I understand now that I must be ready to learn all the time, because you never know where the good stuff can come from.

Inclusive Models of Wellness

Open-mindedness is an important element if we are to move to a more inclusive model of wellness. Honesty and humility are also essential. I will often be talking to a patient, giving them my impression on some health issue. On the one hand, I want them to trust me and to be able to rely on me for information. On the other hand, I never want them to get the idea that I am automatically correct. I will tell them that I, like everyone, am limited by my knowledge and experience up to that moment in time. There are many things I told patients years ago that I now believe to be incorrect. I have seen a number of women in my early career with classic symptoms of thyroid dysfunction, for example, that I told did not have a thyroid problem because a single blood test (TSH) was normal. In retrospect, most or all of them almost certainly would have benefited from iodine and/or thyroid hormone replacement.

The higher a person is on the food chain, the more invested they are in being correct. It is extremely difficult for someone to acknowledge any deficiencies they may have in knowledge and experience. The expert will often give bad advice rather than no advice, or prescribe medication they know will probably not help, just to maintain the illusion that they have all the answers.

As I have alluded to above, the alternative world with its variety of practitioners is not immune to the delusions of expert opinion. In some ways they may be more susceptible to this deficiency because they often have farther to go to earn the client's respect. To this end, they may be less straightforward about when they are incorrect or can't help someone. This has been my experience. The allopathic providers and the naturopathic providers have limitations in what they can offer. I have had alternative providers figure someone out relatively efficiently and resolve an intractable issue that the MDs couldn't sort out. I have also seen them be flat wrong, leading the patient down a path over months and years that ultimately proved to be a dead end. In those scenarios, the patient is even more frustrated by the lack of answers and feels no one in the world is helping them. Most providers remember well their successes and slough off their failures utilizing any number of rationalizations to explain why the person didn't improve. Maybe the person didn't really follow the recommendations prescribed. The MD recommended medication, but they didn't take it. The acupuncturist recommended herbs and they couldn't afford them. The surgeon said to lose weight, but the person was too lazy and that's why the back surgery was unsuccessful. The naturopath said to avoid gluten, but given no improvement, the person must be sneaking pizza at night.

Collaboration is the way through the murk. The empirically trained reductionist allopathic physician would do better to acknowledge the advantages of a broad systemic approach. The spiritual naturopath would do well to acknowledge the many successes of mainstream medicine. Research and studies should provide information to help sort out what is currently the best from both worlds, but they may not be the last word for any complex health issue.

There are major medical institutions scattered around the world that have taken on the task of integrating alternative options into their array of medical services. The Mayo Clinic website says their Integrative Medicine Department was "created to address growing patient interest in wellness-promoting

treatments that are not typically part of the conventional medical care, such as resilience training, meditation, massage therapy and herbal medicine."[98] I admire how open they are regarding their motivation to expand their services. It is based on consumer demand with no reference that these additions provide value. They are conductiong many research studies on herbs like black cohosh, evening of primrose oil, ginseng and others.

The Royal London Hospital for Integrated Medicine seems to have a model several steps closer to true integration. The easiest way to tell is probably to look at the roster of professionals taking care of patients and especially those in leadership roles. If they are all MDs, they may not be getting a wide enough variety of perspectives. The London facility "offers an innovative, patient-centred service integrating the best of conventional and complementary treatments for a wide range of conditions."[99] They have allopaths, naturopaths, herbalists and other practitioners working together. They manage the chronic conditions that, I think, most desperately require a holistic integrated approach, namely chronic fatigue syndrome (CFS), irritable bowel syndrome (IBS) and fibromyalgia. They have departments focusing on diet/nutrition, sleep, and stress management.

How many chronic medical problems are well understood today? Not many. For all of our successes and progress, we barely understand anything about why certain people are sick and others are well. The new, integrative approaches of the Mayo Clinic, the Royal London Hospital, and other institutions may offer the most innovative and promising approaches to cracking open these problems and finding better options for patients, as long as they can adhere to a truly open-minded and unbiased view of the practice of medicine.

Questioning the Paradigm of Evidence-Based Medicine

Evidence-based medicine gives us some answers, but the majority of the funding for research comes from pharmaceutical companies with a very specific agenda. It is well established that the companies will bury studies that do not show benefit for their drug. It is also well understood that the numbers generated in studies can be "cooked" to produce juicy, positive results.

There is an excellent website with short talks from some of the most brilliant, innovative people on earth. The acronym TED comes from a 1984 conference organized to bring together people from three worlds: Technology, Entertainment and Design. Ben Goldacre gave an excellent TED Talk entitled "Battling Bad Science."[100] He noted that industry-funded trials are four times more likely to produce a flattering result than an independently funded study. He stated that in one evaluation, half of all trial data on antidepressants had been withheld by the pharmaceutical industry.

Occasionally, I will have cause to review statistic manipulation with a patient. This could be a younger person with moderately elevated "bad cholesterol" (or LDL) who I'm advising against starting a statin. If the rate of heart attack on some medication goes from 4 out of 10,000 down to 2 out of 10,000, you can say that medication has reduced the risk of heart attack by 50 percent. A 50 percent reduction? Everyone should be on that medication! We should dump it in the water supply. Busy healthcare providers often only have time to read the punch line conclusion of a study in a medical journal.

We must often look for other sources of information. Providers must actively develop more finely-tuned intuition to help guide decision-making. Anecdotes are not fact, but I feel now that they can often provide useful information and should not be dismissed out of hand. I always want to know what a person thinks about what is going on inside their bodies. They can make it easier for me to figure out the problem. Anecdotes and insights leading to well-done studies with minimized bias would be a good model for figuring out some of the more complex health questions.

Respecting a Patient's Wishes

We also need to appreciate that each person has his or her individual preferences. I am currently seeing a 76-year-old, Jane, with paroxysmal atrial fibrillation and elevated blood pressure numbers sometimes up around 180 systolic. The systolic number is the higher of the two blood pressure numbers. For most people, the goal is to have it consistently below 140. Atrial fibrillation is a cardiac rhythm problem where the person's heartbeat is irregular leading to discoordinated muscle contractions within the heart. The erratic heartbeat causes more turbulence as the blood is flowing through the chambers of the heart. This increases the chances of a large clot or thrombus forming inside one of the upper chambers. The combination of atrial fibrillation and high blood pressure puts her at a relatively high risk of a stroke. Despite this, she refuses any blood thinner and will not take a blood pressure pill under any circumstances. This, of course, is her right. For this type of person, where I feel they are making an error in judgment with important potential consequences, I try to assess how readily they will change their mind.

I can usually tease this out quickly and I have had people very resistant to medications who ultimately will agree given a persuasive argument. It helps if they understand that I personally only use pharmaceuticals when I feel there are no better options. One argument that will often sway the person relates to any risk of stroke. Certain medical problems get people's attention no matter what their inclination. This would include stroke and Alzheimer's disease and just about any situation where cancer is possible.

There is a subset of the population that wants to live their way and nobody is going to stop them. They will eat bacon double cheeseburgers for breakfast. They will smoke two packs a day, and double that on Sunday. They have no interest in any form of exercise. They think running on a treadmill going nowhere is for chumps. An underappreciated aspect of health and wellness is that people have the right to make their own decisions even if I, as their health provider, don't agree with them. They would rather live their way and die at 70 than subsist on celery and pea sprouts and die at 75, bitter for not having truly lived life to the fullest. They imagine having a big fat juicy steak for dinner washed down with three Bud Lights in between Marlboros, then drifting off peacefully in their sleep never to wake up again.

I'll remind them that it isn't always that simple. If a person has a stroke, they can live for many more years with a diminished quality of life. If I tell them that uncontrolled hypertension is the number one risk factor for stroke, they usually will start listening. I will then quote them a study that showed that for every 20 points a person's systolic pressure is lowered, their risk of stroke is cut in half. The clincher is to say that if we could reduce their average blood pressure from around 160 to around 120, their risk of stroke may be reduced more than 50 percent. At that point, they are usually more than willing to take a pill once a day.

This 76-year-old I see would not be swayed. She also has advanced degenerative arthritis of her left hip and left knee. She would probably do extremely well with joint replacement but won't even consider it. Half way into a sentence, I see her head is already shaking side to side with a faint grimace on her face. For her, I did not elaborate on any stroke risk relative to her blood pressure and cardiac arrhythmia. I sensed I could not budge her so instead focused on the positives, including her regular yoga and superb diet.

There are many reasons why people want an alternative approach. They are worried about potential side effects and interactions of drugs. Very reasonable. They want proactive options and a better understanding of why people develop certain chronic health problems. Also reasonable. For years, people would tell me they wanted a more "natural" approach to something. As a provider taught that science holds the answer to most questions, I would internally blanch when I heard that. I have come around slowly over my time in practice and now agree that we should work to maximize the body's own capacity to maintain balance and homeostasis.

Dealing with Difficulty

In every medical office in America, and probably the world, there are difficult patients. When I say "difficult" I mean they have many chronic medical issues that are hard to sort out. These people tend to have extreme challenges in their daily life. Many of them are on mental and/or physical disability. Some of them can work but are limited in terms of what they can do on any given day.

These patients have many things in common. They usually have seen many specialists and had extensive testing. They use up a disproportionate amount of time and resources in the healthcare system. They are often on many different medications in a futile effort to gain relief from a myriad of symptoms. They are also, more commonly, women.

This is not sexism. There is something real going on that makes women more susceptible to being a challenging patient. I still see women in this enlightened day and age who see their fourth or fifth specialist and then are told that what they really need is to see a good psychiatrist. Because the venerable specialist with the 140 IQ who graduated from a prestigious medical school cannot figure things out, the only possible explanation is the problems are primarily psychological? The arrogance of this is incredible. This has been going on for many years and still goes on to this day.

Many books have been written describing the differences between men and women. The one I'm most familiar with is *Men are From Mars and Women are From Venus* [101] by John Gray. The book is a little hokey to read, but it touches on many fundamental differences between the genders. On some level, men will never understand or relate to women, and vice versa. One of the gender differences that contributes to bias in medicine is the opposite approaches to communication. It is embedded in human culture, and the male psyche, that men tend to keep to themselves when stressed. From a male perspective, to talk about a problem is to complain. "Complaining" to a male serves no real purpose. It is a sign of weakness. The most extreme version of this is the value placed on playing injured in competitive sports. Professional football players are expected to play through extreme pain without a word.

Women handle stress in a different manner. To females, it is important to talk about what is bothering them so they can garner empathy and support. This, then, is not about complaining, it is about venting. Most of the time the woman just wants someone to listen; the male, on the other hand, will often assume she is asking him to help solve her problems. These discrepancies lead to much frustration in relationships. I suspect these differences also contribute to why women are portrayed in our culture as anxious, hysterical, histrionic and melodramatic. Women with symptoms are often not taken as seriously by a male doctor, or even a female provider, because there is a sense that the patient is probably exaggerating to get support.

There is a presumption embedded in our culture that it's better to be open and talk about our problems. I think this is a good idea most of the time... but not all of the time. For someone stuck in the mindset of being ill, this can be counterproductive. The male approach of willful ignorance and being able to let things go more easily would probably help most with complex chronic medical issues. In this sense, we need integration of female and male approaches to get the best of both worlds.

Moving Forward Toward Integration

So, overall, how could we move forward toward integration? At the International Congress of Naturopathic Medicine conference I attended in 2013, I was impressed by many of the lecturers emphasizing the importance of research. Part of the naturopathic movement, to my surprise, is a push for more investigations into the efficacy of its approaches. Several of the lectures were dedicated to the underlying pathophysiology of disease with an emphasis on immunology. The content was as rigorous as any I had in medical school or have come across at more traditional medical conferences. This should help to convince MDs that naturopaths are working toward a more evidence-based model. My sense, however, is that many physicians will reject any alternative approach no matter what. Thus, patients themselves will probably have to be the primary drivers of change.

My dream is to open a wellness center where a wide variety of practitioners would work collaboratively under one roof. There would be lectures and an open forum to evaluate the relative merits of different options in managing acute and chronic conditions. The model for healthcare would be one of synthesis, with emphasis on a truly proactive approach following many of the principles of naturopathy. The mind, body and spirit would be emphasized in proportional measure. There would be an effort to avoid unnecessary testing. The group would pursue a minimalist approach to pharmaceuticals and use antibiotics sparingly. Every visit would have an element of prevention.

It would be important for the patients to be actively involved in their care. One of the lessons of clinical medicine is that if the provider is putting forth most of the effort, not much will change. We would have group visits with people with similar diagnoses and issues, with a focus on education.

The variety of providers could include MDs, DOs and NDs with an acupuncturist, chiropractor, herbalist, nutritionist, and sleep expert. Potentially, we would also employ or contract with psychologists, addiction experts, personal trainers, massage therapists, life coaches, physical therapists, occupational therapists and others.

The nutritionist would play a central role and have a scope of practice beyond protein, fats and carbohydrates. I remember being excited about taking a food, science and nutrition course in college only to be disappointed by the bland subject matter. The nutritionist would be an expert in food allergies, sensitivities and intolerances, including testing options like Mediator Release Testing, if that turns out to be the most precise way to identify those issues. He or she would have a thorough understanding of insulin resistance, hormonal influences, Paleo and *Wheat Belly*. They could take a person through *The Plan* if a more in-depth, individualized approach to diet was necessary.

In an ideal setting, we would have a fitness center and pool. Aquatherapy and hydrotherapy could be done on the premises. Detoxification programs would be available to address deeply-rooted systemic problems. For the most complicated patient, we would utilize the team approach used by medical doctors in Morbidity and Mortality (M&M) and Tumor Board conferences by medical doctors. In this setting a complex case is presented to a group of providers who then have an intense discussion to find the optimal plan for management. If I have discovered anything in my attempts to help complicated patients, it is that there is no one way out of the chaos. There are common elements, but each person has a unique path to wellness.

New patients would have an incredibly thorough evaluation of their background delving into all aspects of their social and medical history. We would do focused genetic testing, including methylation cycle abnormalities like MTHFR. An attempt would be made to assess the many potential exposures at the patient's home and throughout their occupational history. People could sign a statement of principles at the first visit emphasizing the need for their involvement and participation. This would be an agreement regarding the minimal use of pharmaceuticals and antibiotics. There would be no short-acting opioids like Percocet and Vicodin prescribed for pain control beyond a few weeks.

The center would be open early in the morning and into the evening for convenience. We would have hours on Saturday and Sunday in an effort to treat people efficiently and keep them out of emergency departments. Public and private health insurers should, in theory, be amenable to pay for a wider variety of services with at least partial subsidization of ancillary providers.

The center would work to find the most appropriate and effective vitamin and supplement options. These would be sold at cost to avoid any conflict of interest. There would be an effort to avoid polypharmacy of non-pharmaceuticals as well. Too often I see the holistically-minded patient taking five, ten or more supplements based on recommendations from family, friends and Dr. Oz. Each person requiring pharmaceuticals would have pharmacogenetic testing so we would have the most up-to-date information for safe prescribing. The annual physical would include an individualized, detailed plan to improve lifestyle and maximize prevention. There would be check-ins done on a regular, perhaps monthly, basis to monitor progress and barriers to success. The patient could even have their weight, blood pressure and other information beamed electronically to the office for monitoring.

In short, my dream would be a new, truly holistic model emphasizing pro-active wellness that gets at the deepest levels of care. We would understand each person across all realms including genetic, physical, psychosocial and spiritual. We would find the best options from the mainstream and the alternative world that would help us meet our individualized goals.

11

The Lost Ones

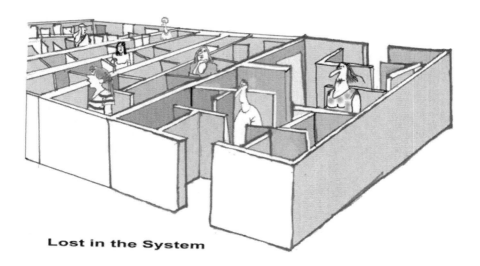

Lost in the System

Every medical office has a cohort of people with complex symptoms that are difficult to manage. These complicated patients will typically have some or all of the diagnoses that are poorly understood or hard to manage. Some of these include irritable bowel syndrome, interstitial cystitis, fibromyalgia and chronic fatigue syndrome. These patients are more likely to have migraines and chronic headaches. They are more likely to be sensitive to medications, requiring lower doses than normally prescribed. They are more likely to be the odd individual who has an opposite or paradoxical side effect from certain medications or OTC drugs. Examples of this would be insomnia from an antihistamine like Benadryl or drowsiness from the decongestant Sudafed. These patients also tend to have more documented allergies to pharmaceuticals. Some of them will have five, six or even 10 medications that have caused reactions or side effects.

If there are numerous side effects to antibiotics, there is an increased likelihood that chronic Lyme disease or some other tick-borne infection is the primary cause for their complex health problems. There is no telling how many people with chronic Lyme disease are put on an antibiotic with worsening of many of their chronic symptoms. The person calls their doctor's office to report "side effects" and this is then documented in the person's medical record. The muscle pains, joint pains, sweat and headaches from the antibiotic were not, in this context, side effects but instead a Herxheimer reaction. This reaction occurs when pathogenic organisms are killed off by antimicrobials, stimulating an intense immune reaction. Getting worse initially can actually be a sign that the person is on the right track.

Irritable bowel syndrome (IBS) is a catch-all diagnosis for any chronic bowel problem mainstream medicine cannot figure out. This was described above in the Trust Your Gut chapter. Patients given this pseudodiagnosis will often have constipation, diarrhea or both. They will have bloating and gas and occasionally abdominal pains that are intense and frequent. Even after blood tests, CT Scans, colonoscopies and gastroenterology consults, the person is left with no effective treatment.

I have already mentioned interstitial cystitis. This could be an autoimmune condition or even a chronic infection of the bladder wall.

Fibromyalgia is a chronic condition characterized primarily by muscle pain and tenderness. Most people with fibromyalgia have issues with insomnia and co-existing mental health problems.

Chronic fatigue syndrome (CFS) was once called the "yuppie flu" and many doctors still think it is a psychosomatic illness with no physical basis. The CFS diagnosis can be a dead end since there are not always options for testing or treatment. That is one element these conditions all seem to have in common.

An optimal healthcare system would include extensive research to discover common elements among these "trainwrecks." Of course, if you believe these patients' problems are mostly psychological, this would be a waste of time. The mainstream medical world keeps plowing along in an effort to come up with the newest, latest pharmaceutical that will hopefully cure some of these medical conditions, or at least effectively manage the related symptoms. I feel investigations so far are just nibbling at the edges with no real understanding of what is going on. The pharmaceutical industry really has no incentive to cure anything. Daily medication for life is a much better strategy for profit.

In these areas where there seem to be systemic issues, the "holistic" world often has more success. Some of these patients may have chronic systemic yeast infections. Many of them could have other chronic, undiagnosed tick-borne infections. Some of these patients more than likely have food intolerances and sensitivities that would never be picked up by standard testing. Many have thyroid dysfunction but their providers rely on a single thyroid tests (TSH) to rule this out and thus the thyroid condition is unmanaged. Many have deficiencies of iodine, vitamin D, magnesium, selenium and other vitamins and minerals. More and more people are building up toxic levels of heavy metals like mercury, lead and arsenic. These are the big ideas and, in my opinion, investigating these possibilities is much more likely to yield a path to wellness for the complex, chronically ill person.

In his book *Io•ine: Why You Nee• It, Why You Can't Live Without It*, David Brownstein, MD, estimates that 90-95% of Americans are deficient in iodine. Iodine is essential for proper thyroid function but also supports all of the other hormones in the body including those produced by the adrenal gland. Brownstein recommends a relatively simple iodine loading test to determine the degree of deficiency for the chronically ill.[102] Iodine replacement can have a dramatic effect on a wide variety of chronic symptoms, especially in those that have not seen benefit from other interventions.

There are probably familial and genetic factors in play as well. It is possible that these complex patients suffered trauma when they were young children. If they were the victims of psychological or physical or sexual abuse as children, that stress may have fundamentally altered the way their bodies respond to infections and other environmental factors. There is no doubt that stress is a major cause and effect keeping them in a chronic state of unwellness. More stress makes magnesium deficiency more likely and Morley Robbins uses the term "Magnesium Burn Rate." Stress uses up the methyl groups required for many of the most important biochemical processes in the cells.

We are entering a new era of healthcare that incorporates genetic testing relevant to the person's tendency toward chronic illness. Decreased activity of the MTHFR enzyme[18] through a genetic anomaly is one of the first major players to be identified. As has already been discussed, the individual with an MTHFR problem and methylation cycle defects[19] is at increased risk of anxiety, depression, bipolar illness, schizophrenia, addiction, blood clots, coronary events, strokes, premature dementia, lymphoma, colon cancer, fibromyalgia, chronic fatigue and other important conditions. Those with MTHFR anomalies have decreased ability for detoxification because of lower levels of glutathione.

A more thorough evaluation of genetic anomalies within the methylation cycle pathways is often required. This is a complex topic and beyond the scope of this book but there are many excellent resources available to providers and patients. Dr. Amy Yasko and Dr. James Roberts are two experts that have a lot of information available online.

Patient Complexity Score

I have come up with my own scoring system for these complicated patients which I will call the Patient Complexity Score. This is to illustrate how difficult they are to manage from a doctor's perspective. Many of these people are suffering all day every day and medical doctors with their pharmaceuticals tend to do little or nothing to help them. The scores are:

- 1 point for each active problem on their problem list
- 2 points for each medication currently prescribed
- 3 points for each drug allergy or drug side effect documented
- 4 points for each of the common, difficult diagnoses like fibromyalgia,

migraines, chronic fatigue syndrome, irritable bowel syndrome, interstitial cystitis, an autoimmune condition, depression or anxiety
• 5 points for each prescribed opioid or abused substance

I have many patients with very high scores. Their symptoms and problems are not, in my opinion, psychosomatic. There is a strong psychological component, but it would be hard to convince me the wide variety of problems is merely mental fabrication. Here's a glimpse into the lives of some of my complicated patients. To most people reading this, these struggles will be hard to imagine. To others, though, they will be all too familiar.

Pam

The first case is 50-year-old Pam who has a long history of medical problems but few satisfactory answers as to why she is chronically ill and struggling. Her Patient Complexity Score comes out at 66. She has 18 active problems, including anxiety, vertigo, headaches and unexplained chronic pain. She only takes one prescription medication, which is a miracle. She has a list of 12 medication "allergies" with corresponding side effects and intolerances. Of these medication intolerances, seven are antibiotics, so there really are almost no antibiotics available for her in case of a bacterial infection. Her intolerance to antibiotics could represent Herxheimer reactions rather than true side effects or allergies, as I have touched on previously.

Pam's situation worsened dramatically in the early part of 2014. She had more intense daily headaches. She had lightheadedness with a fear of passing out that stopped her from driving. She went to the Emergency Department a couple of times. She had a CT scan and then an MRI of the brain. She had pages of bloodwork. She saw one and then a second neurologist to try and find a cause for the headaches. She was started on gabapentin, a medication that can be helpful in suppressing pain from various sources. She saw a rheumatologist who thought she might have a rare condition called temporal arteritis. This poorly understood vasculitis, typically seen in people over 65, causes headaches with tenderness and pain focused along the artery that comes out at the temple. Pam's headaches were more diffuse with no focal tenderness so I thought this diagnosis was a reach. The specialist recommended a biopsy of the temporal artery, but Pam's mediocre health insurance would not cover the $800 procedure. She was already having difficulty covering $300 per week for chiropractic visits and physical therapy sessions. Her eye doctor thought she might have "occipital neuralgia" so referred her to a pain specialist. He thought she had "facet arthritis" to the upper cervical spine instead and performed a cortisone injection to the area. That did not alleviate the pain.

By the time Pam came to me for a visit, she was unable to work. I discussed with her some of the content of the Horowitz book on chronic Lyme disease. I had her do his questionnaire and it lit up like a Christmas tree. The headaches were her primary complaint, but the review of systems showed a wide variety of symptoms involving multiple systems:

- She scored **Mild** for sweats, weight gain, swollen glands, pelvic pain, menstrual irregularities, upset stomach, shortness of breath, heart murmur, muscle twitching, speech difficulty and depression.
- She scored **Moderate** for fatigue, sore throats, breast pain, bladder dysfunction, sexual dysfunction, bowel changes, chest pain, heart palpitations, joint pain, neck stiffness, muscle pain, numbness and tingling, motion sickness, confusion, difficulty reading, forgetfulness and disturbed sleep.
- She scored **Severe** for headaches and lightheadedness.

We were reviewing the list of problems and the potential for a tick-borne illness when she mentioned something that might be relevant. Back in 1990, she had a tick bite and then a flu-like illness with joint pain. She saw her doctor and a Lyme test was ordered. Before she heard the result, she got married and left for her honeymoon in Aruba. She says the honeymoon "sucked" because she was so sick the entire week. The joint pain was so severe her new husband had to carry her from place to place. She improved some after that but told me that may have been the time when her chronic health problems started.

It turns out that she had a positive Lyme blood test and the office called to leave a message for her, but she was away. She never got the message and was never put on antibiotics. She and her doctor at the time did not understand the implications of not managing the infection aggressively early on in its course.

The best explanation for her situation now is chronic Lyme disease with many other interrelated problems requiring a wide variety of mainstream, alternative and individualized options. Pam's blood tests, however, now come up negative, so she and her array of specialist physicians do not accept that as a possible cause. The standard Lyme test has been shown to be unreliable by many credible sources but this is not widely accepted. None of the specialists she has seen can give her an alternative explanation for her chronic symptoms. Their pharmaceuticals and interventions have not provided any lasting benefit. In my opinion, she will never be well unless she pursues a long-term approach against chronic Lyme disease and other related problems.

For all of the brilliance and sophistication in the Horowitz book *Why Can't I Get Better? Solving the Mystery of Lyme & Chronic Disease*, it creates almost as many problems as it solves. Dr. Horowitz sees private pay clients who can afford his services. He orders thousands of dollars of tests and pursues an elaborate variety of interventions in his efforts to cure people of chronic disease. But people like Pam could never afford that path to wellness. My goal is to work within the system, using many of the concepts in Horowitz's book, to find creative solutions that are simple and cost-effective.

Janet, Bonnie, Jill and Darlene

Janet is 49 years old and has 14 active problems involving her gynecologic system, gastrointestinal system, skin and mental health. She has multiple sources of severe chronic pain, including intractable migraines, pelvic pain, "dyesthesia" (with a frequent burning sensation to her extremities) and irritable bowel syndrome. She has six drug allergies and is on three controlled substances. She has a background as a healer. She has a disrupted day/night cycle: she sleeps most of the day and is awake most of the night. She cannot work and is totally disabled by her chronic health problems. She acknowledges openly that many of her problems are psychological in nature and the mind-body connection is working to her detriment. This aspect of Janet's poor health will come up again later in the chapter. Her Patient Complexity Score is 92.

Bonnie is a 46-year-old with 22 active problems in her electronic medical record, including depression, migraines, hypertension, chronic pain from the temporomandibular joint, chronic idiopathic peripheral neuropathy and a history of multiple skin cancers. (Idiopathic is the medical term for "we have no idea what is going on.") She takes 10 medications on a regular basis, including opioids. She only has two drug allergies. Bonnie has almost quit smoking many times. She has worked on pursuing exercise and dietary improvements with only a minor benefit to her overall health. Many of these patients have depression and anxiety, but that begs the chicken and the egg question: Is he/she anxious and depressed because of all of his/her health problems or is an underlying mental health problem playing a major role in his/her subjective experience? Or could it be both?

Bonnie was in relatively good health until she had a child at 40. She developed very high blood pressure inexplicably in the third trimester of the pregnancy. If normal blood pressure is somewhere around 120/80, she got up to 220/100 and required medication. From her perspective, she was never the same after that. She developed palpitations during her menstrual cycles that she had never had before the pregnancy. The palpitations were prominent if laying down on her left side.

Jill is a 54-year-old woman I have seen in the office for over 10 years. She is pleasant, intelligent and works hard but has bounced around in different positions. She also has a relatively low quality of life and every day is difficult for her. She has 15 active problems, 16 medications and three drug allergies. She smokes two packs of cigarettes per day and has progressive chronic lung disease. She is overweight but is working on it all the time and weighs herself at visits. Her Patient Complexity Score comes out at an even 100.

Darlene is 58. She has 19 problems on her list, including depression, seizures, premature osteoporosis, the autoimmune condition Raynaud's, plus hypercoagulability (an increased risk of clotting). She has vitamin D and vitamin B12 deficiencies. She also is the only patient I've seen diagnosed with the rare condition porphyria in 20+ years of being in medicine. She takes 11 medications on a regular basis, including occasional vicodin for chronic pain. She has many sources of chronic pain, including a compression fracture of a thoracic vertebrae. She has a list of 11 medication and food allergies/intolerances. Sadly for her, the list includes caffeine, and that is also rare. She sees multiple specialists and has had tens of thousands of dollars of testing in a vain effort to correct some underlying problem. She cannot work because of her medical problems. Despite all of this, she is very personable and easy to talk to with a good sense of humor. That may be the most incredible aspect of all. Darlene's Patient Complexity Score is 105.

Susan

My sentimental favorite of all of the hypercomplex patients is a woman I have known for over 10 years, Susan Johnson. If anyone understands the limitations of American medicine it's Susan. She has 15 active problems, five drug allergies or sensitivities, and regularly takes 13 medications. She is unique in that she may be the only person I see that meets criteria for just about every murky, difficult-to-manage chronic health condition. Susan has had intractable migraines, chronic fatigue syndrome, irritable bowel syndrome, fibromyalgia and interstitial cystitis for years. More recently, she has started having frequent, unexplainable urticaria (the medical term for hives). I remember her coming in for a visit a few years ago asking why I had never diagnosed her with fibromyalgia. She said she had read up on the diagnosis and it fit perfectly. I didn't really see the point of officially diagnosing her with something that we couldn't easily manage. She seemed disappointed, so I graciously added it to her list.

Susan has issues with depression and regular insomnia. She has had more stress in her life than most of the people I have met. But even with so much stress and so many health conditions, she perseveres. She gets up every day, works her regular job and also works a second, part-time job at night. She supports her two adult daughters as they have had problems of their own.

Susan and I get along well enough that at one point I told her I had come up with a new medical condition for her. Because she had just about all of the complex conditions, I diagnosed her overall state of being as "Susan Johnson Syndrome." It was only partially for humor, because I was trying to emphasize to her that there had to be something systemically wrong in order for her to have all of these diagnoses affecting just about every organ system. Seeing a specialist for each system was a fundamentally flawed approach that did not work.

Susan was doing a lot of research on her own from 2012 into 2013, around the same time my approach to medicine was expanding. We started to have visits centered on issues like leaky gut syndrome, food sensitivities, flora imbalance and yeast overgrowth. She is extremely thin and has had trouble keeping up her weight. When I first talked to her about removing processed carbohydrates and sugars from her diet, she was worried this would lead to weight loss. Her diet was already fairly limited but, as usual, she was willing to do just about anything to be well. She went off carbohydrates and, within a week or so, felt more energy and a decrease in her headaches and diffuse body aches. She said at a follow-up visit that it was the first time in years she was able to stay awake for an entire movie. Unfortunately, she also lost 10 pounds. I had recommended she get off her low dose hormone replacement therapy. She tried, but within a short time had profuse sweats, worsening irritability and almost no sleep.

At a follow-up visit, she admitted she had not started the high-dose, high-quality 25-billion-count probiotic that I had recommended. We healthcare providers have to remember that people have a limited capacity for change. People are busy with their lives and it can be difficult to find the time to make so many changes in a short time. The plan going forward was to try her best with the more limited diet but add Ezekiel bread and whey protein shakes. Ezekiel bread can be a great option. The packaging explains the derivation of the name. "As described in the holy scripture verse: 'Take also unto thee Wheat, and Barley, and Beans, and Lentils and Millet, and Spelt, and put them in one vessel, and make bread of it...' from Ezekiel 4:9." We also cut the hormone dose in half and she planned on starting coenzyme Q10 three times a day for the fibromyalgia symptoms.

Bart

Bart is a 39-year-old who I have been seeing for many years. His mother has fibromyalgia, so there may be some familial component to his chronic issues. Bart's condition is very complicated, involving many systems. He has chronic pain which is not well understood by any of the traditional or alternative specialists he has seen. He saw an alternative provider who diagnosed him with chronic Lyme disease but was skeptical and did not pursue treatment. The tally of Bart's active medical issues comes to 14 and includes pain at the TMJ joint, hypertension, atrial fibrillation, severe esophageal reflux with history of gastritis, profound daily fatigue, frequent headaches, insomnia and psoriasis. He has seen four different cardiologists and they can't give us a good explanation for his cardiac arrythmias. He has had every test they can think of and has been on many different medications to try and control his palpitations.

Bart has also worked with several gastroenterologists. He has had an Upper GI study; two endoscopies into the esophagus, stomach and proximal small intestine; x-rays, CT scans, and too many pages of laboratory studies to count. On a characteristic follow-up visit in October of 2012, he came in on six medications but no active use of any controlled substances. He lived with his wife and 6-year-old daughter. He was out of work and they did their best to get by on his wife's small income as a medical assistant. He told me at that visit "every day I feel like I have the flu." He was having worsening headaches with dizziness. He had chest pains. He had muscle aches so intense he couldn't really do much physically during the day. He had abdominal pain and fatigue. He brought up a new symptom of inexplicable tingling to the face. He also was developing issues with the urinary system with more frequent urination day and night. We had been working on his diet and possible food intolerances and, on a positive note, he mentioned a clear correlation with dairy causing worsening fatigue, bowel problems and headaches.

Now, you can imagine what it's like for the average physician who sees a patient with this many issues at a single visit. It is absolutely overwhelming. I don't feel I can possibly address even half of what Bart or patients like him can bring up at a given visit. At one October visit, I ordered a full complement of blood tests (which will almost certainly not provide any concrete answers), set up a titration study for CPAP for Bart's sleep apnea, arranged for an ENT consult, and doubled his lisinopril to better control his blood pressure. It seems like a lot, but I'm really spinning my wheels in the mud going nowhere, and on some level he knows that.

Sometimes, when I see Bart for a visit, the best I can do is listen to him and be encouraging. If I can keep the polypharmacy to a minimum, that is a worthwhile goal. Bart is not abusing any substances and I do not prescribe any pain medication for him, which is a bonus. He needs a system-wide approach and so my efforts are focusing on food intolerances and potentially systemic candida/fungal overgrowth. I am often trying to decide whether to start a multiple antibiotic regimen for the strong possibility of chronic Lyme disease. He travels far to come to our office and has limited finances, so that makes things more difficult.

At a visit in March of 2014, we discussed his ongoing struggles. In the prior four months, he had seen a new specialist in the areas of psychiatry, cardiology, pain management and rheumatology and was planning to see another rheumatologist, his fourth, in the upcoming weeks after the visit with me. I practically begged him to slow down and see a holistic provider, but he didn't have the resources to pay for an outside opinion and could work only with physicians covered by his insurance.

Toward a Better Understanding

It is easy to see the common elements among these patients. They are mostly middle-aged women with a lot of experience in doctor's offices. They have all seen too many specialists to count. It is harder to find a male with a complexity score over 50, but they are out there and struggling as well. There are many differences among this group as well. Some are married and some live alone. Some are abusing cigarettes and alcohol and some wouldn't touch the stuff. Some have strong family histories of mental health problems, substance abuse and similar problems that are almost certainly relevant. One of the women listed above, though, has a twin sister with almost no overlap in terms of chronic medical issues. Some of these patients come in only occasionally for visits and are relatively low maintenance considering their medical problems. Others are in the office two or three times every month for new complaints and issues that require follow-up.

In addition to the challenges of diagnosis and treatment, I have found that the longer a person is ill, the more they are stuck in the persona of being sick. Everyone has a story to tell. The more we tell that story, including to ourselves, the more it becomes the truth. In the complicated patient's life story, some have created a scenario where they are a victim at the mercy of the world around them. I feel that many of them, in that mindset, really are incapable of pursuing wellness. They have no insight into this and vigorously deny that they are not doing everything possible to get themselves better. I like the following statement by speaker and author Esther Hicks:

Most people do not realize that as they continue to find things to complain about, they disallow their own physical well-being. Many do not realize that before they were complaining about an aching body or a chronic disease, they were complaining about many other things first. It does not matter if the object of your complaint is about someone you are angry with, behavior in others that you believe is wrong, or something wrong with your own physical body. Complaining is complaining, and it disallows improvement.[103]

I have often recommended a course of action that I think could be a breakthrough for the person, only to watch an emotionless, placid response. Either they think this is just another dead-end or they have lost the motivation. In an ideal world I could get them to a psychologist who would assist in the process. This psychologist wouldn't sit patiently and listen to their problems with empathy and compassion, they would yank out all the wiring. It would be a lot of straight talk and maybe a few glasses of cold water in the face. Disrupting the apathy may be the greatest challenge of all.

Now, to be fair, there are many other challenging patients in poor health entrenched in their low quality of life. Many of them are obese, smoke and abuse alcohol. These people can go to the doctor often and utilize a lot of medical resources. Their situations, however, are different in my opinion. They are based primarily on weight and lifestyle. They don't have the unexplained wide range of problems seen in the truly complicated patient.

The person with a high Patient Complexity Score has deeper, more fundamental, causes for their health problems. It is my goal in medicine to understand these "trainwrecks" and help them on a path to being well physically, mentally and spiritually. Currently, the medical system is failing them in every conceivable way. We are not giving them real answers to their problems. We are blasting away with medication after medication. We misrepresent what we know and understand. We are reluctant to think outside of the small allopathic box. If they are difficult to deal with during their 25-minute visit, imagine how life is for them the rest of the time.

Magnesium deficiency has been linked to many chronic processes that are relevant to this group including: fatigue, constipation, dizziness, excessive menstrual pain, facial twitching, headaches, muscle cramps, heart palpitations, mood swings, poor memory, Raynaud's, insomnia, hyperactive bladder, arthritis, osteoporosis, kidney disease, cardiac disease and others. Early on in the work-up, dietary changes and supplementation should be used to get the RBC magnesium levels up around 6.0. This can be done inexpensively through Epsom salts baths as described at the website www.gotmag.org.

My sense is that these hypercomplex patients often have some genetic susceptibility like MTHFR[18] that becomes more important over time, often beginning sometime between adolescence and young adulthood. Perhaps they are under some severe prolonged stress, either from issues at home or because of a medical issue. Maybe they have food intolerances that cause gastrointestinal disruption, making them more susceptible to illness (the leaky gut scenario). It's possible that some of these patients have a chronic infection like Lyme disease. The sequence of repetitive stress probably makes them more vulnerable to other diseases. There is a downward spiral with pain and insomnia causing more stress that leads to more profound medical issues.

A path out of the chaos has to be individualized with a focus on common elements like bowel health, dietary change and the use of supplements like L-methylfolate, vitamin D, omega-3 fatty acids, magnesium, iodine and others. We could ask each of these individuals 100 or more questions and put the data into a computer looking for high correlation coefficients. That may provide some explanation. It would be nice to have access to the databases of groups like the Framingham Heart Study and 23andme. Either way, we need a new paradigm of health to make any real changes.

I would like to develop a protocol for improving the health of these complicated individuals. The starting place, of course, would be an extensive history going back through past medical problems, psychosocial experiences, a detailed family history and a survey of environmental exposures. Testing would include some basic labs: a full thyroid panel including reverse T3, B12, folate, CBC, CRP, complete metabolic profile, RBC magnesium, testing for tick-borne infections, etc.

I would order a hair metal analysis for many patients as I am coming to find that mineral deficiencies and metal toxicities have a significant impact on wellness. The report generated by Great Plains Laboratories, for one example, helps to clarify whether a person is deficient in calcium, magnesium, copper, zinc, manganese, boron, iodine, lithium, selenium, iron and other minerals. Their relatively simple and inexpensive test also checks for abnormally high levels of aluminum, arsenic, lead, mercury and other harmful substances. It is important to think of mineral levels in the context of ratios and balance. Getting the raw number doesn't always tell the whole story. Lithium levels and B12 effectiveness are interrelated. A person needs adequate magnesium and vitamin D levels for calcium to work well. Calcium supplementation is relatively excessive compared to the degree of magnesium deficiency in America. The ratio of zinc/copper and calcium/ phosphorous can be important. Methylfolate and the optimal form of B12 can be essential in combination for those with methylation cycle issues.

We know the gastrointestinal system is the basis for many chronic problems, especially in terms of immune dysfunction. It is estimated that seventy percent of the body's immune system tissue is within the GI tract as gut associated lymphoid tissue (GALT). Our microbiome interacts with our immune system and our brain in complex ways forming a triad that needs to be managed accordingly. Some with refractory bowel problems would have a comprehensive stool analysis that goes far beyond what can be done in mainstream labs.

I would run a full methylation cycle genetic profile for everyone. The website 23andme, even though it seems to be for ancestry use only, will process a saliva sample for DNA for $99. The raw data then needs to be uploaded from 23andme to another website like geneticgenie, livewello or mthfrsupport to generate a report on methylation cycle abnormalities. This report would be different for each person. This information can be among the most important for the chronically ill person. It can provide the foundation for a path to wellness but, right now, there are too few providers knowledgeable in the area of methylation cycle defects. The patient who pursues this testing will have to do a lot of research on their own and become an expert. They could then try to find an open-minded provider willing to take on the project.

For some of the tests above, it matters which laboratory is used, especially when it comes to Lyme tests. Most patients would get an iodine loading test to check for iodine deficiency. Stage I would include patients starting a high-quality, daily probiotic, increasing water intake to at least 30-40 ounces per day, improving diet and starting to wean off any and all substances including coffee. Stage II would be taking each patient through The Plan, or an elimination diet, to identify the foods and food types that may be triggering internal inflammation. This could involve a shift to a Paleo diet. Stage III would be to address polypharmacy and gradually pull back on their medications. I would try to optimize supplementation for each person and avoid the "shot gun" approach as much as possible.

At that point I would reassess each patient in terms of their quality of life. The process is almost always difficult but is definitely worth our efforts because of the ripple effect from these patients outward to friends, family, co-workers and others involved in their lives. As Clarence says in the classic holiday movie *It's a Wonderful Life*: "Each man's life touches so many other lives." The complex patient may not have as much impact as George Bailey, but their poor health always has a collateral effect on the other people in their life.

It is possible that the most important aspect in managing the complicated patient is addressing the mind/body connection and the deeper spiritual deficits. I suspect we could address diet, lifestyle and substance abuse optimally and the person would still be ill. We could put the complex person on supplements like vitamin D, coenzyme Q10, probiotics and many others and we would only be part way to healing. The underlying anger and frustration of the chronically ill person is probably the densest barrier to penetrate.

The second complex patient I mentioned, Janet, was possibly the hardest person I have ever managed. It was frustrating for both of us from the first visit. She would come in once a month for a follow-up visit. Every visit was about the same—she was desperately tired and experiencing severe, debilitating pain from multiple sources. She had penetrating migraines, severe abdominal and pelvic pain and other constitutional symptoms. I would see her as the last patient in an extended visit and we would typically run over. She had seen numerous mainstream and alternative providers but none of them really helped her. Her work-up did show a malabsorption pattern on a CT scan of the abdomen and she did have some other abnormalities revealed through lab testing, but there was no test that could represent her level of "dis-ease." We talked about diet and supplements. She would often find a new book and review it with me at the visit. I tried to be honest and convey that I really didn't understand why she was so sick. Although I wanted to help her, she eventually understood that I did not have the tools, experience or insight to move her forward.

After more than a year, she saw a naturopathic provider. To the provider's credit, he did not talk to her about avoiding gluten or adding another vitamin. He focused immediately on the mind-body aspect of her situation. She emailed me a summary of the visit:

He thinks I need to basically tune in to the flow of life, nature, etc. start meditating 3 times per day, walking every day, release all thoughts about illness and disease and treatment, etc. It's profound and also very simplistic... We're all students in the class of life. One thing he suggested was for me to resume doing reiki on other people, but not charge money for it, as a way to separate the ego and return myself to a giving, selfless state. I can appreciate it from a karmic perspective, but it's not easy to do when you're broke.[104]

My instincts aligned with hers. I suspected those interventions were the most crucial for her. She started following the naturopath's advice, walking and meditating, and did reiki on someone for 20 minutes. The day after, she felt worse in her joints and her abdomen. She had a severe migraine rated at "15 out of 10" and pounded several narcotic pills to try and get relief. It's easy for me or someone else to fault her for turning to narcotics. It would be easy for someone to fault me for even giving her a prescription for them. To be in that much pain, however, no matter what the cause, is something most people will never experience.

12

Finn's Story

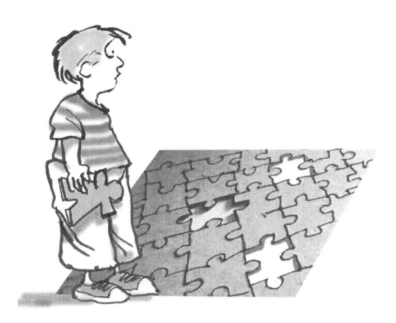

In terms of the potential impact of alternative approaches, Finn's story dramatically illustrates the deficiencies of both mainstream and alternative options. I first saw him in the office when he was about twelve months old.

He was born full-term following an uneventful pregnancy and was bottlefed. He had many ear infections with multiple courses of antibiotics starting before six months of age. He had recurrent pulmonary infections and saw several specialists leading to a working diagnosis of asthma. He had a sweat test at eight months old negative for cystic fibrosis. He eventually had his tonsils and adenoids removed with multiples sets of tubes placed in his eardrums to reduce his risk of infection.

In terms of development, Finn started talking at a relatively young age and by two could speak in full sentences, but his speech was somewhat difficult to understand. There was a question about whether this was related to having so many ear infections with persistent congestion inside his middle ear space. The Early Intervention person saw him once a week for about four months, ultimately deciding he no longer needed services. They did comment in their evaluation on some degree of poor muscle tone in his trunk, but otherwise they found no concerns.

Finn continued to have sinus issues, ear problems and respiratory infections until he was four years old. He was on antibiotics, and occasionally oral steroids, to get the infections under control. At 3 years, 11 months, Finn was diagnosed with Lyme disease. He was once again put on antibiotics. It was around this time that things started to change. Finn attended two different preschools and the teachers at both schools commented that he was sluggish and couldn't sit up during circle time. They said he was less social and played more by himself. He was evaluated with a variety of blood tests that came back normal.

Finn's health gradually deteriorated. He saw a respected pediatric neurologist at Boston's Children's Hospital, considered one of the top pediatric hospitals in the world. The specialist noted the change in muscle tone and the report that he was a bit withdrawn from his peers, although Finn was still interactive and spoke well during the visit. The doctor ultimately said he might have Attention Deficit Disorder (ADD) or possibly Asperger's, a high-functioning form of autism. People will often say a child is "on the spectrum," meaning on the spectrum of Autism. The neurologist said Finn would likely "grow out of it" and recommended the family return in six months if there was further regression.

Two months after that visit, Finn started making strange eye movements. The parents reported he was becoming more "naughty" and difficult to control. He would try to open the car door when they were driving. He had a compulsion to touch fire if he saw it, which was new for him. The mom says that around this time he was extremely hard to care for and was "driving [them] nuts!" She figured maybe she was doing something wrong as a parent. This is very typical of parents, especially mothers, who blame themselves when something goes wrong with their child.

Around that same time, Finn's grandfather came to stay with the family for five weeks. Finn and his grandfather got along well with a strong emotional bond. The grandfather went home and unexpectedly died a week later. Finn started saying that he was "scared for [his] life" and was afraid of dying. He asked a lot of questions about death and, according to his mom, became "consumed" with the topic. Finn's dad went back to his childhood home by himself to attend to things. While his father was away Finn changed the most dramatically.

He became more quiet and less responsive. When Finn's dad came home after being away two weeks, he immediately noticed the changes and asked what was wrong. Finn had almost completely stopped talking and begun making weird noises. He spent a lot of time spinning or just standing alone in the corner by himself. He would stay there as long as his parents let him.

The parents arranged for an evaluation at Project Chilld, a group I have discussed before. Their initial assessment was that Finn was not autistic. They wondered about a condition called Landau-Kleffner Syndrome (LKS). In this condition a child will manifest signs of autism from recurrent seizures. The mom contacted the pediatric neurologist and described what was happening. She said he still did not seem very concerned. A visit was scheduled for several months later.

Finn had also regressed in terms of potty training, refusing to go to the bathroom. He experienced severe constipation. He had a habit of lying on whatever hard object he could find so that his abdomen was pressing on it. One time, I saw him in the office and he moved around the room trying to find something to lay his stomach on. A few times, without any recognition of me, he laid across my thigh as if I were an object. As he was lying across me, he was making odd vocalizations. Finn saw a pediatric gastroenterologist and was put on daily laxatives with no benefit.

Finn's mom did a lot of reading on the Internet trying to figure out why her son was exhibiting so many signs of autism at a relatively advanced age. She came across a lot of suggestions that diet could contribute to or be the cause of his problems. In particular, she found many references to a gluten-free, casein-free diet. With nothing to lose she tried it, and by the fourth day Finn started to talk again. It seemed like a miracle at the time.

Finn went back to the neurologist for a follow-up visit. By that time he had improved, especially in terms of his ability to use expressive language. The neurologist did an evaluation and concluded that the dramatic decline in Finn's status was caused by his grieving the death of his grandfather. To be thorough, though, Finn had a hearing test, MRI of the brain, blood work and an Electroencephalogram, or EEG. All of these tests were normal, probably reinforcing the specialist's overall impression.

The parents were still not satisfied with how things were going. Shortly after Finn turned five, I recommended he see Gloria, the medical intuitive and certified nutritionist I had worked with over the prior few years.

Gloria had a transformative personal experience of her own with some similarities to Finn's story. She was a schoolteacher when, out of nowhere, her young son started having seizures. They were so frequent and debilitating, her son would have episodes when out playing with his friends and have to run in before he soiled himself. Her son saw several of the top pediatric neurologists in Boston and was put on different medications that caused side effects. At one point—which I think Gloria would view as a turning point in her life—she said "Enough!" Gloria did her own investigations and thought that her son's diet might be causing the seizures. She went into her cupboard with a garbage bag and cleaned it out. She remembers driving all over eastern New England trying to find the healthiest organic foods for him. This was in the 1970s when organic foods were hard to come by.

Gloria overhauled her son's diet and the seizures resolved. She says that was over 30 years ago and he hasn't had a seizure since then. This started her on a path where she spent years as an apprentice to a medical intuitive based in Arizona. She had the passion to learn and some natural ability and, a new career blossomed. Early on in her solo practice, Gloria made contact with an allergist/immunologist at a hospital near to where she lived. He was the chief of the hospital's Department of Medicine. He was also remarkably open-minded. He had heard that she was helping a lot of people that could not get help otherwise. He had a small group of patients that were complicated and, despite his best efforts, he found he could not help them. He was an intelligent, well-educated and respected individual secure enough to say that he did not understand why a subset of his patients would not improve.

He told Gloria, the medical intuitive, she could work with this group of patients to see if they would get better. By her account, within a few months 21 out of 22 were significantly improved. She had made recommendations regarding their diets and added certain supplements and vitamins.

Finn went to see Gloria for his recurrent stomach pains and constipation. She recommended a stricter diet, including one without yeast. She recommended a group of vitamins, supplements and probiotics. His mother now says in retrospect, "This was the most anyone helped Finn in his [up to then] five years of life." After that visit he got better and better. He was talking more and interacting with people around him.

Soon after, he had a follow-up visit with the same pediatric neurologist. At the visit, his mom says he was "talking up a storm." She told the neurologist about the dietary changes and he shrugged it off as nothing more than a coincidence. He also said that the EEG had ruled out Landau Kleffner Syndrome. The mom knew from her reading that it often took more than a standard EEG to rule out LKS. The doctor said once again they should call if Finn regressed and come back in six months. The mom had no intention of returning for another visit. There's an unspoken notion that if you just keep putting people off, and schedule one six month follow-up after another, that many people will just get better on their own. This is often the case, of course, because of the body's innate potential to heal itself.

In the four months after seeing Gloria, Finn continued to improve and was nearly back to his baseline. He was in school and doing well. The teachers reported he was doing "above average" work. In February of 2012, his mom started to introduce new foods and he quickly went downhill. They traveled to Florida to see a physician that worked primarily with autistic children. The physician put Finn on a series of strong medications that Finn could not handle very well. He got worse and worse. The eye fluttering and strange eye movements had never completely resolved and he started having episodes where he would roll his eyes back and stare off into space.

They went back to Gloria and she recommended stopping the medications that had been started by the doctor in Florida. She returned Finn to a lot of the same supplements she had recommended at the initial visit. By then they had seen a neurologist who specialized in LKS and Finn had a more intensive 24-hour ambulatory EEG study. This was normal, so LKS was more clearly ruled out.

Finn came in for a well visit with me and I noted that his language was meager compared to where it had been. His parents and older sister had to force him to talk and he would typically only repeat what they said or give short, one- or two-word answers. Finn's mom, willing to try anything to help him, was about to start TSO therapy. This is a radical approach where Trichuris Suis Ova (TSO), or the eggs of a certain porcine whipworm, are ingested by the patient. This has been studied for the treatment of autoimmune inflammatory bowel disease, Crohn's disease and ulcerative colitis. In a study in 2005 with 29 patients with "moderately severe" Crohn's disease, 72.4% of them went into remission with TSO therapy.

The concept is an offshoot of the hygiene hypothesis mentioned earlier in the book. Over millions of years we have co-evolved with a wide variety of species including, of course, microorganisms and worms. The gut plays a primary role in a high percentage of complex medical conditions, including autoimmune conditions. The idea is to return the bowel, as much as possible, to its natural state. The gastrointestinal system is an essential but underappreciated element of the immune system. Thus, by restoring worms to our gut, the more balanced bowel flora enhance the immunoregulatory functions that then ameliorate any autoimmune interaction. The symptoms of autism, as an autoimmune condition, might then improve. There is some research and many anecdotal reports on the success of this approach. Finn and his family went to New Jersey to see a practitioner utilizing TSO. They pursued it for several months without dramatic benefit. It was a testament to the level of frustration people experience trying to negotiate through alternative medical options. It also likely reflects the complexity and variation among children with autism.

In the summer of 2013, there was a fascinating turn of events. Finn's mother's blog describes what happened when, inexplicably, Finn started eating plants in their yard:

Pica is a disorder in many children and adults with Autism. It's called a non-food disorder. People who eat inedible things like: chalk, dirt, coins, clay and more…If you look it up on the internet, you would immediately see that it is directly correlated to a vitamin or mineral deficiency.

Ah Hah!!! Of course it is! Because the body knows what it needs! If you look at what these people are eating (the non edible items) you will surely see that they are looking for replacements of the minerals and vitamins their body needs. They aren't choosing to eat a couch or the curtains in your living room for god's sake! They are eating things with substance. This really should be obvious! And with so many autistic children having terrible gut and digestion issues, this all really makes sense. When you have poor digestion and stomach problems you aren't fully absorbing any vitamins and nutrients. And especially when your child is on a GMO filled, gluten filled, dairy glazed diet.

Finn started presenting signs of having Pica last year. He puts many things in his mouth to explore them and for sensory reason but doesn't eat them all. He has, however, become obsessed with eating the plants in our yard. I have looked up every single one of them to make sure they aren't poisonous. And like a bird foraging for food in the forest he is not eating the poisonous plants. The main plant Finn is obsessed with is called 'Arborvitae'. He will, in fact, leap tall buildings in a single bound to get one! You should see the impressive show in our backyard every afternoon. His dad put up an awesome fence a few months back with chicken wire to conceal the Arborvitae's that are lining our yard. Finn has found a way to get to those damned bushes every time!

A few weeks back, I decided to ask our nutritionist what was in this plant and why is Finn so incredibly obsessed with it. When we looked up Arborvitae on the internet something really interesting came up. The natural agent for detoxifying the body of heavy metals and other toxins is called Thuja. Thuja is in the Arborvitae bush naturally. Ah-Hah!!! Both of us got the goose bumps all over our bodies when we read this. Finn's body was telling us what he needed! And does he ever !!!"[105]

Finn's parents pursued detoxification programs to simulate the arborvitae, but it did not lead to significant improvement. Some time after that blog post, the mom emailed me about another option. This would potentially be another unique solution: cholesterol supplements helping children with autism. Cholesterol has become a villain in our culture. All of the negative associations with cholesterol have helped the pharmaceutical industry make hundreds of millions on cholesterol-lowering medication. I have already countered some of the erroneous assumptions we make about cholesterol: foods high in cholesterol raise blood cholesterol; any medication that lowers blood cholesterol will lower cardiovascular risk, etc. The reality is that cholesterol is essential to us. It is used to build cell walls. Fat and cholesterol are important in the development of our nervous system.

The conceptual framework that a cholesterol supplement could enhance the nervous system made sense. I researched it, but did acknowledge to Finn's mother that this was out of the box with uncertain implications for his long-term health. The main source of information on this approach came from William Shaw, PhD, who wrote an article entitled "The Role of Cholesterol in Autistic Behaviors."[106]

Weighing the pros and cons, I could see no obvious harm for Finn in taking a cholesterol supplement. Within a couple of weeks of a low dose cholesterol supplement, Finn showed marked improvement in his language and behaviors with more eye contact and focus. His teachers noticed significant improvement in his participation in the class and commented to his mother even though they were not aware that any new supplement had been started. As with many of our successes with Finn, there was eventually a plateau.

Finn is fortunate that his parents are so doggedly pursuing any and every option to help him, whether mainstream or alternative. Their case and others like it show that we need a better system of collaboration where any idea, even ones as radical as TSO and cholesterol supplementation, are considered and evaluated thoroughly.

In summary, there was a clear relationship between Finn's diet and bowel health and his late development of autistic symptoms. He did not follow the more typical pattern of autism but he developed the signs relatively late, with slow development at first and then rapid deterioration just after five years old. I think it is likely that, for Finn, it was the perfect storm of a genetically susceptible individual and a constant barrage of environmental factors. He was bottlefed which may have contributed. It is well established that breastfed babies have fewer ear infections and allergies and less asthma. Finn's allergic issues and recurrent infections led to many courses of antibiotics and steroids. These medications almost certainly hammered away at his internal balance of flora. Perhaps, with less protection from his good bacteria, he had permeability of his intestines, the "leaky gut syndrome." The disruption of this barrier made him vulnerable to a whole host of systemic toxins. The cascade continued with food intolerances that increased inflammation. It would explain why he improved when his diet was changed. Finn represents many of the most important aspects of wellness that are only slowly being recognized.

There are many researchers working on the causes, treatments and potential cures for children on the autism spectrum. These include Elizabeth Mumper and Ken Bock, among others. It is not clear whether mainstream physicians will accept their conclusions, but I think eventually they will have no choice.

A Connecticut naturopath, Jared Skowron, has written books on pediatric health and works with many children with autism. Vice president of the Pediatric Association of Naturopathic Physicians, he spoke at the International Congress of Naturopathic Medicine in July of 2013. I followed up with him after the conference to get his perspective on several aspects of autism. He agrees that environmental toxicity is a major contributor and references immunizations as likely playing a significant role. To suggest that immunizations might have a role in autism and other autoimmune conditions is the third rail of medicine. For many years, I have reinforced to parents that the massive studies done in several countries have found no link. In researching for this book, however, I have had to question my own opinion on the subject. This shift is based mostly on *The Autoimmune Epidemic* book that is, itself, based on hundreds of references. The author, Donna Nazakawa, shows solid, mounting research from many sources that indicates autism is an autoimmune condition and that immunizations play a role for the vulnerable individual. Nazakawa does not conclude that people should not be immunized. From her research, the benefits outweigh the risks for the general population. She suggests, however, that it may be worth limiting the number of immunizations or pursuing an alternative or delayed schedule for a child with increased risk.

Dr. Skowron, to his credit, mentions postponing immunizations until the child is older. Many in the alternative world view immunizations as singularly harmful and propose to eliminate them completely. I think a more individualized, intermediate option makes more sense. If I were the all-powerful Health Czar and could impose my will on the American people, at this point in my career, with my current level of understanding, I would probably alter the immunization schedule. A prime example of a poorly-designed system developed for the masses is the imperative by which babies get immunized for the Hepatitis B virus.

Since I've been in medicine, there has been a shift from giving the first shot shortly after birth to at two months of age. Neither really makes any sense. After coming in contact with probably more than 5,000 different patients, I have had one person with chronic Hepatitis B. The primary modes of transmission would be IV drug use, unprotected sexual activity and mother-to-baby in utero. Perinatal infection is a major problem in developing countries but relatively rare in the United States. All women who get prenatal care in America get screened for the Hepatitis B virus. So, in this example, we are immunizing 100% of babies shortly after birth to try and prevent the rare scenario where a pregnant woman picks up the Hepatitis B virus during pregnancy *after she has been screened.*

To recommend all immunizations to all individuals according to the same schedule may not be optimal, but for us to discontinue our immunization programs because of a small risk to a limited group of individuals would be foolhardy. It seems to be human nature for people to dig in and drift to the extremes, ignoring any information that disrupts their worldview.

Dr. Skowron also wrote in an email about the potential benefits of detoxing women before they became pregnant. Detoxification programs are not in any way, shape or form part of traditional medicine. They are a major component, though, of the alternative world's approach. It would be fascinating to perform a study where women with children on the autism spectrum went through some standardized detoxification program before giving birth to a second child. We know that there is a strong genetic component to autism and Asperger's, so we could compare the rates of autism in subsequent children between the detoxification group and the control group. The results of such a study could dramatically change both our understanding of overall health and our approach to immunizations.

The most relevant genetic anomaly may be the methylene tetrahydrofolate (MTHFR) defect. I have found a strong correlation with this anomaly and the risk of autism. If we pursued more widespread genetic testing of this type for those at higher risk, treating a pregnant mother and a young child with supplements like methylfolate, an optimal form of B12 (which can vary based on an individual's genetics—methylB12, adenosylB12 or hydroxyB12), and others, it could significantly reduce the rates of autism. This is an area that deserves a bolus of resources. Bill and Melinda Gates, where are you?

13

The Fungus Among Us

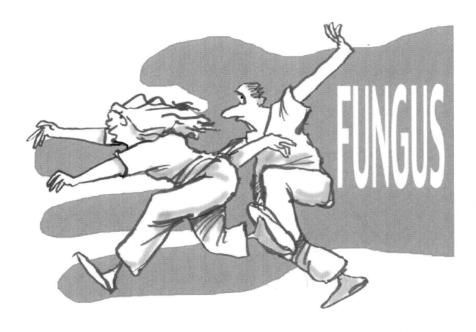

I often see patients that are a challenge to figure out. I assume this is the norm for most practicing physicians. I have had somewhere over 80,000 patient visits at this point over 20+ years in medicine so my ignorance is not from a lack of experience. In the early part of my career, I accepted the fact that I would probably never sort out these complicated patients. These are the lost ones discussed in the previous chapter. But I no longer accept that premise. I can see a way through now and am increasingly determined to help them. One development in my practice that has led to some success for the complex patient is exploring the area of systemic fungal overgrowth or imbalance.

The idea of a person's internal flora being out of balance and causing a systemic yeast infection is one I've heard for many years. I went through my own Kubler-Ross changes with this issue. The five stages of denial, anger, bargaining, depression and acceptance can apply to more than just grieving. I first thought it was preposterous. I then thought it made little or no sense, because I assumed that the body should be able to maintain an adequate internal balance of its micro-organisms. Patients tried to teach me about the issue for years, but I wasn't ready as there was no basis for it in all of my medical training. It took much open-mindedness before I altered my thinking. Today, I believe gut flora and intestinal health are paramount factors of long-term health and wellness.

Agnes

For many years I have been seeing a woman who is now in her 70s. Agnes is married to a retired executive and has four children and multiple grand-children, all scattered around the country. Typically, I see her once a year for a blood pressure check and maybe for the occasional sinus infection or bronchitis. She has well-controlled hypertension on a single blood pressure pill. She is followed by a gastroenterology specialist for some ill-defined chronic form of pancreatitis. She may be the only person I see with that par-ticular issue which, alone, is a reason to take a step back. The GI specialist is well respected in my area and has the pancreatitis issue under control, even though I don't think he has a solid understanding of the underlying cause. He maintains her on a pancreatic enzyme supplement.

Agnes had also been followed by a urologist for many years. She had frequent urination, up to every hour on some days, with bladder discomfort. She had burning with urination, but the urine cultures did not show any bacterial urinary infections. For a while she had undiagnosable pelvic pain. She had chronic daily right flank and right-sided abdominal discomfort. She often felt "red and raw and sore" in the vaginal area. She had extensive testing of her genitourinary system, including urine studies, x-rays, CT scans and MRI scans. One of the scan reports commented on a "kink" in her right ureter. This was not mentioned, however, in subsequent scans, so everyone blew it off as an irrelevant finding. She was convinced it was important, though, because it was an abnormal result involving the right side where she had her symptoms.

Over the years she tried many different medications for these symptoms but none helped. She was on hormone replacement. She was on pharmaceuticals for overactive bladder. One urologist tried gabapentin in an effort to quell her discomfort. Gabapentin is a seizure medication that can be used for chronic pain. It is often the lamest of options, one that suppresses the symptoms but does not address the underlying cause. The only thing that seemed to work for her was an oral antifungal, fluconazole.

She saw me at one point because the specialists did not feel comfortable prescribing oral antifungal medication long-term. The urologist had sent her to an infectious disease specialist who really could not explain why she responded so well to an oral antifungal. He did not think it was appropriate for her to stay on oral antifungals because of the potential that she would develop a resistant organism that would be difficult to treat. This is an important principle, and she and I discussed that possibility as well.

At these earlier visits, when we were discussing the benefits of oral antifungal medication, I really had no basis for what was going on. I had heard patients mention systemic fungal issues here and there but, as I have mentioned before, this was not an issue that had ever once been mentioned in my medical training. From my perspective, based on the knowledge I had for much of my medical career, a person could get a fungal skin infection from excessive moisture or they could get a vaginal yeast infection after taking antibiotics. The skin issue is relatively common, especially to the groin as "jock itch" or the feet as "athlete's foot." Almost every doctor just recommends an OTC antifungal cream and then some measures to try and prevent recurrence. The vaginal issue is likewise managed with an OTC cream or a single dose of the oral antifungal fluconazole.

I do remember addressing the question of systemic yeast infections early on. I typically would dismiss it, saying that the body should be able to maintain its internal balance. I would occasionally get a bit testy, implying that the idea was borderline absurd. I might mention to some of those holistically-inclined patients that the only systemic fungal infections I was familiar with were those in severely immuno-compromised patients in the hospital who had positive blood cultures for fungal elements, a.k.a. fungemia. Those patients needed hardcore intravenous antifungal medications. I think it made me uncomfortable to think that the patient may have more knowledge than me on some subject. The easiest thing to do at the time was to convincingly discount their concern and move on quickly.

By the time Agnes came in to ask whether I would prescribe the oral fluconazole I was on the verge of being persuaded that a systemic yeast infection could be the explanation. I asked the lab person if we could do a urine culture for fungus. I don't think I had ever ordered that test before. She looked into it and the test was available. I recommended to Agnes we do that test first to try and clarify the issue. To my surprise, a week later the test came back positive for a species of candida yeast. That was somewhat of a revelation to me and, in retrospect, was an important positive finding. After that I ordered multiple urine fungal cultures on her. Some were positive but more were negative, so it was fortunate that her first urine culture was positive, otherwise I may not have started treatment.

I agreed to initiate long-term fluconazole for her. She responded very well. Any time I would see her for a visit, she would say that the medication worked extremely well at keeping her symptoms under control. She would take half a pill two, three or even four times per day. If she missed the pill for even a day, her vaginal and urinary discomfort would quickly return. Although this wasn't an ideal long-term strategy, and I was worried we could create a "superbug," I felt her quality of life was worth the potential downside. She had absolutely no reservations about taking the fluconazole as she was relatively miserable without it.

After a while, I started working with Agnes to try and clear the problem rather than just suppress the internal fungal organisms. This approach typically involves several fundamental changes for the person. A high level of hydration is beneficial and I will often recommend 40-50 ounces of water per day. Some people propose half an ounce of water per pound of body weight, but this really isn't practical because people would be drinking water all day, running back and forth to the bathroom. The patient needs to minimize, or eliminate, the food types that cause the yeast/fungus to bloom internally and grow out of control. Sugar and foods that break down to sugar, like bread, crackers, etc., should be avoided. Early on, most fruits should also be removed from the diet as they are typically high in sugar. The person should consume little or no alcohol. The final initial strategy is a high-dose, high-quality probiotic with a 10+ billion count per day and at least 10 different strains. There are probiotics like Florastor with the beneficial form of yeast sacchromyces boulardi which can be useful as well.

The person with a systemic yeast infection will often have a multitude of other problems related to the issue, including gastrointestinal disorders, chronic fatigue, depression, allergies, headaches, and impaired immune function. The basic principle that now guides my practice is utterly simple: the more systems that are involved, the more we need to search for a broad systemic cause like candida overgrowth. There are times when yeast over-growth is the only important issue contributing to poor health, but this is uncommon. Managing this problem is typically only one of many strategies needed to help get the complicated patient well.

In *The Yeast Connection* by Dr. William Crook, the author recommends a series of basic questions as a start:

1. Have you ever taken a broad-spectrum antibiotic?
2. Have you ever taken antibiotics for two months or longer, or at various times during the course of a single year?
3. Have you ever used tetracycline or other drugs to treat acne for one month or longer?
4. Do you now suffer, or have you suffered in the past, from prostatitis, vaginitis, or other conditions affecting your reproductive organs?
5. Have you ever taken birth control pills?
6. Have you ever taken cortisone-type drugs (prednisone, etc.)?
7. Are you sensitive to perfumes, insecticides and/or other chemical odors?
8. Do your symptoms worsen during damp, humid weather, or when you are in places with mold?
9. Have you ever suffered from athlete's foot, ringworm, or other infections of the skin or nails?
10. Do you crave sugar, breads, and/or alcoholic beverages?

11. Are you severely bothered by tobacco smoke?[107]

The answers to these questions, of course, need to be put into context. Anyone can get athlete's foot or a vaginal yeast infection. To me, it's the frequency and severity of the symptoms that is more relevant. If I see an adult with conjunctivitis, I'll ask how often they are getting the episodes. If it is an isolated event, they probably have simple conjunctivitis from a virus. If they are getting episodes several times per year, they probably have some other process ongoing, like allergies or ocular rosacea. I find the question of craving sugar and carbs particularly interesting. Most of the resources about yeast overgrowth mention this as a potential sign of imbalance. If this is true, it implies the candida has co-evolved with humans developing some mechanism to influence our brains and dietary choices. We may be craving the foods they need to flourish within our bodies. It only takes a small degree of skepticism to question the idea that all people with sugar cravings have yeast overgrowth. With these complex issues, though, it is by evaluating a wide variety of signs, symptoms and test results that we are nudged toward or away from a diagnosis like yeast overgrowth. I tell patients that each positive piece of information moves us closer to that diagnosis and each opposing piece backs us farther away.

The primary cause for yeast overgrowth may be antibiotics that blitz the good internal flora, but there are many other factors, including steroids, birth control pills, environmental pollutants and a devitalized American diet. The hormone progesterone has been shown to stimulate candida overgrowth. Acid blockers used for acid reflux and other gastrointestinal conditions reduce the acidity of the stomach, altering the pH. This can help to tip the balance, creating an environment more suited for candida growth.

The topic of relative acidity and alkalinity in the body is yet another that has never come up in any aspect of my medical training. I have never seen reference to it in medical journals or specialists' notes. I think it is worth attention and can be an important factor if we are to improve the whole body. Different parts of the body have different optimal pH values. The stomach needs an extremely acidic environment (with pH somewhere between 2 and 4) to function properly. The normal pH range in the colon is slightly acidic, between 5.5 and 7. Research suggests that candida will convert from a relatively benign form to a more pathogenic hyphal form with increased alkalinity of the intestines. The organism flourishes and then produces ammonia as a byproduct that increases the alkalinity further. Probiotics can tilt the balance of power with the good bacteria competing with the candida but also producing lactic and acetic acid to lower the pH back toward the normal healthy level.

Conscious Eating by Gabriel Cousens, MD, describes how to balance pH. As a means of monitoring pH, Cousens recommends a 24-hour urine test starting with the second urine of the morning and concluding with the first urine of the next day. A pH paper dipped in the urine will ideally read 6.3-6.9 for non-vegetarians and 6.3-7.2 for vegetarians. The best way to balance pH is to eat the right foods/herbs (and you may need digestive enzymes to get the benefit of the foods).[108] But you can also help alkalinize the system by using unfiltered, unpasteurized apple cider vinegar. This stimulates digestion if taken five minutes before meals. One can take a few drops in water with honey, two teaspoons of apple cider vinegar to one teaspoon honey, or two tablespoons can be taken with a meal. Cousens devotes sections to individualizing the diet.

Candida yeast is a normal inhabitant of the human gastrointestinal and genitourinary tracts. It should not be pathogenic and for most people is kept in check by a high volume of "good bacteria." If a person's internal environment shifts and the overgrowth develops, this can lead to a cascade of effects within the body. It is hypothesized in much of the alternative literature that candida can penetrate through the walls of the bowel, contributing to or causing "leaky gut syndrome." When the barrier is compromised, much material that is better off confined to the gut makes its way into the bloodstream and other tissues.

This process may explain the steady increase in food sensitivities and food intolerances and why there is so much variation of this problem among individuals. These foods making it through the unhealthy bowel into the blood stream may be the reason why one person is more sensitive to wheat and another cannot tolerate soy. The body would view these substances as foreign, provoking a response from the immune system. This would explain why some have mild reactions and others more intense. If there is a cumulative effect over time, it would explain the findings in the book *The Plan* where the average person has three or four food intolerances by the time they are around forty years old.

Tricia

I've been seeing Tricia for many years. She tends to be overweight with a body mass index over 35. She has steadily gained weight each year and developed type 2 diabetes. She has chronic headaches and chronic back pain requiring occasional prescriptions for Percocet, a controlled narcotic. She has a stressful life with two children from her first marriage and a third, from the current marriage, on the autism spectrum. Her current husband has many health issues of his own but perseveres and works hard to support the family.

Tricia, somewhat unhealthy in the big picture, got much worse relatively quickly. In July of 2012, she developed extreme fatigue and needed to sleep much of the time. Her headaches worsened. She developed severe muscle, joint and bone pain. She specifically complained about pain in her hands. There had been multiple family members with strep throat, including Tricia, one month prior to the onset of the systemic symptoms. One of the first tests I checked was an ASO, or anti-streptolysin O test, measuring antibody levels against the subtype of strep that causes throat infections.

Tricia's ASO result was extremely elevated—more than five times normal. She went on several rounds of antibiotics with the working diagnosis of a strep infection actively causing her joint and muscle pain, lethargy and other symptoms. She initially responded well, but with each round of antibiotic she had a less vigorous response. The pain responded very well to the oral steroid prednisone but worsened again when the dosage was decreased. (Oral steroids are very potent at reducing inflammation from any source, so a positive response does not typically help in clarifying the underlying cause for the inflammation.)

Tricia required strong narcotics to give her relief during the day, and that led to a number of difficult conversations regarding appropriate pain management. The desperate person will do just about anything to relieve pain. They do not necessarily care if they cause any longer term issues. Because Tricia was in steady decline and I really couldn't provide her with any concrete answers, I sent her to an excellent infectious disease specialist in the area.

His initial impression was that she had post-streptococcal arthritis. He ordered other lab tests, but there were no compelling results. Tricia's C-reactive protein (CRP), a marker of internal inflammation, was completely normal. He wanted other family members to get cultures to make sure one of the other four in the house wasn't a carrier. Tricia was put on yet another round of amoxicillin, but that did not seem to make much of a difference. The throat cultures for the other family members all came back negative. At the follow-up visit where the specialist ultimately had a "very, very long discussion" with Tricia and her husband, he still didn't seem clear on what was causing her issues but mentioned in his note it could possibly be "an active infection which could be strep or just a virus." The specialist's recommendation was to see a rheumatologist for another opinion. Tricia's husband, in particular, was frantic to get some answers and help for her. He called our office every few days to give us updates and ask what else could be done to make her more comfortable.

By the time Tricia saw the rheumatology specialist, things had progressed further and she had extreme sensitivity to touch. She was having night sweats with a cough, sinus and throat irritation as well. Rheumatologists are by their nature incredibly thorough, so the specialist went through a long series of questions. But no further clues were found. This special-ist's lab tests included some to rule out tick-borne infections and a chest x-ray to rule out the relatively rare condition of sarcoidosis. In the end, the rheumatologist did not think Tricia should be taking narcotics or steroids and recommended Tylenol, with a preliminary diagnosis of fibromyalgia/myofascial pain syndrome.

This was not much of a breakthrough. I am often frustrated when trying to manage severe pain and the specialist says the patient shouldn't be on nar-cotics. Tramadol is often recommended, which is by prescription and could be called "narcotic lite" because it works similarly but is technically in a dif-ferent class. In this case, the specialist recommended Tylenol. When I read her note, I knew I'd be getting a call within a day or two. The fibromyalgia diagnosis was just another way of saying you have muscle-based pain and we have no idea why. Good luck with that. See your primary care doctor.

At Tricia's next follow-up visit with me, I was doing an exam and Tricia stuck out her tongue. "Ahhhhh...," she said without prompt. I took one look at that tongue and, kapow, I thought I knew what was going on! Her tongue had a thick coating of whitish-brownish-grayish schmutz. It looked awful, like she had just eaten an old shoe filled with garbage. Around that time I was pursuing a crash course on yeast overgrowth, and there it was right in front of me. I sat down and discussed with her and her husband what I thought was going on.

By that point I thought yeast/fungal overgrowth was an important element of what was causing Tricia's symptoms, but I really couldn't be sure if it was the primary issue or a secondary issue. They were motivated to do just about anything. Tricia apparently did not drink water very often and lived her life in a chronically dehydrated state. She consumed above average amounts of sugar, starch and carbohydrates. I recommended making some radical changes in these areas and started her on a high-dose probiotic. I cultured her tongue and she started working on her side of it. Within a few days Tricia was remarkably improved. It seemed we were on the right track. She was able to cut back on her narcotic pain medication intake as her pain was much lower. The "scrambledness" of her head was the area that improved most dramatically.

I saw Tricia for a follow-up visit and told her that if she got better, she would always be my index case for systemic yeast. I could not know how important this would be for my practice overall. The culture of her tongue grew massive amounts of candida and a positive result came back relatively quickly. Her pain improved but persisted. Her energy improved, but she was still tired. In an unexpected turn of events, her sugars normalized over the two-week period since making the changes. She started getting low sugars so stopped both of her diabetes medications and the sugar numbers stayed in a normal, non-diabetic range. Tricia specifically commented on joint pain being worse after eating any bread or cereal with milk.

But let's not get ahead of ourselves. It was possible that being better hydrated was why she felt better. It could have been the improvements in her diet. It would be predictable that with fewer carbohydrates and less sugar in her diet, and with better hydration, her frequent hyperglycemia resolved and that was the primary reason for her improvement. Tricia's improvement could even have resulted from the probiotic, independent of any effect on yeast overgrowth. For us to really know if a yeast overgrowth problem existed and then was improved, we would have to have a reliable test to identify if she had it and when it was resolved. We would also need this to be somewhat reproducible for a larger group of people. In an ideal world, we would randomize a sample of people and have some placebo group going forward in a more rigorous test. You can see arranging this would be nearly impossible in a busy primary care office.

As with many complicated patients, Tricia improved, but for years afterward I was unable to get her symptoms completely under control. At follow-up visits I would check to make sure she was following the lifestyle recommendations and taking her probiotic and other supplements. I tried to get her in with an alternative provider, but they could not continue beyond the first visit because of cost.

At later visits we began to put together other pieces of the puzzle for Tricia. Even with negative blood tests, there was a strong possibility that she had a tick-borne illness like chronic Lyme disease. I started antibiotics and for more than a week after that she worsened with more muscle aches, joint pain and low grade fevers. This seemed to represent a Herxheimer reaction, so the likelihood was higher that she had another chronic infection contributing. On the antiobiotics, over several months, she improved but still had a variety of frustrating symptoms, including migratory muscle and joint pain, extreme debilitating fatigue and depression. It was a long process to get out of bed every morning.

At one point, I ran MTHFR testing and Tricia came up with two genetic anomalies. I started L-methylfolate, methylB12 with other B vitamins and SAMe. As has been mentioned previously, an abnormally functioning MTHFR enzyme from genetic abnormalities can lead to insufficient levels of many neurotransmitters, including serotonin, dopamine, melatonin, norepinephrine and epinephrine. The person can also have low levels of glutathione, a potent naturally-occurring antioxidant and detoxifier in the body. For the complex MTHFR pathways to work well, a process called methylation is required. I talked with Tricia and her husband about using SAMe on a regular basis because it is one of the primary donors of methyl groups. Stress from any source will use up methyl groups. From my perspective, she would need the methylated B vitamins and co-factors, but she also needed SAMe to compensate for her high level of daily stress. I told her to take between one and three of the supplements depending on how much stress she was under on a given day.

Managing her MTHFR issue may have been the breakthrough we needed. Within a month or so of adding those supplements, she began to improve. By 3-4 months her health was dramatically better. At a follow-up visit in the fall of 2014, she was vigorous and alert. Her chronic pain had mostly resolved and she no longer required prescription pain medication. It took more than two years to significantly improve Tricia's health. We had to overhaul her diet, balance her flora, improve hydration, correct yeast over-growth, suppress probable chronic Lyme disease and manage an important underlying genetic anomaly.

Rob

Rob, an astronomer, had not been feeling well for several years. It was hard for him to remember how long he had been having symptoms. He described a cyclic pattern with a one-week flare-up about once a month. He had moderate discomfort to his upper abdomen. When he had the abdominal pain, he would subconsciously rub his upper abdomen. He showed me an area where he had rubbed the hair completely off. He often had a sour taste in his mouth. He had chest pains. He described a "prickly" sensation to his legs and torso. Those sensations felt like someone was "poking [him] with needles." He would typically have flare-ups of acne as well, even though he was in his late 30s. He described bouts of dizziness and intense fatigue. He noticed a yellow film on his tongue for much of the flare-up. He could have bowel changes as well, most of them unexplained constipation. In his words: "It felt like there [was] a battle going on inside me."

Rob had the standard laboratory work-up for fatigue. This includes screening for anemia, iron deficiency, an underactive thyroid gland, and B12 deficiency. Many providers will also check a complete metabolic profile that includes kidney and liver function. The two most common causes of chronic fatigue may be chronic insomnia and obstructive sleep apnea, neither of which show up in a blood test.

Rob slept well and already had a normal sleep study ruling out sleep apnea. He had had other testing by various specialists and no one could explain his constellation of problems. He was beginning to look for a more systemic holistic explanation. We discussed the potential for fungal overgrowth and imbalance. I knew he was a scientist, so I was careful with my wording and recommended he do some reading on the subject. I also encouraged him to cut out carbs and sugar and alcohol as much as possible and then come back in a few weeks to discuss the matter further.

At the follow-up visit, he had done his homework. His wife was even more motivated and had read extensively on the issue. Rob thought the diagnosis fit and was willing to start treatment. He had not, however, made any changes to his diet yet. It can be frustrating for a provider to come up with what they feel is the path to wellness only to have the patient blow it off. A patient's level of commitment typically reflects the level of illness, but not always. Rob was unwell but skeptical and had difficulty altering his diet.

With continued encouragement he began avoiding flour, sugar and alcohol. He improved his hydration. He took a good probiotic. Within a few months Rob dramatically improved. His energy was restored and he no longer went through the cycles of intense symptoms. More than a year later, he had lost almost 50 pounds. He still had occasional flare-ups, but this related to an inconsistent diet.

One online resource, Wellness Watchers, describes a four-stage process for correcting yeast overgrowth and the related health problems: "(I) Killing the yeast overgrowth, (II) Eliminating the fuel for the growth of candida through a yeast-free diet, (III) Restoring the normal friendly bacteria in the bowel, and (IV) strengthening the immune system."[109] Often during yeast die-off the person will have a Herxheimer reaction. The parts of the organism stimulate a massive immune response and people will feel much worse for a few days or sometimes up to a few weeks. This reaction is more typically associated with blowing up the Borrelia Bergdorferi bacteria during treatment of chronic Lyme disease, but it is pertinent in any scenario where a chronic infection is being treated with antibiotics.

I remember seeing a new patient many years ago. He had heard I had some degree of open-mindedness in regards to chronic Lyme disease. By that time, he had seen just about every mainstream and alternative provider who had anything to do with chronic Lyme disease across New England, New York and New Jersey. I rattled off seven or eight of them and he had seen them all: Donta, Horowitz, Raxlen, Rothfeld, Hecht, Burrascano, Hubbuch and others. He said he didn't understand what all of the fuss was about. According to him, it was easy to figure out if someone had chronic Lyme disease: just give them a strong antibiotic against Borrelia Burgdorferi and if the person gets a lot worse, they likely have it. Even for me, this didn't seem quite reliable enough to make that elusive of a diagnosis, but he was assured.

For yeast overgrowth, the Herxheimer reaction can be very intense. I forewarn patients that they may feel much worse before they get better. If they are not aware of this phenomenon, they often assume they are having some reaction to the antifungal or antibacterial treatment. They call the office, telling one of our nurses to put the antibiotic on their allergy list because they cannot tolerate it.

Vanessa

Vanessa is a travel agent in her 50s that I have been seeing for many years. She has had a wide range of symptoms most of that time, including fatigue, joint pain, frequent headaches and cognitive deficits. She works as an executive, but for years has had problems with focus and short-term memory loss. She has even developed some dyslexia as an adult. I did a broad work-up and couldn't come up with an explanation for her diverse problems.

Vanessa was referred to a neurologist. She reported headaches most days of the week that felt to her like her head was in a vice. The specialist did a standard work-up, including an MRI of the brain. The MRI showed an abnormal focus related to either a small stroke, the effects of chronic migraines or possibly some other source. Different medications were tried but did not control her headaches very well. The neurologist was unable to explain Vanessa's particular cognitive changes so referred her for intensive neuropsychological testing.

The testing included a summary of her life going back to childhood. She reported frequently misplacing items as a child and some degree of restlessness and inattention, but nothing else significant. She managed her way through school, ultimately finishing college with a bachelor's degree in education. As part of the evaluation, it came out that she had a traumatic brain injury from a motor vehicle accident in 1987. Vanessa wondered if that was the cause for her cognitive deficits. As part of the neuropsychological testing, Vanessa did a Beck Depression Inventory-II that did not show any signs of clinical depression. She did a mini-mental status exam scoring 29 out of 30. She had some planning difficulties in the clock drawing task. The various tests ultimately confirmed a wide variety of cognitive impairments, but the psychologist could offer no explanation for why they had developed in her 50s. Early onset Alzheimer's wouldn't encompass the big picture.

Shortly after I started seeing Vanessa, I told her she might have chronic Lyme disease or some other chronic infection. I typically tell people that a diagnosis of chronic Lyme disease is very controversial. In my time, I have not seen a medical issue so divisive. The mainstream providers—which would include most infectious disease specialists at major teaching hospitals—believe either that chronic Lyme is rare or that it doesn't exist. The primary rationale for this belief is their reliance on what I believe is an utterly inferior and almost useless lab test. Time and time again, patients at an infectious disease specialist's office have been told flat out they did not have Lyme disease because the ELISA antibody titer test was negative.

The alternative world, on the other hand, would say that chronic Lyme disease is vastly under-diagnosed. "Lyme-literate" doctors say that the standard Lyme blood tests can't be trusted and that a special lab in California (Igenex) or some other labs around the country need to be used. If this is true, there is no telling how many people have been falsely diagnosed with some other chronic condition like seronegative rheumatoid arthritis or multiple sclerosis. What I have found more often in those I suspect have chronic Lyme disease is that they have struggled with symptoms for many years and have seen a wide variety of specialists with no clear diagnosis given. They see specialists in infectious disease, rheumatology, neurology, orthopedics and maybe even cardiology. The specialists can't tell them what is wrong or provide any plan for improvement. They only tell them one thing for sure: they do not have Lyme disease.

Each time I would see Vanessa, we would discuss the possibility of chronic Lyme disease. I always made it clear that I was not saying she had this problem, but that, in my opinion, it was possible. One wrinkle in all of this is that even if we confirm that a person has Lyme disease, it is not so easy to treat. I tell people the longer they have the chronic infection, the harder it is to clear up. I have treated a group of people with antibiotics, one or, more often, a combination, for up to a year or longer. Some patients have responded relatively quickly. Others have not. In the documentary "Under our Skin," a woman with advanced, debilitating chronic Lyme disease, who can barely walk because of the profound impact on her nervous system, ultimately gets better after more than two years of antibiotics.

At one visit Vanessa came in and told me she had the name of an infectious disease person specializing in Lyme disease. I had never heard of the person, but I was fully supportive. Beautiful, I told her. Make a visit and let's see what she has to say.

About a month later I saw Vanessa for a follow-up visit. I was curious about what the ID specialist had to say. Apparently, this specialist used the entire visit to get on her soapbox and harangue Vanessa about the bogusness of chronic Lyme disease. She said that doctors like me were irresponsible. She said I was in some way trying to take advantage of Vanessa. The specialist recommended she go on thyroid hormone replacement, even though her thyroid panel was normal. Sometimes, the standard thyroid level, or TSH, can be a bit misleading. Some percentage of people will have a TSH on the high side of normal and this will represent an underactive thyroid. I agreed to a trial of hormone replacement and at the next visit, a month or two later, Vanessa said her fatigue was a bit better. The other symptoms were about the same.

I had tried several times to steer Vanessa toward the alternative practitioner I use for chronic Lyme. Vanessa was somewhat reluctant in terms of the time and money that would be required to go down that path. I never push people hard to go down that road because they really have to be completely committed. They have to be prepared for the process of muscle testing which will seem bizarre and unlike anything they have encountered. They need to be ready for radical changes to their diet and recommendations for many supplements to be taken each day.

Vanessa's life went forward and I would see her occasionally. She was typically about the same. She managed reasonably well, but her quality of life was poor overall. She saw a rheumatologist and was diagnosed with fibromyalgia, but none of the prescribed medications seemed to help her chronic pain. At one visit, she seemed very positive and said things had improved. She was reluctant to talk about it because she was afraid it would jinx her success. She had seen a new neurologist who prescribed Topamax for her chronic headaches. Her headaches had nearly resolved and she was feeling better overall. I was glad the headaches were improved, but didn't feel at that time we had really uncovered the bulk of her problems. I still thought chronic Lyme disease was probable. I have seen many people with similar symptoms to Vanessa pursue therapy for chronic Lyme disease and get better.

She came in for a visit months later. The headaches were still reasonably well controlled with the Topamax, but she had severe fatigue, rashes and bowel problems. She still had a foggy head with focus problems and cognitive deficits that no one could explain. I began an investigation regarding the possibility of chronic fungal overgrowth. Vanessa consumed a lot of sugar and carbohydrates as well as regular alcohol. She was overweight. On review of systems, she was getting vaginal yeast infections with no apparent cause.

I did some blood work and, boom, her labs showed positive IgG and IgM antibodies for candida. The usual testing for an acute or chronic infection involves blood tests for antibodies. Ig is short for immunoglobulin. IgG is a type of antibody associated with a chronic infection or chronic immunity. IgM is a type of antibody associated with a recent infection or exposure. Thus, if someone has a positive IgM and a negative IgG, they are assumed to have a new infection. If they have a negative IgM and a positive IgG, this is most often chronic immunity after immunizations. But this can also correlate with a chronic infection. If the person tests positive for both anti-bodies, this can mean that they have a chronic active infection. As is often the case, these tests are not always reliable and doctors can, in my opinion, draw erroneous conclusions from positive or negative results.

Vanessa's positive IgG and IgM levels in the context of her chronic symptoms were an important finding. She would need to make some radical changes to her diet—virtually eliminating sugars, carbohydrates and alcohol. She would need high-dose, high-quality probiotics, and she might need an indef-inite course of an oral antifungal, fluconazole or nystatin. We reviewed the plan and Vanessa did not seem inclined to make the changes. She seemed skeptical that yeast overgrowth could explain her health problems. She had never heard of that problem from any of the doctors she had seen.

I did not see her for about a year after that. Once, I was walking through our waiting room and saw her sitting there, waiting for a visit with one of the other providers. She waved at me and I waved back. "Vanessa..." she said meekly. "You remember me?" Yes, of course, I remembered her. She stood out because she was a kind, hard-working person lost in a medical system that could not get her well. Some time after that, shortly after reading one of David Brownstein's thyroid books, I saw Vanessa's husband for a physical. He told me she was still struggling with many of her chronic symptoms. I asked him to have her set up a follow-up visit with me so we could do a more thorough work-up of her thyroid function. Between the time I saw her husband and the time she came in for the visit, I had worked my way through most of the Horowitz book on chronic Lyme disease.

At that visit she started by saying that her chronic asthma was well-con-trolled. She wanted to focus on the positives first. She believed in the power of the mind to enhance the positives and suppress any negative issues. Her pulmonologist had her on a twice-a-day, high-dose inhaled steroid that kept her from developing bronchitis. (I didn't mention that the steroid could be exacerbating an underlying yeast overgrowth problem.) In other areas, she wasn't doing as well. Her "fibromyalgia" continued to flare-up intermittently with moderately intense muscle and joint pain. She was using OTC Tylenol PM to help with insomnia. Her memory problems were getting progressively worse. She said there were times when she would go to a store and then couldn't remember how to get out of the parking lot.

Vanessa also had a new pattern of symptoms to discuss. For a few weeks before the visit with me, she would have one or two days a week where she would wake up with an intense headache. It would start in the morning and last all day. On those days she would cry for no reason and had more difficulty with her focus. It was almost impossible to work. She said she was "in a black hole" and any negative thoughts she might normally have were more prominent. She would think repeatedly about what would happen to her husband and her business if she died. I told her about the Horowitz book. I thought it made more sense that she had chronic Lyme, chronic yeast overgrowth and thyroid dysfunction with other areas that needed attention.

She then mentioned for the first time an incident back in the late 1980s. She was walking on Crane's Beach in Ipswich, Massachusetts, with a close friend and found a tick on her body a few days later. She developed a red, swollen area on her right thigh. She saw a doctor who told her it was an allergic reaction of some sort and should resolve without treatment. She couldn't be sure, but wondered in retrospect if the majority of her chronic symptoms started around that time. This was our 30th visit together and we had discussed the possibility of chronic Lyme before on multiple occasions, but I had never questioned her about specific tick exposures. I assumed she would have mentioned any tick encounters of significance. She also said that the friend she was walking with on that fateful day developed a flu-like illness shortly afterwards. He joked back then that spending time with her apparently made him ill. Vanessa told me that, to this day, he suffers from chronic headaches, fatigue and muscle pain. Her friend has seen many doctors and was diagnosed with fibromyalgia but none of the standard treatments seemed to help.

I had Vanessa do the questionnaire from page 35 of the Horowitz book. The results were dramatic. She scored "Mild" for the symptoms of unexplained weight gain, swollen glands, chest pain, blurry vision, vertigo and disorientation. She scored "Moderate" for changes in bowels, joint pain, muscle cramps, neck stiffness, lightheadedness, confusion, difficulty with concentration, forgetfulness and mood swings. She scored "Severe" for fatigue, back pain and headaches. Horowitz says that a score over 46 represents a "high probability of a tick-borne disorder." Vanessa scored 60 points.

As of the writing of this book, I am just starting the process of trying to sort our Vanessa's problems. I feel we can get her well again with the help of the Horowitz book, but it will be a long, arduous process. An update on Vanessa's path to wellness will have to come in my next book.

14

Polypharmacy

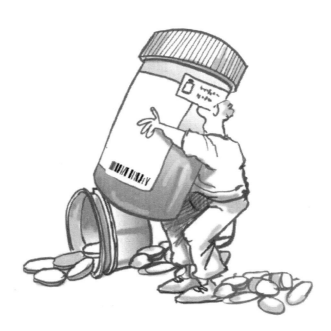

Over the past 100 years in America, we have become increasingly dependent on pharmaceuticals to manage our problems. This is embedded in our culture now. Like a vine that has wrapped itself around us, insinuating itself into every crevice, we are under the spell of prescription drugs. It is hard to imagine a world of health without pharmaceuticals at the center.

The Capital Steps song "Take Ten Pills" says it all:
Round like a circle that is forming, made of television ads
More and more I see the warning of the conditions I might have
I have countless new disorders that have finally been revealed
I have dry eye, spastic bladder and that one with Sally Field
I take drugs for every syndrome, I'm like a powder keg
When I kick my spouse at bedtime, now I claim it's restless leg
If your health is in decline
Just take ten pills and you're fine
Like the lithium I'm taking with a dose of estrogen
Mixed with Demerol and Prozac, now I've got hair on my chin
Son's on Ritalin and Bextra, we thought he had ADD
But it turns out that the whole time he is just an SOB
I need Ambien, Lunesta, to help me sleep allright
'Cause Levitra and Cialis keep my husband up all night
If your life's as bad as mine
At least ten pills come to mind
Lasix, Cruex, Metamucil, Celebrex and Naproxen
Then I take a few Vytorin that I wash down with some gin
Now my ears are always ringing, I think Lipitor's to blame
There's no reason that I take it, I just really like the name
I mix Lidocaine with high balls, and the side effects were queer
I was hearing through my eyeballs, and I'm tasting through my rear
And that giant nose of Claritin is something I must try
And I take Ginkgo Biloba, but can't remember why
So I quit those pills cold turkey, it was all a big mistake
And I swear there is no supplement or medicine I'll take
And though lately I have found, though depressed and feeling down
Thanks to Botox I can't frown[110]

There are many reasons why we are overly reliant on medications. I am referring not just to prescriptions, but also to many of the over-the-counter options as well. This is big business with billions of dollars involved and many standing to gain or lose, including drug companies, pharmacies and doctors.

As I have mentioned before, much of medical training involves the memorization of hundreds of different medications. Budding doctors and other healthcare providers have to learn the brand name, generic name, dosages, potential side effects and the potential interactions with other medications. We have multiple pharmaceutical options for just about every condition or symptom imaginable. No wonder there is so little time spent on nutrition and other non-pharmacologic options. There is so much drug information to learn that the idealistic medical student doesn't have any time to spend on the wishy-washy alternative options. We may not understand what causes or cures the condition, but we have three, five or even ten medications we can try that may or may not work, that may have side effects, and that may work but you need to be on them for life.

There is often a certain degree of laziness involved here as well, both for the patient and often for the healthcare provider. For the person with heartburn, the doctor can go into details of their lifestyle and investigate barriers to change, or they can just give them a script for Prilosec. The patient can cut back on coffee, stop having pepperoni pizza and lose 10 pounds, or they can just take Prilosec. The drug prescription makes for a relatively quick visit and it helps a busy primary care provider plow through twenty or more patients per day. I can imagine most PCPs have this regular internal debate: "Well, I can spend five minutes explaining why I think the infection is probably viral and why an antibiotic won't help, or I can save the five minutes, give this patient the antibiotic, and send them home satisfied."

With the growing scarcity of primary care providers and the growing need for cost-effective, high-quality primary care, there are going to be more and more patients seeking out a smaller and smaller group of doctors. This trend will only put more pressure on PCPs to see more people. It is a nice concept to close off the patient panel and have lots of time for a relatively small group, but there is a high demand. People need to be seen somewhere.

Another contributor to overprescribing is the dreaded "standard of care." Whenever you read "standard of care", I want you to imagine it being said by a deep male voice like the almighty God in *Monty Python and the Holy Grail.* The cartoon God's jaw drops slightly out of sync with his words. This standard of care is the assumed standard by which a primary care provider or any other doctor would be judged, notably in a court of law. If a doctor is sued and the case goes to court, expert witnesses are often brought in to give their opinion about how the doctor involved diverged from the standard of care.

Most doctors working in a practice have an undercurrent of fear that pervades every decision they make and affects how they document each visit. Almost every day we see people who could have an important acute medical problem or serious chronic diagnosis. It is presumed that doing lots of tests and prescribing lots of medications will lower the provider's risk of being sued. At least we did something, and that has to be better than doing nothing. Right?

We could go through just about every class of medication prescribed and it would be easy to show that most, if not all, are over-utilized. An IMS report from 2010 lists the top ten prescriptions in America by volume. (I will review the top ten by cost in the "Cost of Doing Business" chapter.) When drugs are studied, the pharmaceutical industry almost always presents the results in terms of relative risk reduction. This is no coincidence. It is the easiest way to come up with a positive conclusion.

If taking a certain medication reduces the rate of stroke from ten out of one billion to seven out of one billion, the stroke risk has gone down by 30%. A much better way to summarize clinical studies is the Number Needed to Treat (NNT). This tells us how many people have to take the medication for a certain period of time to prevent one bad outcome. In the preposterous stroke example just noted, the NNT would be 333 million, meaning that many people would have to take the medication to prevent one stroke. Doesn't sound quite as good as saying the stroke risk is reduced by 30%.

If our political leaders truly represented us, they could mandate that drug companies publish all of their studies, not just the ones that show benefit. There are many people currently addressing this issue, including *Overdosed America* author John Abramson, MD. In a reasonable healthcare system we would have an independent researcher review the statistics. They would present the results in many ways, including NNT. The government has recently compelled credit card companies to give more information regarding how long it would take to pay off a bill if the person only paid the minimum. Is this so different?

The Prescription Hit Parade

Which medications are prescribed the most? *Opioids*, including Vicodin, are among the most popular. In 2010, there were 131 million prescriptions given for opioids. We are not managing pain well if our primary solution is a narcotic. This also reflects, of course, the epidemic of prescription drug abuse.

Statins were the second most prescribed medication type in 2010 at 94 million prescriptions. I think statins do have a place in American medicine: for selected individuals they reduce risk, typically in the setting of secondary prevention. I do think, however, we have lost our way when it comes to managing the most important health problem—cardiovascular health. Somewhere deep in the recesses of the American brain is the idea that we're free and we can do whatever we want. The scientists and the doctors will take care of us. They will always come up with some new medication or procedure to keep us fat and happy. Wrong.

On a positive note, there do seem to be a number of trends toward improving lifestyle. Many health insurance companies are utilizing wellness coaches to work with people over the phone. This will help supplement the efforts of busy primary care providers if done well. More and more employers are focusing resources on keeping their workers healthy. They have their own doctors and nurse practitioners. They are checking blood pressures and running lab tests. They are carving out time for people to exercise at the gym down the hall. The employees have monetary incentives if they can meet certain wellness goals. If this trend continues, it should have a tremendous impact on prevention. Regular exercise significantly improves the functioning of the immune systems.

Numbers 3, 5 and 10 on the list of most-prescribed pharmaceuticals are all *medications for hypertension.* They are ace inhibitors, norvasc/amlodipine (a type of calcium channel blocker) and thiazide diuretics, respectively. For years I thought that hypertension was perhaps the one and only area where medications may be under-prescribed in America. The standard for blood pressure may be loosening, however, to 150/90 for those over 60 years old. It may turn out that blood pressure is also overmanaged, especially in older patients.

It is estimated that one out of three Americans has hypertension, and the incidence goes up steadily with age. There is a familial aspect as well. I have seen many patients in their 40s with superb lifestyles and low BMIs (body mass indexes) starting to get borderline numbers. They are, of course, frustrated by the idea that despite their best efforts their blood pressure may still go up and medication will be recommended. The stakes are too high to ignore, however, as poorly controlled hypertension is the number one risk factor for stroke and a major risk factor for heart attack. In addition, it plays a major role in chronic kidney disease.

The order of these antihypertensives is somewhat telling. In a fantasy world of cost-conscious, effective healthcare, the diuretic would be the most commonly prescribed medication in this class. One of the rare times the federal government actually did a study with benefit in primary care took place in 2002. The National Heart Lung and Blood Institute (NHLBI) ran a study called The Antihypertensive and Lipid-Lowering Treatment to Prevent Heart Attack Trial or ALLHAT. This study used the gold standard of being a randomized, double-blind, multi-center clinical trial. It was, at that time, the largest clinical trial conducted, with 42,418 participants over 55 years old followed for over five years. Researchers compared several classes of antihypertensive including the calcium channel blocker amlodipine, the ace inhibitor lisinopril, the alpha blocker doxazosin, and the runt of the litter, the thiazide diuretic chlorthalidone. In the end, they were all comparable in terms of controlling blood pressure and lowering risk of heart attack and stroke.

The best medication is no medication, but if one were to conjure up the ideal medication, it would be the thiazide diuretic. It only needs to be taken once a day. There are minimal, if any, side effects. It is extremely effective and, maybe best of all, is incredibly inexpensive—it typically costs under $5 per month. It is one of the few bargains in American medicine today.

The study came out in 2002 but it wasn't until 2010 that the thiazide diuretics squeaked their way into the top ten of all prescription drugs. For those zealots of evidence-based medicine, why didn't this hard evidence change the prescribing practices of America's physicians? It is extremely difficult to get people to change what they do. This may be especially true of a western-trained physician who is expected to have all the answers. A person will accept certain ideas as fact. It makes life much more difficult to have to always question everything.

On a side note, the one clear scenario where the hypertensive person may be overtreated is when they have underlying obstructive sleep apnea. There are millions and millions of Americans with undiagnosed sleep apnea. (See the Pulmonary chapter "Breathing Room for the Spirit"). For many of them, if we managed their sleep apnea, they might be able to get off of the medications that lower their blood pressure.

The fourth most prescribed medication is the family of pharmaceuticals used for *thyroid replacement*. These came in at 70.5 million prescriptions written. The alternative world offers many options for managing an underactive thyroid gland without prescription medication, including iodine supplementation, natural thyroid replacement and dietary change. David Brownstein, MD, outlines alternative options very well in *Overcoming Thyroid Dysfunction*.

In her book *The Plan*, Lyn-Genet Recitas offers a non-prescription approach to boosting thyroid function. I am increasingly optimistic about the ideas her book offers and feel these could have a major impact on my patients' chronic health issues. I wish I were independently wealthy. I fantasize about being able to fund well-done studies that would answer some of these questions that bridge the mainstream and alternative worlds of health. What if millions of women could control their thyroid with dietary changes and supplements? What if a study showed that Brownstein's and Recitas' approaches were more successful at managing related symptoms and thyroid blood levels than the status quo? It could change the way we manage this chronic problem. Bill and Melinda Gates, where are you?

Coming in at sixth on the hit parade are the blockbuster medications *proton pump inhibitors*. Americans filled over 50 million prescriptions for these medications in 2010. Let's give 'em a big hand. I have reviewed my concerns and frustrations with these medications in earlier pages. It was estimated in the IMS report that twenty percent of Americans get heartburn at least once a week. Supersize everything and fill the stomach with lots of mediocre food and what happens? It backs up! Your poor stomach can't handle all of that. Some of the partially digested food will go downstream into the small intestine, but much will go back the other way. There are really only two ways for it to go.

The next two medications by volume are both antibiotics, Zithromax at number 7 and amoxicillin at number 8. In terms of antibiotics, we're doing better but we are still using them in excess. I have seen estimates as high as

98% in terms of what percentage of coughs, colds and sore throats are viral vs. bacterial. Over 90% of ear infections resolve without antibiotics. Over 90% of bronchitis is viral with no response to antibiotics. We now know that the majority of sinus infections resolve without antibiotics as well. In terms of these sorts of infections, we basically have bacterial pneumonia and strep throat left.

In 2011, antidepressants were the group with the most prescriptions, but none of them individually got into the top ten. These include sertraline (Zoloft), paroxetine (Paxil), fluoxetine (Prozac), citalopram (Celexa), venlexafine (Effexor) and buproprion (Wellbutrin). Some of the SSRI benefit for depression may be placebo effect. In my experience, the SSRI medications are very effective for chronic anxiety. They are almost certainly more effective for generalized anxiety disorder than they are for depression. This does not mean, however, that lifelong medication is necessarily the best answer. My sense, at this point in my career, is that by identifying and managing genetic MTHFR abnormalities we may be able to manage chronic mental health issues at a deeper, more profound level.

OTC Options

We shouldn't let our friends hucking OTC (over-the-counter) medications get out of this either. There was a study done years ago where participants took each and every cough medication they could find in the local pharmacy.[111] This included Delsym, Triaminic and all 14 varieties of Robitussin. When the average person goes down the cough and cold medication aisle, they can't help but think what a great country we live in where we have so many options. But if you read labels for most OTC medications, it doesn't take long to realize there are usually only a few different active ingredients that have been put together in every possible combination.

In the above study, not one of the OTC options purported to help with cough was more effective than placebo. The only cough medicine more effective than placebo was a prescription syrup with codeine. Yet Americans spent 4.2 billion dollars on OTC cough and cold remedies in 2011. This is one of the great unknown shams perpetuated on the American people.

I see many patients on three, four, five or more prescription medications. Some take ten or more. For those on more than 10, we would need a supercomputer to sort out all of the potential interactions. I don't intend to be critical of other providers, since many of these medications are also prescribed by me. It gets tricky, however, as people age and experience a growing number of medical issues. My path is to find better alternatives to pharmaceuticals and gradually work back off the polypharmacy gravy train.

Many elderly people have a stable of physicians looking after them. The minimum is usually the primary care doctor, dentist, eye doctor, orthopedist and dermatologist. Each provider, other than the dentist, is managing their own organ system and prescribing medications. Like most PCPs I am reluctant to change or micromanage another doctor's stuff. Over the years I have been prescribing less and less of just about every pharmaceutical, yet the polypharmacy just keeps on rolling.

There have been a few times when I thought a person was overmedicated and took matters into my own hands. In my practice I see a lot of patients from group homes. The people that live in these homes have an incredible diversity of intellectual, physical and social disabilities. Their limitations affect their ability to advocate for themselves. Many of these patients are nonverbal or minimally verbal. Most are unable to give much if any history. This makes it challenging both to come up with an accurate diagnosis and to manage their health well.

One of my favorite group home patients is Ben, now in his 70s. Ben has come a long way from when I first saw him in the office. He was a victim of polypharmacy and, like many group home patients, overmedicated. Ben has mental health issues in addition to other chronic medical problems. Because patients like Ben are unable to give detailed histories, my impression is that many of them are loosely diagnosed by psychiatry. If someone has a labile mood, they might be diagnosed with bipolar. If someone is sleeping a lot during the day, they must have major chronic depression.

For the first several years I was seeing Ben, he was drowsy and often confused. He was confined to a wheelchair. I noticed repeatedly that he was on a variety of psychotropic medications with high likelihood of the side effect of drowsiness or fatigue. I sent his psychiatrist a note a couple of times politely requesting we cut back on some of Ben's medication. The primary care doctor questioning the almighty specialist does not always go well, especially given I have little or no personal contact with the specialists that I send people to. They could be mild mannered and reasonable or they could be egomaniacal tyrants.

Ben's psychiatrist told the group home staff that he did not want to reduce or eliminate any medications because he was worried that the patient's behavior would worsen. To the credit of the staff that worked with Ben every day, they eventually came to me and said they didn't care if the behavior got worse. They said they were willing to deal with it and could always increase the doses if Ben really got out of control.

I began reducing Ben's psychiatric medications. I did this on my own because, to me, the quality of life of the patient was more important than my stepping on the toes of another physician. At each successive follow-up visit, he was more alert and interactive. His personality came out more and more. He wasn't a lump sitting in the chair waiting for his next meal. It turned out he is quite the womanizer. He has the roving eye and will gawk at just about any female nearby. He is a master of flattery, always with a nice compliment for the ladies. The nurses in my office now know to shoo him away as he tries to kiss the back of their hands.

The most touching moment came when Ben went to his younger sister's birthday party. She had been very involved with him for most of his life and they were close. She had gradually grown to accept his relatively poor quality of life. At the party, Ben had improved to the point where he was out of the wheel chair. He walked in and it was the first time his sister had seen him walk in over 10 years.

15

The Cost of Doing Business

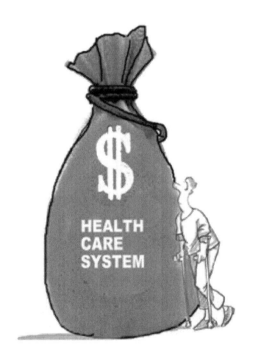

To state the obvious, Americans spend too much on healthcare. Most have read reports that we spend much more than any other industrialized nation on earth. Despite this, the U.S. tends to be toward the middle or bottom of the spectrum on what many agree is the most important measure of health. In 2010, healthcare in America cost an estimated $2.6 trillion dollars. This is a staggering sum of money. Like the national debt, the higher these numbers get, the harder it is to appreciate. To put it in perspective, we spend about $8,000 per year for each man, woman and child. The average charge for someone to be in the hospital is $18,000 per discharge. This is unsustainable. This is also not a liberal or a conservative issue. Healthcare costs are choking everyone—individuals, small business owners, and corporations as well as local, state and federal government.

Healthcare dollars are largely spent in three areas: hospital care (31%), physician and clinical services (28%), and pharmaceuticals (10%). Many have analyzed ways to save money in our current system. My own perspective of cost savings, relative to primary care, follows.

I would argue that an important yet underappreciated aspect of being a good primary care physician is having some consideration for expenses. There are many ways that a primary care physician can reduce costs. Any service that a primary care physician does well in lieu of specialty care is reducing cost. Any visit that can be made in a primary care environment, rather than an emergency department, is saving money. Specialists are paid more overall, but there is also a fundamentally different philosophy when it comes to evaluating the patient.

The specialist is the end of the line and likely feels considerable pressure to make a correct diagnosis. For this reason they often order extensive tests. The textbook example of this is the rheumatology consult. Due to the complexity of the patients they see, rheumatologists typically order several pages of blood tests and a series of x-rays. I am in no way criticizing specialists for over-ordering tests, since they are working hard to make what is often an elusive diagnosis. Assuming there are competent primary care physicians, the specialists get only the most challenging cases.

In the current CYA (cover your you-know-what) health environment, even specialist referrals are very often CYA. There are four main reasons why I personally utilize specialists. The first is CYA. A patient with rate-controlled atrial fibrillation on the blood thinner Coumadin, who is asymptomatic with perfect blood pressure, may be well managed, but the standard of care is for that person to see a cardiologist on a regular basis. There are, in fact, many chronic medical conditions where it is the standard of care for the person to be followed by a specialist.

"Dr. Lenhardt" An imaginary lawyer approaches me on the stand. "Your patient with asthma had an attack that caused them to be admitted to the ICU. Did you consider consulting a pulmonologist?"

"No." Here, I think he's trying to trick me. If I say I considered it, then I clearly made the wrong choice by ultimately choosing not to. If I say I didn't consider it, then I may be a flake, but I didn't actually make an error in medical decision-making.

"Which type of specialist," the lawyer presses forward, "would you consider to be the expert in asthma management?"

"Um, a pulmonologist."

"Yes, I agree. So, you are aware that a pulmonologist is an expert in asthma? Do you think you know more than a pulmonologist when it comes to asthma?"

"No, I guess not."

"Well then, why wouldn't you consult one? Wouldn't it seem to be in the best interest of your patient to get the best advice possible?"

The next reason for a specialist consult is that I am stumped regarding a diagnosis or an effective option for management. The third is that they can do a test or a procedure of which I am not capable. The fourth is the patient requests the visit to get a second opinion. Primary care physicians certainly need a wide variety of specialists to help provide quality care across the board, but if we eliminated the pure CYA reason, it would save on expenses.

Emergency Department Costs

Emergency department (ED)/emergency room (ER) charges will almost always be more costly. The Health Care Cost Institute noted that the average cost for an ED visit in America in 2010 was $1,327. The same year, the average cost for a primary care visit was $86. This is obviously a bit of apples and oranges, but I will go through a number of consecutive ED visits below to try and see how much could be saved if primary care access were improved.

On the anecdotal side of things, I'll never forget one of my first experiences working in the ED as a medical student. I saw a young woman who had a sore throat and cough for a few days. I presented the case to the attending physician, saying it was likely viral, but a rapid strep test was probably a good idea and, if negative, she could be sent home. I remember thinking the strep test was probably unnecessary, but I wanted to make a good impression.

The attending physician chuckled softly, putting his hand on my shoulder as if I had made a joke. "Oh, no. We'll do a urine pregnancy test, complete blood count, chest x-ray, and then, if it's all normal, send her home with a z-pak [antibiotic]." Ah, the naive medical student.

To reduce ED visits, primary care providers should keep up with the cultural trends. There are 5:30 a.m. spinning classes and evening/weekend master's degrees. I would argue that to ask a primary care provider to work early mornings, weeknights and weekends should be incentivized by the insurance industry. The trend toward 24-hour walk-in clinics is a step in the right direction.

I read a review that estimated only five percent of ED visit were unnecessary. It would seem the person that did the study probably had some angle, some inherent bias, because that seems to be a dramatic underestimate. As an exercise, I looked at notes from 20 consecutive ER visits that came across my desk over 3-4 weeks:

1. 13-year-old with a viral syndrome
2. 40-year-old with shoulder injury, negative x-rays
3. 35-year-old with knee injury, negative x-rays
4. 82-year-old with aspiration pneumonia, admitted to the hospital
5. 21-year-old with chest pain and shortness of breath, normal work-up including CXR and EKG
6. 17-year-old female with flank pain and fever, ruled out for a kidney infection
7. 39-year-old female with intermittent fast heart rate or "tachycardia" for a couple of months
8. 62-year-old female with underlying coronary artery disease complaining of chest pains
9. 25-year-old with a fall and a forehead laceration

10. 83-year-old with dementia with increasing agitation and combative behavior

11. 3-year-old with severe abdominal pains; CT scan showed constipation but transferred into Boston to rule out a rare, serious condition called a volvulus; ultimately found to be constipation alone

12. 31-year-old group home patient with scalp laceration related to self-injurious behavior

13. 57-year-old female with a bacterial skin infection of the right arm cellulitis with negative testing for a more important type of cellulitis caused by the resistant bacteria MRSA (pronounced "Mursa")

14. 2-year-old with influenza and secondary pneumonia

15. 59-year-old with change in mental status admitted with delirium secondary to lobar pneumonia

16. 55-year-old male with a neck strain

17. 37-year-old male with testicular pain after a fall

18. 48-year-old male with chest pain, part of a recurring pattern of chest pain that had already been thoroughly worked up; no serious cause identified

19. 49-year-old wheelchair-bound group home member with mental retardation, cough and fever; found to have left lower lobe pneumonia

20. 52-year-old female with history of brain tumor and epilepsy with change in mental status and dizziness

I would propose breaking down ED visits into three categories. The first is a true emergency or a situation with a genuine likelihood of an emergency. These are the visits that belong in an ED and are what EDs are designed for. Of the 20 cases just listed, I'd say only six fall into this category: the 82-year-old with pneumonia, the 62-year-old with chest pain, the 83-year-old with change in mental status, the 3-year-old with severe abdominal pain, the 59-year-old with delirium and pneumonia, and the 52-year-old with a brain tumor.

The next category is judgment calls. The ED serves a genuine role in these cases but, as they are not technically emergencies, the person ideally would have been seen either that day or the next in a primary care office. Of the twenty, I would put seven in this category.

The last category is the cases that absolutely do not belong in an emergency department. They are the domain of the "worried well" and a waste of the taxpayer's money. This would include the viral syndrome, the shoulder and knee injuries, the 17-year-old with flank pain, the cellulitis case, the neck strain and the testicular pain. These total seven out of 20.

Not everyone would agree with how I triaged this group of 20, but the overall point would be the same. There is no doubt that the percentage of inappropriate visits to an ED is relatively high. I am not necessarily besmirching the good people who usually have no idea what is emergent, urgent or commonplace. My point, overall, is that if we expanded access to primary care and minute clinics, it would save the U.S. a tremendous amount of money.

In 2009, the CDC ran statistics for emergency departments in America. The total number of ED visits that year was 136.1 million. The average ED visit cost $1,327. Of these visits, 12.6% of the patients were admitted to the hospital.

In my hometown estimates above, 30% were true emergencies, 35% were reasonable for the ER but not true emergencies, and 35% did not belong in the ER at all. I would say these 20 patients are fairly representative of the ER notes I review in my office. If we were just to keep out the third category (assuming the 35% is close and a differential of $1,327 to $86 average charge), the estimated savings would be just over $55 billion dollars. If we really expanded non-urgent provider availability, then 70% of the visits would be unnecessary. In 2009 dollars, this represents a potential savings of $116 billion dollars.

Now, some of you may have already spotted several flaws in this scenario. The first is that we are facing a shortage of primary care providers, so to expand access to PCPs is next to impossible. Even if there were financial incentives for providers to work nights and weekends, there is a large void to fill. A move in this direction is also dependent on patients having a clearer understanding of protocol. Patients would discuss the borderline cases with some provider and then follow the recommendations. If I'm talking to someone on the phone and they tell me they want to go to the ER, I don't often tell them they can't go. Finally, the cases that were less emergent probably have lower costs, so it really isn't reasonable to use the $1,327 average charge for those. Even with all of these flaws to the scheme there are billions of dollars to be saved if we improve the system.

Pharmaceutical Inflation

Pharmaceuticals are a massive contributor to excessive costs in the system. In 2010, it was estimated that 18% of all healthcare costs were from pharmaceuticals. In a report by IMS for 2010, they listed the top drugs in terms of cost. For the first time ever, all of the top ten prescription drugs by volume were generics. Obviously, none of the medications with the highest costs were generic. This sounds encouraging, but the cost savings from drugs going generic did not keep up with cost increases from new name-brand options.

One of my greatest frustrations in medicine is that we seem to realize most of the negatives of capitalism with very few of the positives. In the capitalist model profit is the primary motivation. It's hard to argue that profit is not a major player in American medicine. Everyone is clambering to get a piece of the pie. We often spend more than double what other industrialized countries in the world spend, yet we are not near the top in the most relevant measures of health, like longevity.

There are many positives of capitalism and you would think that the American healthcare system would be more efficient. Wrong. We probably have one of the least efficient healthcare systems in the world due to our exorbitant administrative costs.

You would think that capitalism would spur great innovation. In the area of new pharmaceuticals and medical devices, this is almost certainly true. The drug development angle, though, is a bit of a scam. The pharmaceutical industry often says it has to charge so much in order to fund research for the next great medication. With respect, they inflate their research numbers by adding marketing expenses, like drug reps hawking medications to unsuspecting physicians. The industry also comes up with many drugs annually with little or no real impact on health. This would include the 6th proton pump inhibitor or the 10th ace inhibitor or the 7th statin. Newer is almost never better, just much more costly.

There are times when the industry does come up with some novel medication that has a dramatic impact on health in America. I would put Singulair on that list. Singulair came out over 15 years ago but, to this day, is often not covered by most insurance companies. I would also put Chantix on that list.

This drug for smoking cessation is completely different from anything that came before it and, if people can tolerate it, is probably the best option for quitting. There are many chemotherapeutic agents that have had dramatic effects for cancer patients. For those drugs and a few others, I have no problem with the pharmaceutical company making a few hundred million.

Perhaps the main way that capitalism could work well in healthcare is by keeping costs down by way of some good old-fashioned competition. Why do gas stations have prices within a few cents of one another? Competition. Why do most of the cereals in the grocery store have similar prices? Competition. The more competition, the lower the prices and the more razor thin the profit margin. But competition in healthcare is a myth.

Take proton pump inhibitors, for example. For many years these included Prilosec, Nexium (its evil twin), Prevacid, Protonix and Aciphex. The pharmaceutical industry does not tend to do head-to-head trials which would produce a winner and a loser. In our healthcare system they can all be winners. Plenty to go around. So, with no head-to-head trials we can assume that the proton pump inhibitors are probably roughly comparable. Aciphex had the lowest market share year after year. Now, wouldn't you think that in a normal capitalist model the makers of Aciphex would cut the price to increase market share? You don't need a master's in economics to figure that one out. They don't, though. All of the companies charge a high price for their PPIs, somewhere over $80/month.

A fundamental factor in healthcare that changes the ethical landscape is that there are four major players, not two. In a regular free-market situation there is the producer and the consumer. The consumer chooses which item to buy based on price, quality and other factors. In medicine, it's primarily the physician that makes most of the decisions for the patient. The insurance company pays the bulk of the bill. The pharmaceutical company will charge as much as possible with little or no competitive pricing, while the drug reps take care of lunch, dinner, sports tickets, gifts, trips and anything else. The conflict of interest seems obvious. Yet many physicians would say, "Oh, just because the rep takes me out to Morton's for Caesar salad, martinis, prime rib and flourless chocolate cake doesn't mean I will prescribe the medication more often."

We cannot generalize this effect to all individuals, but studies done on this issue show that the more the reps spend on the doctor, the more they can shift the doctor's prescribing habits. What most people, and even most physicians, don't realize is that the drug companies pay the pharmacies for information on what doctors are prescribing. They can do a very simple analysis: I gave Dr. Smith two tickets to the Red Sox for a charge of $200 and his prescribing of Viagra went up 85% for the two months after that (for a net gain of $14,500).

Let's go through the top ten drugs in terms of price:

1. Lipitor ($7.2 billion in sales): Since this study was done, Lipitor has gone generic. Thus, it is appropriately a first line option with simvastatin, the generic for Zocor.

2. Nexium ($6.3 billion): Proton pump inhibitor. It works well but is really only generic omeprazole at double the dose. There are often better alternatives to chronic stomach acid suppression.

3. Plavix ($6.1 billion): There is benefit after a heart attack so plavix is probably worth the hefty price for up to 12 months after the event. Other than that, it is barely more effective than aspirin. Plavix is over $3 per pill while aspirin is a mere four cents per tablet.

4. Advair ($4.7 billion): The problem with Advair is two-fold. It is effective for asthma, as both treatment and prevention, but it should have gone generic many years ago. To still make 4.7 billion is an affront to the American people. The second issue is that there is scant evidence for its benefit in COPD, the chronic lung disease usually associated with long-term smoking. I remember the studies being done when I was in residency in the late 1990s. That there is only mediocre benefit has been mostly ignored.

5. Abilify ($4.6 billion): This medication is an antipsychotic and, for the most part, was developed for schizophrenia. The problem for the pharmaceutical industry is there are not enough schizophrenics to keep the money flowing. It has been successfully promoted for the management of bipolar and, in my experience, can be beneficial. It is also pushed for depressed patients with irritability or agitation. This is, in my opinion, a bit of a stretch.

6. Seroquel ($4.4 billion): This is used in several mental health scenarios but also to help people sleep. There are many ways to address insomnia without medication, yet too often we resign ourselves to medications for this problem. When prescription medications are used, it would be more ideal to use them for a short time or only occasionally. Many prescription

options for sleep are as effective as Seroquel and much less expensive for the cost-conscious.

7. Singulair ($4.1 billion): As I have mentioned, this is an excellent medication, effective with minimal side effects, but it should have gone generic many years ago.

8. Crestor ($3.8 billion): This newest statin is powerful but unnecessary as there is no evidence that it is more effective or offers fewer side effects than the generic simvastatin. Crestor lowers cholesterol numbers at lower doses, but that's just smoke and mirrors. What would make Crestor worth the cost is if it significantly lowered the risk of heart attack and stroke more than the other statins. It likely doesn't so really has no business being prescribed at all.

9. Actos ($3.5 billion): Typically a third-line agent for type 2 diabetes, its days may be numbered as its cousin Avandia (with a similar mechanism of action) has already been shown to significantly increase the risk of congestive heart failure.

10. Epogen ($3.3 Billion): Used to stimulate red blood cell production idin people with cancer, especially if undergoing chemotherapy. Epogen has some value in those with anemia related to advanced chronic kidney disease. No argument from me, this medication was a major development. But I fear it will remain expensive for my grandchildren.

Generics are obviously important in keeping pharmaceutical costs down, so I am pleased to note the trend away from the bogus medicines conjured up by the pharmaceutical industry that bolster their revenue but offer no real impact on health or wellness. We desperately need evidence-based comparison studies, but the only group with the funds to do the research is the one with no incentive to do so. There is an unstated agreement between the pharmaceutical industry and the American people: develop new drugs and maximize profit for a period of time, then slip quietly away so the generic drugs can be made to lower health care costs. Yet there are many examples of where this trust has been broken.

The first questionable strategy is when the drug companies take a successful drug that is going generic and flip the molecule around or isolate its mirror image to create a new drug. This bit of chemical hocus pocus probably requires some intense lobbying with strategic campaign contributions. I would love to be a member of whatever group decides whether to allow a new pharmaceutical to be considered a new and unique drug that can stand alone. Here's me on that board…

The representative from the drug company starts his presentation: "So, we've come to present Zyxovox, a new drug to help people resolve hang-nails more quickly." You need a lot of z's and x's these days to have a winner. "Our research has shown that 1% of people with hangnails will have them clear 15 minutes earlier when compared to placebo." At this point the rep is really just going through the motions because he and his company have never had a new medication turned down before.

"Denied!" I say, slamming down my gavel. "Next."

"What?" The rep is dumbfounded. "What do you mean 'denied'?"

"I mean your new drug is ridiculous on so many levels that I'm denying you the opportunity to fleece the American people of millions of dollars."

"Now wait just a minute…"

"Your new medication, all x'ed and z'd out, is practically identical to the one you're replacing. It has minimal benefit for a minor problem. You only created it because your old blockbuster will be going generic next year. You must think we're pretty thick to approve that drug. Goodbye."

The rep raises a hand in objection. "But this is America. People should have the right to any medications available. It's not proper for you to choose for them."

This is true and there is a right to free speech. As with most things, however, we need to find the proper balance for these issues of health and economics.

One example of the mirror image chemical scam is Lexapro. Celexa was developed in 1989 and I remember it being relatively new while I was in residency. It quickly became a favorite. It was touted as the Selective Serotonin Reuptake Inhibitor (or SSRI) with the fewest side effects. It was popular but limited in use because it was new and expensive. In 2003, Celexa went generic as citalopram and became a much bigger seller. For many years it has been my drug of choice for chronic anxiety and sometimes for depression.

Just before Celexa was going generic, in 2002, the same company came out with the isolated S-version of citalopram, Lexapro. There was no evidence that the medication was more effective that citalopram. That doesn't matter, though. They pushed it hard and it has done well commercially.

The pharmaceutical industry actually used this mirror image new drug isomer strategy in another way to go from one of the biggest blockbuster drugs to a second, even bigger money maker. I have discussed the problems with acid blockers in prior pages. Prilosec came out and sales skyrocketed because it was the simplest solution to a common problem (heartburn). While Prilosec was headed toward generic status as omeprazole, the company developed Nexium. They took the mirror image chemical and then doubled the dose.

Americans just keep shoveling the potent acid blockers down their throats. Larry the Cable Guy is pushing that stuff all day long. If he's the spokesperson for managing heartburn you know we're in tough shape. It seems to be the go-to medication for almost any gastrointestinal problem. Heartburn? Of course. Upset stomach? Sure. Hoarseness? Yes. Bowel changes? Let's give it a shot. What harm can it do?

When a drug gets classified as new and unique, it can be name-branded with a much higher price tag. If they can push this new drug through at the federal level, that leaves the easy part—convincing doctors that the new drug is an improvement. One of the main problems with keeping health-care costs down is that the doctor or nurse practitioner, historically, has no financial stake in their decisions. They are making decisions for the patient. If the insurance company covers a medication, then neither the doctor nor the patient have any financial stake. In that case the average person usually wants the newest and latest option.

The next bogus "new drug" strategy didn't really catch on much, but I bring it up because of how grossly insulting it is to both doctors and consumers. You take a medication that is already once a day and lasts about 24 hours and make it a controlled release version. I remember seeing a shelf in our sample closet overflowing with Paxil CR. This was such a pathetic attempt to extend profits after the generic was allowed, it burned me.

Yet another money-making strategy is for a drug company to exaggerate the difference between a new class and an existing class of drugs. About 15 years ago, a new class was developed called the COX-2 inhibitors. There were three in the class: Vioxx, Celebrex and Bextra, all developed to have fewer gastrointestinal side effects and a lower risk of bleeding. Intended to replace ibuprofen (Advil, Motrin), naprosyn (Aleve) and other NSAIDs, they were extremely expensive and almost always required paperwork to try and get them approved. If the patient had a history of a bleeding ulcer, the doctor had a shot.

In the end, there was a major scandal with Vioxx because it was found, years after it was on the market, to be increasing people's risk of cardiac events. That and Bextra were yanked off the market. Celebrex is still around. It turns out that the difference in gastrointestinal risk is relatively low. The COX-2 inhibitors also were never promoted as being more effective than the older anti-inflammatories. It must be the power of the mind, though, because many people are utterly convinced it is the only pain reliever that works for them. I have to say I'm not exactly crushed that they've been able to keep Celebrex from going generic, even though it should be way past time.

The next scenario is in relation to the drug Aricept. This is the first-line agent for Alzheimer's dementia. I am not necessarily criticizing the drug industry when it comes to Aricept. With Alzheimer's you have a devastating health condition that affects the person and their family in many ways. When people come in to discuss options, they are typically desperate for any help. Unfortunately, there is typically not much help available. Aricept overall has minimal benefit.

The most common way to assess a person with memory problems and cognitive deficits is the Mini-Mental Status Examination (MMSE). This measures many different areas of mental functioning. A perfect score would be 30/30. The person with dementia will typically be 24 or below. The process is slow and people will decline by 1 or 2 points per year. Aricept can increase a person's score by 1 point on average. Only in a country like ours with lots of resources would a medication like Aricept ever be used.

For a more thorough analysis of the slippery ethics of the pharmaceutical industry, I would recommend reading *The Truth About the Drug Companies* by Marcia Angell. Beware, though, because reading the book will likely add a healthy dose of negativity to your life. I read a chapter from the book each night before going to bed and became so aggravated I would rant and rave for half an hour. I carried on to such a degree my wife finally told me to stop reading the book because it was driving me crazy and keeping her up.

Medical Testing

Cutting back on unnecessary medical tests would certainly save money. Many different tests have been cited as being overused, including CT scans for headaches, MRI scans for back pain, EKG for asymptomatic patients, and on and on. Despite the prevailing idea that American people are spoiled and unreasonable, I have found most patients are willing to discuss the issue of cost. They understand that we're all in it together and that healthcare costs have been out of control for many years. There are some that will insist on the page of lab results and the lumbar MRI following a week of low back pain, but they are a minority.

Old-school annual physicals included regular urinalysis and EKGs. People, especially those over 65 years old, will often ask about these tests and imply they are getting inferior care if they don't get the full battery of tests. These days, though, insurance companies typically won't cover tests without a specific reason. Yet another old-school practice is bone density studies for all women over 50.

I took an informal survey of the primary care providers in my office, asking them the percentage of tests they ordered that they felt were unnecessary (meaning the tests were ordered as defensive medicine or to make the patient happy). The results were 90%, 80%, 80%, 60%, 40%, 50% and 80%.

The total estimated cost savings from eliminating even the average number of unnecessary tests would be gargantuan, yet this would take a fundamental shift in the culture. It would require some sophisticated tort reform where doctors and nurse practitioners as a group could test less without fear of lawsuits. The American people would have to understand their individual role in cutting costs.

There is a model that would potentially work. For parents who decide to homeschool their children (who win the national spelling bee competition), there is a legal fund set up. Each family puts in a small amount of money, maybe $100 per year. If some family has an altercation or disagreement with their school district, they can use money from the fund to pay legal fees. In the same way, why don't we have doctors sign a pledge to not order unnecessary CYA tests and, instead, put money in a fund that would be used for their defense, if needed? There is malpractice insurance, but that does not seem to serve this purpose.

Hospital Expenses

Statistics show hospital care is the greatest expense in the system, topping out at $800 billion for 2010. Primary care is crucial in reducing the admission rate. In the more comprehensive view of primary care, the provider looks for opportunities everywhere to prevent visits to the outpatient office and to the hospital.

We finally seem to be shifting to a healthcare model that emphasizes prevention. Primary care providers are incentivized to see people within 14 days after discharge to minimize risk of readmission. Private employers are rapidly developing in-house wellness programs to keep their employees healthy.

End-of-Life Care

Another area where we could reduce cost is end-of-life care. This is a sensitive issue. Any hint that cost is a consideration when deciding about level of care toward the end of a person's life will get an immediate reaction from most people. Doctors need to be having conversations with people about their goals for the end of their life. If we can be clear on what an individual wants, in terms of level of care, then everything else will fall into place. Why spend an exorbitant amount of money on an intensive level of care if that person would not have wanted it?

During a discussion on the issue, a provider will review living wills, health care proxies, and when and if the patient would want to become DNR/DNI. DNR/DNI stands for "do not resuscitate/do not intubate." I encourage patients to discuss all of their wishes with any and all relevant family members so that everyone understands. There are too many scenarios where one sibling from the west coast is left out of conversation and then, toward the end of life, there are battles within the family over level of care. It is optimal, although rarely done by me or others, to have a family meeting to review everything. Hopefully this will be easier in the future as health care providers work more collaboratively.

I had several profound experiences with end-of-life issues while in residency. We spent a lot of our time in the hospital taking care of inpatients on the medical floor. There was a man I had seen several times on the wards. He was in his late 60s with advanced chronic obstructive pulmonary disease. He had quit smoking but still yearned for a cigarette. Some people give up cigarettes and three days later couldn't care less. Others still crave them 20 years after quitting.

This patient was on all the medications available for COPD. He was followed closely by a solid pulmonologist. The last two options for the COPD patient typically are continuous oxygen by nasal cannula and an oral steroid, like prednisone, every day to reduce airway inflammation. He was on 2.0 liters of oxygen day and night plus a relatively high dose of prednisone. Long-term use of prednisone has a lengthy list of associated problems, but when it comes to helping someone breathe, doctors have few options.

Each stay in the hospital for this man was more difficult. I would sit on the edge of his bed and talk with him about sports or politics. He would be sitting up, working for each breath even with free-flowing oxygen. One time, he said he wanted to ask me something. I could tell by his tone that it was something important. He asked if I would help him end his life. I was utterly unprepared for that and I didn't know what to say to him. I told him I'd have to think about it and we'd talk the next day during rounds.

It is much easier to have an opinion on some issue when you're not in the thick of it. The topic of euthanasia would come up occasionally in discussions with other residents. The average person has an opinion and can blather on about it. In principle, I am in favor of euthanasia. It was a very different matter, however, for me to actively participate in helping a person die. I realized I didn't know much about the process. I had read something vague about a potassium infusion. I imagined what it would take for me to do it. I would have to read up on the details from some bootleg website. I would have to procure the necessary materials somehow. I would then have to sneak into his room off hours, maybe in the middle of the night, and do it.

I talked with him the next day and apologized, but said I really couldn't go through with it. It was illegal and I didn't want to put my medical license in jeopardy. He understood. He wasn't upset. I talked with him about a hospice consult, but he respectfully declined because he didn't think they could help him.

As part of my training in family medicine, I also spent time working in nursing homes. Each resident was assigned a small group of nursing home residents to follow and look after. One of the patients assigned to me was an African American woman in her 80s. She had end-stage dementia. I read through her background information and went to see her for the first time.

I found her in a darkened room full of beds, a few beds down on the right side of the room. She was resting comfortably on her back and didn't stir while I checked her heart, lungs, pulse and abdomen. She had been in the same bed for several years. The nurses said she hadn't moved or had any change the entire time she had been there. Regular feedings through a feeding tube into her stomach were keeping her alive.

I wondered if this was how she would have wanted to live out her life. I looked through her records again and found that her health care proxy was a niece living relatively close to the facility. I checked with the nurses, but none of them ever remembered seeing her. I thought it would be best to reach out to the niece to discuss things, so I called her.

I said I was a doctor involved in her aunt's care. I reviewed the case and shared that her aunt was stable. I then gently tried to ascertain whether the niece knew anything about her aunt's wishes. The niece told me she hadn't been that involved in her aunt's life, but there were no other family members, so some years prior a lawyer had contacted her so that they could have someone on record. I probed further to see if she could make any guesses about what her aunt would have wanted for the end of her life. The neice didn't seem comfortable making any judgments, so I hung up and went back to my rounds.

I saw the patient several more times during weekly visits. Her status didn't change and there was no reasonable expectation it ever would change. She was in a "persistent vegetative state." I couldn't shake the idea that this probably was not how she would have wanted to live her life. I called the niece again to discuss the aunt's level of care.

I asked the niece if she had ever considered withholding the tube feedings. She didn't understand what I was driving at. I said that perhaps her aunt wouldn't have wanted to live like this, that we could try to make a guess or a "substituted judgment" on what she would have wanted. I said that if the niece had a clear sense that her aunt would not have wanted to live in this state, one option would be to remove the artificial feeding tube. The niece became very upset at that point and said we would be killing her. I responded that, in my opinion, we wouldn't be killing her, we would be letting her die peacefully. We were actually keeping her aunt alive by artificial means. If it weren't for the tube feedings, she probably would have died naturally many years ago.

I remember a sense of pride that I went out of my way to do the right thing. It seemed obvious to me that no one would want to live in this state with no meaningful hope of recovery. But the niece was appalled. She said, "Who do you think you are wanting to end her life? You've been seeing her for, what, three weeks now? You have no business interfering in her care in this way!" That ended the conversation and it was an important lesson for me on how some people perceive what is appropriate at the end of life.

These days I try to go over things as thoroughly as I can with patients and their families to avoid scenarios such as this. There is a nice resource called *The Five Wishes* at the website www.agingwithdignity.org. It provides a framework for individuals to clarify in detail what they will want at the end of their life. When appropriate I get hospice involved, since they are the experts in end-of-life comfort care. Even if the patient has a terminal illness with no defined time frame, hospice can be tremendously helpful to both the patient and the family. Given the high cost of long-term medical care and the spectrum of personal beliefs, such conversations only make sense.

16

The Path to Righteousness

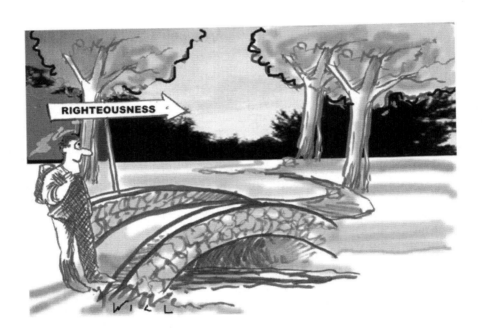

A growing number of my patients have improved their health by utilizing both mainstream and alternative options. This represents the best of both sides. Sean, a 40-year-old art teacher originally from Ireland. Married and the father of three daughters, came in to see me a few years ago. He was having recurrent episodes at work with lightheadedness on the verge of fainting. His chiropractor sent him to me on an urgent basis. By that initial visit with me, Sean had seen his previous primary care doctor on several occasions and had seen many specialists in Boston. All of the providers to that point were well-educated, intelligent and motivated, but they could not provide him with many answers. The work-up was thorough, including pages of blood tests, urine tests, an EKG, cardiac monitoring, chest x-ray, echocardiogram, MRI of the brain plus CT scans of his lungs, abdomen and pelvis. His wife came to the initial visit and said he was "not himself." I could see right away that he was sluggish, glassy-eyed and not completely there. He described it as feeling "fuzzy in the head." He had recurrent pain with urination with no obvious cause, night sweats, mild joint pain and some trouble with his vision.

He had regular tick exposure, so my initial working diagnosis for Sean was chronic Lyme disease. This would not have easily explained all of his symptoms, but it can cause a wide variety of effects including havoc within the neurologic system. The Lyme blood tests done through most mainstream labs are not reliable enough to rule out the chronic infection so I started him on empiric antibiotics in combination. I made some other recommendations in terms of vitamins and supplements as well.

The changes I made for Sean, including the antibiotics, did not improve his symptoms much, but he didn't get terribly worse either, so I referred him to one, then later another, non-mainstream provider. Both alternative providers came up with the same conclusion independently: he had an intestinal parasite. This would explain why his wife had similar, milder symptoms that started around the same time. She improved and he worsened. Her body had been able to clear the parasite and his had not. With treatment that included herbs and supplements, most of Sean's symptoms improved. His fatigue and foggy-headedness resolved. He continued to have intense episodes at work, however, where he would feel anxious and experience sweats and lightheadedness. The episodes would usually happen early in his workday and not very often at home or on the weekends.

We discussed that he might be having panic attacks. Sean was a somewhat uptight person and easily acknowledged that. His father also had issues with anxiety. For me, the presence or absence of a positive family history (especially in first-degree relatives) can help differentiate something innate from something acquired. I started him on an SSRI medication, Celexa. I worked up the dose gradually and the episodes almost completely resolved. He would still get an occasional milder sensation early on during some workdays where he would feel the urge to leave the room, but he was finally satisfied. With this person and many others in my practice, we see that it takes both sides of the equation to figure out and manage an individual's complex medical issues.

Barbara, a patient I have seen for many years, has a slightly different story. She is in her 40s with short, sandy-brown hair and works as a personal trainer. She developed autoimmune type 1 diabetes when she was a young girl. Her pancreas was attacked by her immune system and the islet cells that produce insulin were slowly destroyed. Before the development of synthetic insulin, all type 1 diabetic patients would die. Barbara had been maintained on insulin injections for her life until a few years prior when she was changed to an insulin pump. The pump measures her sugars and more finely regulates her insulin requirements in an effort to mimic the sophisticated feedback mechanisms of the human body.

Late in 2013, Barbara came in to see me wanting to discuss her experiences at a wellness institute in Florida. She spent over $5,000 for 10 days at the institute with the lure that they might be able to get her completely off insulin and cure her type 1 diabetes. They told her that roughly three out of ten diabetics who came to the institute got off insulin. They were going to accomplish this feat of magic through dietary changes and supplements. My first response was that this was absurd. I wondered if they had success with type 2 diabetes patients and lumped the two types together in a dishonest ploy to increase revenue. A minority of type 2 diabetes patients progress and ultimately require insulin to lower their sugars. For that group, it would not be surprising if the majority would get off insulin with exercise, dietary changes and weight loss.

They had Barbara stop caffeine and switch to mostly raw foods. They gave her intravenous vitamin C treatments that caused her sugars to go up dramatically. When she told the staff at the institute about the blood sugar increase, they told her that didn't happen and the numbers must be inaccurate. They recommended hormone supplementation with no clear rationale. She purchased a wide variety of supplements from the institute. She lost 12 pounds and her insulin requirements decreased slightly, but she was not cured. Mainstream medicine has been working on real potential cures for many years, including transplantation of islet cells and pancreases.

In addition to the diabetes plan, the institute told her she had problems with her thyroid, liver and right ovary. They wanted her to come in to see her primary care doctor right away so that imaging studies could be ordered. I would not order CT scans that would expose her to unnecessary radiation but agreed to targeted ultrasounds. Her blood tests and the ultrasound studies of her thyroid, liver and ovaries eventually came back normal.

Overall, she spent a large amount of money and I ordered a cluster of unnecessary tests. Mainstream medicine has kept her alive and reasonably well. The alternative group likely helped with some of the fine-tuning of her health and wellness, but at a relatively high costs. The primary provider at the institute drove a $120,000 car that he parked in his private spot near the front door. He has likely passed the tipping point where the spoils of his labor influence his clinical decisions.

In the first case study, Sean's story, we see a person with complicated symptoms who had most issues corrected by alternative practitioners when mainstream doctors had no answers or solutions. But Sean also did very well on a prescription medication to alleviate chronic anxiety with panic attacks. In the second case study, Barbara's story, a woman's life has been saved and maintained by modern medicine with its focus on pharmacology and technology. The alternative world had some benefit, but it was limited. In both cases, we see an inefficient process that makes it difficult for the patient to find the best option and avoid exorbitant cost.

To review the obvious, we need a shift in our healthcare system. It needs to focus more on prevention and proactive approaches. It needs to devote resources to pinpointing the underlying causes for chronic disease processes. But this shift will only come about from the ground up, person-by-person. We will need to recruit open-minded physicians and ignore the entrenched. We would save tremendous amounts of money if the system shifted toward more primary care providers, fewer pharmaceuticals and a decrease in unnecessary testing. There also needs to be some overarching tort reform that would protect physicians in such a way that they could practice without fear.

But people are not inclined to change. Most feel more comfortable staying with the status quo. In my medical career I have found a dense resistance to any new ideas that diverge from allopathic principles and approaches. If we are ever to move beyond our place in time and space, it will take a minority to push the envelope. The naturopaths are in that minority and their influence is quietly growing in America.

Naturopathy and Functional Medicine Cost Less

The naturopaths have worked out many of the details for us already. If we truly followed the naturopathic principles outlined in the chapter "Toward Integration", with a smattering of strategically used pharmaceuticals and the occasional surgery, we could have a healthcare system that served the people well. This could happen and, for several reasons, I believe we *can* move to a better system. Why? People themselves are becoming more aware of the need. If insurance companies realize that the naturopathic model is as effective but at significantly lower cost, they will start to reimburse and fund naturopaths and other alternative providers with more enthusiasm.

Naturopathic medicine costs less than conventional care. In other words, the use of natural health products has the potential to improve health outcomes and reduce costs. A 2006 University of Washington study and summary of various studies found that, in Washington State, naturopathic care cost insurers $9.00 per enrollee vs. $686.00 for conventional care. One year of lifestyle intervention for patients with coronary artery disease not only improved all health outcomes and reduced the need for surgery but also cost significantly less than conventional treatment ($7,000 vs. $31,000–$46,000). It was estimated that if the current level of medical intervention continues, the U.S. will end up spending $9.5 trillion dollars over the next 30 years caring for cardiovascular disease, diabetes and congestive heart disease alone. By adding in greater preventive strategies to improve patients' health, costs could be reduced approximately $904 billion, or by almost 10%. In just one year, patients who received intensive lifestyle modification and naturopathic therapy for type 2 diabetes improved all health scores (lipids, % body fat, etc.) and decreased medication requirements, compared to those on standard therapy. Total expenditure on health care by insured Complementary and Alternative Medicine (CAM) users is less than non-CAM users ($3,797 vs. $4,153); this is approximately $9.4 million in savings for just 26,466 CAM-users. But CAM's most significant reduction in total medical expenditures is seen in patients with the greatest disease burden, usually the most expensive patients.

Another offshoot of the movement comes from the functional medicine group. I had written most of this book and was discussing it with a like-minded patient. He made some reference to me practicing functional medicine. I had never heard the term before, but when I looked it up I found that functional medicine described well the changes I was trying to make in my daily work. The functionalmedicine.org website lists six core principles that are similar to many of the basic tenets of naturopathy.

1. An understanding of the biochemical individuality of each human being, based on the concepts of genetic and environmental uniqueness;
2. Awareness of the evidence that supports a patient-centered rather than a disease-centered approach to treatment;
3. Search for a dynamic balance among the internal and external body, mind, and spirit;
4. Interconnections of internal physiological factors;
5. Identification of health as a positive vitality, not merely the absence of disease, and emphasizing those factors that encourage the enhancement of a vigorous physiology;
6. Promotion of organ reserve as the means to enhance the health span, not just the lifespan, of each patient.

Naturopathic and functional medicine providers typically put more emphasis on bowel health and an individual's microbiome.

The Importance of Probiotics

For the common chronic gastrointestinal ailments, we should be using more probiotics and digestive enzymes. The best probiotic has a wide variety of flora, maintains the viability of the good bacteria over time after manufacturing, is delivered to the small intestine and colon in high quantities, and includes "prebiotics" which are the food the probiotic bacteria need to survive. One of the best probiotics available is Prescript-Assist. It meets all of these criteria and has been studied for effectiveness. Friends of ours, a husband and wife, are very savvy about these issues. They are frequently providing me with some of the best, most up-to-date information on diet and wellness. A Christmas present from them was a bottle of the Prescript-Assist probiotic and a bag of Bob's Red Mill All Natural Potato Starch. The potato starch survives through the stomach to provide nourishment to the good bacteria. This resistant starch helps maintain the health and volume of the good bacteria. Another excellent probiotic comes from Dr. Ohhira. His include the prebiotic nutrients that will help maximize the viability and effect of the good bacteria in the body.

We may eventually take an inventory of the volume and variety of each person's gut flora. A new technique called high-throughput sequencing enables us to catalog the trillions of bacteria in a person's gastrointestinal tract. Individualized probiotics could more finely optimize the ideal balance of flora, creating a new approach for the prevention and treatment of illness. Naturopaths sometimes utilize fasting to decrease the bacterial load in the intestinal tract. If you kill off 100 million bacteria with a fast and 10% of those are pathogenic or otherwise harmful, supplementing with "good bacteria" through a probiotic improves your ratio and percentage of good/bad bacteria.

Probiotics need to be used on a more regular basis, especially for people taking antibiotics for acute infections. Some would likely benefit from daily probiotics to help regulate their immune system, mood and other important aspects of wellness. We need to be aggressive with probiotics in young children. It is clear from my medical practice that a disrupted microbiome is a major risk factor for pediatric behavioral problems and the development of autism. I feel that any child on antibiotics or steroids should be on an extended course of probiotics. Any child with signs of a dysregulated immune system should be on regular probiotics. Any child deemed to be at higher risk of autism, either from genetics or environment, needs to have their microbiome tended judiciously. One good option is Garden of Life's probiotic powder for kids. This can be started at a dose of ¼ teaspoon added to water, or some other approved liquid, for children as young as three months of age.

Simple dietary modifications would work for many patients, but not for others. From my time in medicine, I have found that the more complicated the patient, the more individualized any dietary intervention needs to be. The alternative providers are more likely to tailor their dietary recommendations to an individual's particular issues. Traditional providers and alternative providers should collaborate more often. We need a source to fund well-designed placebo-controlled trials without pharmaceutical company bias to answer the most important clinical questions.

When I first heard of the National Center for Complementary and Alternative Medicine (NCCAM), as an offshoot of the National Institutes of Health, I was optimistic the department would be a step toward integration. I was also hopeful this group would have access to the massive financial resources of the federal government to fund studies that evaluate alternative options. Ah, those wistful days of unblanching optimism in our leaders...

In retrospect, I'm not sure the center (renamed the National Center for Complementary and Integrative Health, or NCCIH, in 2014) has lived up to that standard. The studies done early on focused on several of the darlings of the alternative world, including St. John's wort for depression,[14] saw palmetto for an enlarged prostate,[112] and glucosamine for arthritis.[113] The St. John's Wort study was referenced in an earlier chapter. When I reviewed the patient populations used in these studies I felt that they were set up to fail, though I doubt this was a conspiracy. As far as I can tell from the website, the department is comprised of PhDs and MDs. Not surprisingly, there may be a mainstream bias if there are no alternative providers involved in decision-making.

On the NCCIH website the review of naturopathic medicine is one negative comment after another. Their "Key Points" are as follows:

- Although some of the individual therapies used in naturopathy have been studied for efficacy and safety, naturopathy as a general approach to health care has not been widely researched.

- "Natural" does not necessarily mean "safe." Some therapies used in naturopathy, such as herbal supplements and restrictive or unconventional diets, have the potential to be harmful if not used under the direction of a well-trained [i.e. MD] practitioner.

- Some beliefs and approaches of naturopathic practitioners are not consistent with conventional medicine, and their safety may not be supported by scientific evidence. For example, some practitioners may not recommend childhood vaccinations. The benefits of vaccination in preventing illness and death have been repeatedly proven and greatly outweigh the risks.

- Tell all your health care providers about any complementary health practices you use. Give them a full picture of what you do to manage your health. This will help ensure coordinated and safe care [to protect you all from the witch doctors].

In a perfect world where access and cost did not matter, the U.S. would gradually shift away from low-quality, processed carbohydrates toward locally-grown fruits and vegetables with regular intake of high-quality lean protein. The Paleo diet, or something in the neighborhood like the South Beach diet, would probably have the most dramatic impact on the general population given the rates of obesity, diabetes, heart disease, headaches, bowel problems and other chronic health issues. A vegetarian diet is likely optimal for many (but not all) people because there is a dark side to vegetarianism. Someone avoiding animal protein can feel free to binge on bread, pasta, cakes and cookies and still maintain some degree of righteousness. They would also be prone to iron and B^{12} deficiency without supplementation. A simple aspect of eating better is for each person to be more mindful of what they are consuming and assess how they feel afterwards. If you have four slices of meatball pizza for lunch and are in a stupor all afternoon, it may not be the best option for you. It's stunning how most people mindlessly cram food into their gullet day after day, ignoring the effects on their mind and body.

In terms of the obesity epidemic, our assumption is that weight gain is caused primarily by overeating. In this model the weight gain increases insulin resistance putting the person at risk of metabolic diseases like type 2 diabetes. There is building evidence that we may have that sequence out of order. Certain foods, chemicals and toxins in our environment may be causing insulin resistance that then causes weight gain and obesity.

There is a TED talk by Peter Attia from 2013 on this subject. He and others are doing intensive research on obesity. As is often the case, it was a personal experience that forced him to question his assumptions. He was a young surgeon who regarded overweight people with arrogance and contempt. Out of nowhere, as a young fit male, he developed insulin resistance. He realized the simple formula that blames people for bad habits was incorrect. Dr. Attia says there are about 30 million obese Americans with no signs of insulin resistance. These people do not seem to have increased risk of diabetes or cardiovascular disease. He says there are about six million people with normal weight that have, for some reason, developed insulin resistance and are at relatively high risk of chronic health problems. His primary hypothesis is that refined sugars, starches and grains are driving insulin resistance and secondary obesity.

Exercise needs to be a focal point of our society. If we invested in life coaches to work with people on a regular basis we could individualize long-term intervention, finding the most appropriate mode of physical activity for each individual: take the stairs, park as far away as possible, use a bike as part of a commute, find a pool near the house. We know physical activity done on a regular basis, in just about any form, increases daily quality of life, improves the functioning of the immune system and lowers the risk of almost every important common chronic medical problem.

The optimal form of physical activity for an individual would depend on their goals. Any form of vigorous exercise seems to help with mood. For weight loss, the most important thing is likely to be standing up or moving around at least once every 20-30 minutes. Our metabolisms slow down the longer we are sedentary. Pursuing some form of resistance training is also helpful for weight loss as more muscle leads to a more active metabolism all day long. If the goal is fitness, the best approach is probably some form of high intensity interval training over relatively short periods of time. If a person were to choose the one form of exercise with the greatest benefits, it would almost certainly be yoga. There is no other form of physical activity that so effectively incorporates conditioning, balance, strength, flexibility and mindfulness.

We need to systematically reduce our exposure to environmental chemicals and toxins. The potential effects of so many chemicals and toxins is so utterly complex, with so many variables, we will probably not have firm toxin-disease correlations any time soon. *The Autoimmune Epidemic* by Nazakawa makes a strong argument for cleaning up our exposures as thoroughly as possible to reduce the risk of autoimmune and other chronic conditions.

The logical question for anyone reading this book is: What can I do to minimize exposures and maximize health and wellness? An excellent website, www.ewg.org summarizes the research and findings of the Environmental Working Group. The website is frequently updated, providing a wide variety of information on chemical and toxin exposures for the general public. Eating fresh, organic food is probably the first step. Making sure the water is filtered, possibly through a filter with reverse osmosis, is important. Consider testing your water supply for heavy metals and halides like chlorine and fluoride. Avoiding plastic food containers and using glass baby bottles, including one by Evenflo, would decrease the BPA and phthalate exposure. Of note, "BPA-free" plastic is not phthalate-free so can still cause harm. Using high-efficiency particulate absorption (HEPA) filters, including on your vacuum cleaner, would reduce fire retardant and airborne chemicals in the home environment. If excessive mold in the home is a possibility, there are inexpensive test kits available at hardware stores.

We should use technology and genetic testing to our advantage. Pharmacogenetic testing is available now from several labs around the country. This allows us to do a simple swab of the inside of the mouth and quickly get a report giving us precise information on how any individual will process hundreds of pharmaceuticals. This should be done for everyone. It would reduce the current trial-and-error method for those that require pharmaceuticals. It should reduce the incidence of mild side effects and more severe drug reactions. There is also a high likelihood that the genetic testing will become a means for profit. Each person that gets their individualized genetic profile taken will need visits and interpretation. The pharmaceutical giants will likely see opportunity in these profiles. The millions of people determined to have a higher risk of Alzheimer's could be put on a medication like Aricept. Economic realities, however, will keep a lid on this kind of polypharmacy as the insurance companies will do anything and everything to avoid paying that bill.

The best care in the 21st century will likely include an evaluation of a person's single nuceotide polymorphisms (SNPs). The SNPs are an individual's genetic variations and many of these anomalies are implicated in chronic medical conditions. The group 23andme will do DNA analysis from a bolus of saliva for $99. The raw data then needs to be run through another website like genetic genie, livewello, Yasko's knowyourgenetics. com or Ledowsky's mthfrsupport.com. These reports will provide several pages on many of the most important genetic anomalies relevant to most important chronic medical conditions. The relatively common MTHFR anomaly, for one, can increase the risk of autism, bipolar illness, depression, blood clots, miscarriages, premature coronary events and strokes, early dementia and certain cancers among other important health issues.

Americans love technology but, in my experience, the majority of people appreciate the big picture and are willing to do their part to reduce costs. When the debate over healthcare reform was in the public forum, in the runup to the Affordable Care Act, there was a (temporary) wave of cost-consciousness among my patients. A main focus of the discussion was the need to cut healthcare costs and so, for some time, people in my office would say that I should use my best judgment. If the MRI or CT scan or other expensive test wasn't really necessary, then we should wait. I had never heard so many people express that sentiment, and I have seldom heard it since then. But it showed me that many Americans are reasonable.

We need low-cost, efficient technology that enhances communication between patients and providers and empowers the patient to improve their own health. Smartphones and, potentially, some even more convenient and more powerful devices will allow people to do urine, blood, sweat, and saliva testing by themselves. An individual can check his or her vital signs and heart rhythm. Nanotechnology could see sensors transmitting information from inside. We could have tiny robots cleaning our arteries like the little fish that routinely clean the teeth of larger fish.

We are almost to the point where we will grow tissue in a lab using a person's cells for the original matrix. 3D printers have been used to make an artificial trachea to maintain the airway for an infant born with a collapsed bronchial tube. Organ transplantation from donors could become obsolete.

But even in the future, technology will probably still be secondary to the most basic of interventions. The simplest approach often remains the best approach. Many doctor's visits and chronic problems would be minimized or disappear simply with good hydration, a high quality mattress, a solid diet with minimal processed foods, regular physical activity and an emphasis on strengthening our interpersonal relationships. That short list would make most mainstream and alternative options unnecessary.

The options available to people for improving their health are absolutely overwhelming today. A new diet comes out once a month. There are hundreds of different vitamins. There are thousands of herbs and alternative dietary supplements. It is almost impossible for private citizens and healthcare providers to sort through it all and identify the best options. Collaboration would help but solid research will be needed as well. The group "Natural Standard" provides high-quality, evidence-based information about complementary and alternative therapies. This has been used as a reference throughout the book.

Top Ten American Health Scams

In summary, the top 10 health-related scams perpetuated on the American people are (in David Letterman's count-down style):

10. *Got Milk*: The milk industry has done a masterful job over the past 100 years of convincing the American people, and especially parents, that cow's milk is crucial for the bone development and general health of our children. Some people do extremely well with cow's milk but many cannot tolerate it, and the benefits for bone health are marginal.

9. *Nutrition Bars*: Nutrigrain bars are the poster child for this group. Despite the healthy-sounding name, they are sweetened with high fructose corn syrup and brightened with artificial dyes. Most of the protein bars/health bars are just hyped candy bars.

8. *Soy*: One would think soy is a healthy staple in the American diet, but it depends on the form. Most mass-produced soy in America has low nutrient density and is a poor option for maintaining protein intake. Sensitivity and intolerance to soy is likely underappreciated and underdiagnosed.

7. *Pork, The Other White Meat*: It's really not true, but brilliant in its simplicity. Right around the time Americans were pulling away from red meat toward chicken, turkey and fish, the pork industry developed this marketing campaign. They knew if they could nudge pork over into the white meat category they would be set. Yes, pork looks white, but in terms of health, it should be grouped with red meat.

6. *Yogurt*: Plain yogurt can be an excellent source of protein, calcium and vitamin D. Mass-produced yogurts like Chobani, however, often have high amounts of processed sugar. People think that yogurt is helping to maintain the balance of good bacteria, but yogurt in the grocery store does not typically have the variety or the quantity of good bacteria required to enhance the microbiome. Most of the good bacteria from yogurt is destroyed before it gets to the small intestine and colon where it is needed.

5. *Diets*: The effective ones all work back to something close to Paleo or the Mediterranean diet. Forget the tabloids and stick to the basics. People need to find an optimal way of eating that they can pursue for life.

4. *Science & Technology*: We rely on them to save us. It will always be a major part of our lives providing tremendous benefit, but we can't rely on doctors, scientists and high technology to provide us with the answers to all of our questions.

3. *Statins*: This is not to say that statins don't have value, but their importance

is greatly exaggerated.

2. *Plastics*: In the movie *The Graduate,* Dustin Hoffman's character (Benjamin) is at his high school graduation party and a pair of family friends initiate a serious conversation about Benjamin's future:

Benjamin: "I'm just..."

Mr. Braddock: "...worried?"

Benjamin: "Well..."

Mr. Braddock: "About what?"

Benjamin: "I guess about my future."

Mr. Braddock: "What about it?"

Benjamin: "I don't know. I want it to be..."

Mr. Braddock: "...to be what?"

Benjamin: "...Different."

Mr. McGuire: "I want to say one word to you. Just one word."

Benjamin: "Yes, sir."

Mr. McGuire: "Are you listening?"

Benjamin: "Yes, I am."

Mr. McGuire: "*Plastics.*

Benjamin: "Exactly how do you mean?"

Mr. McGuire: "There's a great future in plastics. Think about it. Will you think about it?"

There is growing evidence that plastics, phthalates and other related chemicals are harmful to us.

And the #1 scam perpetuated on the American people is...

1. *Whole Wheat and Whole Grains*: We have been told by the food manufacturers for many years that these are good for us. The government's food pyramid reinforced the idea. More books like *Wheatbellly* and *Grain Brain* are coming out all the time exposing this hoax.

Moving Forward

To maintain optimism, let's run through the Top 10 Ways to Maintain Health, again David Letterman style:

10. Avoid unnecessary pharmaceuticals, vitamins and supplements. Some that are most likely to be beneficial include vitamin D, fish oil, iodine, magnesium and a probiotic, but the quality of the brand of each supplement is important.

9. Hydrate well, primarily with filtered or other high quality water.

8. Be mindful. Pursue meditation or yoga or some other regular activity to spend more time in the present moment.

7. Invest in a high-quality mattress.

6. Get enough sleep pursuing principles from someone like Kirk Parsley, MD.

5. Eat quality food in moderate quantities with a focus on fruits, vegetables, nuts and lean protein.

4. Avoid harmful substances, notably cigarettes.

3. Get regular exercise and stay active during the day, avoiding any prolonged sedentary stretches.

2. Stay connected to other people and the world.

1. Tend your microbiome.

Sometimes we find simple solutions to health problems. I have countless patients that had a wide variety of problems resolve by eliminating a food or food type from their diet. I had a 35-year-old male with recurrent anal fissures for 10 years get resolution by removing gluten from his diet. Gluten has become a villain and I believe that many people do have issues attributed to gluten intake. The *Wheat Belly* crowd would say that wheat is the problem but wheat and gluten are often interchangeable. David Brownstein, MD, asserts that thyroid disorders and iodine deficiency explain many poorly understood chronic diagnoses like chronic fatigue syndrome and fibromyalgia. Some would probably say that improving internal pH levels would facilitate improvement for a wide variety of health problems. We know that the balance of internal flora is crucial. Morley Robbins, the "Magnesium Man," feels that addressing magnesium deficiency is the most important option for the management and prevention of chronic health problems. Experts like William Crook, MD, who wrote *The Yeast Connection*, link a long list of symptoms to fungal overgrowth.

What I have found in my research and in practice is that they are all correct in some sense, but each patient is different. One of the great lessons of my medical career is that everyone requires a unique approach to diagnosis and treatment. Richard Horowitz, of all sources of information known to me, seems to have captured this better than anyone. He has done much of the groundwork for me in my ongoing efforts to more successfully help the complicated patients that I see every day in my office. In Dr. Horowitz's landmark book *Why Can't I Get Better? Solving the Mystery of Lyme & Chronic Disease,* he describes what it took to help one of his patients:

The keys to getting Chris better were aggressive treatment for the Lyme disease and babesiosis, getting him to sleep, treating his low adrenal function, avoiding the food allergens, stopping the blood sugar swings with a hypoglycemic diet, chelating his heavy metals, mitochondrial support, detoxing him properly, and shutting down the production of inflammatory cytokines responsible for the Jarisch-Herxheimer flares. These were the essential components that led to his successful treatment.[114]

What do methylation cycle SNP genetic testing, dysbiosis (microbial imbalance), yeast overgrowth, immune dysfunction, chronic Lyme disease, thyroid dysfunction, magnesium deficiency, iodine deficiency, adrenal fatigue, pH balance, food sensitivities, heavy metal toxicity and other important subjects have in common? They are not part of standard medical training? Yes. They need more research before most medical professionals will accept them as important? Yes. They require testing not performed in mainstream laboratories? Typically, yes. There is also no accepted mainstream standard of care.

Perhaps the most important distinction, however, among this list of "alternative" health issues is that there is no pharmaceutical solution. Dietary changes, stress management, environmental controls, detoxification, herbs, vitamins and supplements are the primary modalities of treatment for most of them. The mainstream juggernaut is so conditioned to a pharmaceutical approach that many providers never question whether this is an optimal approach to wellness.

For those of you with chronic intractable symptoms involving multiple systems that have not responded to a multitude of pharmaceuticals pre-scribed by a wide variety of doctors, I would research these different approaches and try to find those that fit best with your issues. I would then find an open-minded primary care physician who is willing to work with alternative providers to find an individualized path to wellness. That will probably be a difficult task, but working with an MD can help to minimize expenses as the insurance companies will typically cover the majority of tests ordered by mainstream allopathic providers.

Americans are gradually coming to recognize the flaws in our healthcare system. As much as we would like it to be, it is not in fact a well-organized system designed to efficiently maintain wellness and prevent disease from occurring. On the homefront, more and more people are becoming aware of the low-quality, low-cost food we consume. Documentaries like "Food, Inc." and books like *The Autoimmune Epidemic* will hopefully educate us a little at a time, slowly redirecting the course of our country's healthcare. The process is incredibly slow and laborious, like turning an ocean liner. But we have no choice. We must keep moving forward for our own health and the health of future generations.

Appendix A

The Quick and Dirty Approach

This is not just one of those disclaimers you buzz through. Truly, these short blurbs are oversimplifications of what are often complex medical issues. See a reliable healthcare professional to discuss all options for diagnosis and management. Many individuals require a unique approach.

Allergies and Asthma: Try to figure out environmental triggers. If unable to control symptoms adequately, consider acupuncture if symptoms chronic and problematic. For severe, acute symptoms seek medical care. Inhaled and oral steroids are typically the most effective short-term options.

Anxiety: If short-term or occasional, consider cognitive behavioral therapy techniques, self-hypnosis, meditation and other relaxation techniques. Yoga is probably the best form of exercise as it incorporates mindfulness. If chronic, difficult to manage, and affecting relationships, pursue a holistic approach with vigorous exercise, a diet without processed glutamate-based foods, and good sleep; consider an SSRI medication like Celexa or Zoloft.

Arthritis (Osteoarthritis): Staying active is crucial. Maintaining good muscle strength helps keep the joints stable, minimizing mechanical wear and tear. Lose weight. Try Omegaberry for several weeks. If it doesn't work, try SAMe for 1-2 weeks. If that doesn't work, try glucosamine for 1-2 months. Maintain any of these supplements alone or in combination that seem to decrease joint pain.

Autistic Disorders: Do a lot of research. Become an expert. Seek alternative opinions liberally. Improvement is probable with diligence, dietary change, optimal supplementation, patience and the right practitioners. The best information may be found through Amy Yasko. There is a free online copy of her *Pathways to Recovery* at the website dramyyasko.com. Her other website, knowyourgenetics.com, and her book *Feel Good* are excellent resources as well.

Attention Deficit Disorder (ADD/ADHD): Improve diet, especially by avoiding artificial colors/dyes and minimizing sugar and processed foods; increase amount of sleep and minimize screen time. Consider other factors that are contributing and get a complete work-up including neuropsychological testing if possible. Important to rule out co-existing problems like sensory integration dysfunction (especially auditory processing issues that make it seem like a child has focus problems), hearing problems, anxiety and learning disabilities. Deanol may be as effective as stimulants like Ritalin but research is lacking. As a last option, the stimulants can be incredibly effective and improve academic performance and self-esteem. William Shaw, PhD, has useful information about other causes and relevant testing through Great Plains Laboratories.

Behavioral Issues (Pediatrics): Do not accept an opinion or diagnosis that doesn't seem to fit. Be wary of advice; you know your child best. Become an expert. The solution may be as simple as improving the child's diet or may require a wide variety of changes and interventions.

Coronary Artery Disease: Focus on exercise, paleo or similar diet with minimal sugar/wheat, and maintain a healthy weight. Take a beta-blocker, a statin and 81mg aspirin unless contraindicated. Drink at least five cups of water per day to decrease blood viscosity. If there is a strong family history of premature coronary disease, do research on genetic methylation cycle anomalies and try to find a practitioner who is an expert in the area.

Chronic back pain: Work on core strengthening of the back, buttocks, abdomen and legs via yoga, pilates, TRX, personal trainer, physical therapy or other modality. If there are other musculoskeletal problems and/or there is asymmetry (i.e. one shoulder higher than the other, one hip lower than the other, etc.) consider working with a chiropractor.

Chronic Fatigue: Pursue standard work-up and make sure that a full thyroid panel is done. Find ways to maintain adequate sleep, hydration and a quality diet. Consider a sleep study to rule out sleep apnea and assess amount of time in deep restorative sleep. Read Horowitz's *Why Can't I Get Better?* book. For persistent fatigue, consider seeing an alternative provider. Look at the Youtube videos and books from David Brownstein, MD, because thyroid dysfunction and iodine deficiency may be the underlying cause even if your thyroid screening blood test (TSH) is normal. Consider magnesium supplementation with information from www.gotmag.org. Review the SHINE protocol.

Chronic Knee Pain: Quadriceps strengthening and weight loss are key. If not improving and you cannot do what you want physically, see your doctor.

Depression: Do whatever possible to be physically active on a regular basis. Avoid substances. Consider seeing a therapist. Consider fish oil supplement.

Discuss with providers whether medication is appropriate. Consider the book *Chemistry of Joy* for a holistic approach to long-term improvement. Read Yasko's *Feel Good* book and get methylation cycle testing through 23andme.com. The raw data from that website then needs to be processed through a website like geneticgenie, livewello, knowyourgenetics or mthfrsupport.

Diabetes (Type 2): Focus on exercise, paleo or similar diet with minimal sugar/wheat, and maintain a healthy weight. Use medication if necessary to keep A1C number around 7.0% and see your provider at least every six months to monitor potential effects of the diabetes on your eyes, kidneys, heart, circulation and feet.

Gout: Drink lots of water every day to flush the uric acid out of your system. Keep animal protein and beer to a minimum. If you're having frequent flare-ups, discuss with your doctor taking allopurinol every day. It is very effective with minimal side effects or interactions.

Headaches: Focus on the common triggers first. Hydrate well, manage stress, get more sleep and avoid artificial sweeteners, cold cuts and MSG. If not improved, wean off caffeine and alcohol. After these changes, a more radical dietary overhaul may be needed. Going off wheat or gluten may work. MSG and glutamate are found in a wide variety of processed foods under many different names. If these interventions fail, get the *Heal Your Headache* book by Buchholz. Last option would be a daily preventative medication like amitryptiline, propranolol, verapamil or Topamax. Consider magnesium. If all else fails, try to find a chiropractor who specializes in upper cervical manipulation.

Heartburn/Esophageal Reflux: Do not accept long-term acid suppression as the only strategy. Chew thoroughly, eat slowly and minimize acidic foods, fatty foods, caffeine, alcohol, chocolate, mint and other provocative foods. Don't eat late. Lose weight. Consider digestive enzymes before meals but you may need to try more than one to find an effective option.

High Cholesterol: Focus on exercise, paleo or similar diet with minimal sugar/wheat, and maintain a healthy weight. Fish oil, flaxseed oil and krill oil will not change the numbers much but are probably worth taking for the wide variety of benefits to joints, heart, brain, etc. If you have diabetes (even if well-controlled), a history of coronary disease or are considered high risk when putting your numbers into a risk calculator like the one from the

Framingham Heart Study, consider a daily statin.

Hypertension: If lifestyle has been maximized and blood pressure is still consistently over 140 for the top number, consider either prescription medication or meditation/acupuncture/relaxation techniques. DASH diet reduces blood pressure about 10 points on average. Some alternative options like beet root juice, hawthorn root and others may help, but research may be insufficient. Consider magnesium.

Irritable Bowel Syndrome: Do not accept this as a real diagnosis. Do an elimination diet in some form to try and identify food types contributing to your symptoms. Try a Paleo diet with no wheat, gluten, dairy, sugar or processed food. Take a good probiotic every day. Consider a digestive enzyme like Digest Gold up to three times per day. Consider fiber supplement daily. If still not resolved, try to find holistic-minded primary care provider to arrange for food sensitivity testing, intestinal permeability testing, gut flora evaluation and other relevant evaluations. Consider magnesium.

Kidney Stones: Drink a lot of water every day. Find out what type of stone you had. Calcium oxalate is the most common. For calcium oxalate, maintain calcium in the diet, but avoid oxalate. Some of the most common forms of oxalate are tea, cola and dark green vegetables. It may be worth taking steps to alter the pH of your urine by diet, supplements or medication.

Muscle Cramps: Start with better hydration and some regular stretching. Muscle relaxers like cyclobenzaprine 5mg can help reduce severe pain. Best option may be a daily magnesium supplement. A good source on magnesium replacement can be found with the Magnesium Advocacy Group.

Prostate Enlargement: If obstructive voiding symptoms come on abruptly over a short period of time, it is most likely prostatitis and will respond to 2-4 weeks of antibiotics. For chronic symptoms, the first priority is to evaluate for prostate cancer. If PSA blood test and rectal exam are reassuring, there are several options. Saw palmetto can help with younger males, i.e. 50-60. Flomax or tamsulosin usually work as the next option and the patient will typically know within a week if it works. If chronic and interfering with quality of life, prostate surgery is generally safe and effective. Most men I see that have the procedure wish they had done it 10 years before.

Rheumatoid Arthritis: If seronegative, meaning a normal rheumatoid factor blood test, consider full work-up for chronic Lyme disease by an enlightened practitioner before starting TNF agents. If you have a wide variety of chronic symptoms beyond joint pain, read the Horowitz book. If sero-positive, the TNF prescription medications often have amazing positive benefits on long-term joint pain and disability. Thyroid hormone insuffi-ciency, as described in David Brownstein's book, may also be the underlying cause.

Stroke Prevention: Blood pressure control is paramount. Some anti-platelet blood thinner like aspirin is standard of care. Lifestyle and stress manage-ment are crucial.

Urinary Tract Infections: For treatment, short courses of antibiotics usually work well. If recurrent, make sure cultures are positive. If not, you may have interstitial cystitis or some other urologic condition. For prevention, stay hydrated and possibly try a daily D-mannose supplement.

Appendix B

Natural Standard

The following information is from naturalmedicines.com (formerly health. naturalstandard.com), a website designed by healthcare providers and researchers to offer evidence-based information about complementary and alternative medicine, supplements and therapies. Grades reflect the level of available scientific data for or against the use of each therapy for a specific medical condition.

A = Strong Positive Scientific Evidence

B = Positive Scientific Evidence

C = Unclear Scientific Evidence

D = Negative Scientific Evidence

E = Strong Negative Scientific Evidence

By Option

apple cider vinegar	Not evaluated.
andrographis	A for upper respiratory infections; B for ulcerative colitis
artichoke	B for bile secretion stimulant and elevated cholesterol
banderol	Not evaluated.
barley	B for high cholesterol
bilberry	Nothing in the A or B category. Not enough research.

bitter melon	Nothing in the A or B category. Not enough research.
candex	Nothing in the A or B category. Not enough research.
chamomile	Nothing in the A or B category. Not enough research.
chaste tree berry	B for hyperprolactinemia and premenstrual syndrome
chromium	B for low blood sugar and high blood sugars associated with polycystic ovarian syndrome (PCOS)
cinnamon	Nothing in the A or B category. Not enough research.
coenzyme Q10	B for hypertension
coleus forskohlii	B for asthma, cardiomyopathy and glaucoma
corosolic acid	Nothing in the A or B category. Not enough research.
cranberry	Nothing in the A or B category. Not enough research.
cumanda	Nothing in the A or B category. Not enough research.

deer antler	Nothing in the A or B category. Not enough research.
digestive enzymes	Not evaluated as a group.
echinacea root	B for common cold.
elderberry	B for influenza.
fish oil	A for coronary artery disease; A for hypertension
french lilac	Not evaluated.
garlic	A for high blood pressure and high cholesterol; B for heart disease
ginkgo	B for cerebral insufficiency; B for dementia; B for generalized anxiety disorder (GAD) and B for schizophrenia
glucosamine	B for knee osteoarthritis and B for generalized osteoarthritis
green tea	B for genital warts and B for high cholesterol
gugulipid	B for high cholesterol
hawthorn root	A for congestive heart failure.
huckleberry	Nothing in the A or B category. Not enough research.

hydrastis (goldenseal) | Nothing in the A or B category. Not enough research.

hydrogen peroxide | Not evaluated.

lavender oil | Nothing in the A or B category. Not enough research.

maca | Not evaluated.

magnesium | A for abnormal heart rhythms and hypertension in pregnancy; B for asthma, type 2 diabetes, hearing loss and pain

melatonin | B for pediatric insomnia, elderly insomnia and jet lag

mistletoe | Nothing in the A or B category. Not enough research.

myomin | Nothing in the A or B category. Not enough research.

oat bran | B for heart disease, high cholesterol, diabetes and gastric cancer.

olive leaf extract | Nothing in the A or B category. Not enough research.

orchex | Nothing in the A or B category. Not enough research.

probiotics	A for acute diarrhea, atopic dermatitis; B for cirrhosis, IBS, UC, sinusitis, "immune enhancement," growth
propolis	Nothing in the A or B category. Not enough research.
psyllium	A for high cholesterol; B for constipation
rauwolfia	Nothing in the A or B category. Many warnings in the D and F categories regarding safety.
red yeast rice	B for high cholesterol
SAMe	B for osteoarthritis
samento	Nothing in the A or B category. Not enough research.
simplex M	Nothing in the A or B category. Not enough research.
St. John's wort	A for mild-moderate depression; B for somatoform disorders.
trehalose	Not evaluated.
tribulius	Not evaluated.
umcka	A for bronchitis; B for acute pharyngitis and the common cold

vitamin C	B for common cold prevention, iron absorption enhancement and urinary tract infections
vitamin D	A for kidney disease, psoriasis, thyroid conditions; B for dental cavities, muscle pain and osteoporosis
wheat germ oil	Nothing in the A or B category. Not enough research.
zinc	A for diarrhea in children and stomach ulcers; B for acne, herpes simplex virus and immune function

By Condition	Those with "Strong Scientific Evidence" (but not including those with "Good Scientific Evidence")
Acne	vitamin A
Allergic rhinitis	whey protein
Alopecia	none in the strong scientific evidence category
Anxiety	kava, music therapy
Autism	none in the strong scientific evidence category

Alzheimer's dementia	gingko biloba
Asthma	boswellia, buteyko breathing technique, choline, coleus, ephedra, psychotherapy, pycnogenol, yoga
Attention deficit disorder	none in the strong scientific evidence category
Back pain	none in the strong scientific evidence category
Chronic fatigue syndrome	none in the strong scientific evidence category
Chronic obstructive pulmonary disease	none in the strong scientific evidence category
Common cold	andrographis
Coronary artery disease	beta-glucan, beta sitosterol, niacin, omega-3 fatty acids, psyllium, red yeast rice, soy
Depression	light therapy, music therapy, St. John's wort
Diabetes	alpha-lipoic acid
Ear infections	none in the strong scientific evidence category
Fibromyalgia	none in the strong scientific evidence category

High blood pressure	garlic, omega-3 fatty acids, yoga
High cholesterol	beta-glucan, beta sitosterol, folate, garlic, glucomannan, niacin, omega-3 fatty acids, plant sterols, psyllium, red yeast rice, soy
Inflammatory bowel disease	none in the strong scientific evidence category
Irritable bowel syndrome	none in the strong scientific evidence category
Menopause	calcium, vitamin D
Migraine	feverfew
Nausea, vomiting	acupressure, shiatsu
Obesity	ephedra
Obsessive compulsive disorder	none in the strong scientific evidence category
Osteoarthritis	acupuncture, chondroitin, glucosamine, willow bark
Osteoporosis	calcium, vitamin D
Parkinson's disease	none in the strong scientific evidence category
Restless legs syndrome	none in the strong scientific evidence category

Sinusitis	whey protein
Sleep disorders	melatonin
Thyroid disorders	iodine, vitamin D

End Notes

1. http://usgovernmentspending.com/
federal_budget_detail_fy13bs12013n

2. http://www.who.int/whr/2000/en/whr00_en.pdf

3. "US Health in International Perspective Shorter Lives, Poorer Health" The introductory paragraph: The United States is among the wealthiest nations in the world, but it is far from the healthiest. Although Americans' life expectancy and health have improved over the past century, these gains have lagged behind those in other high-income countries. This health disadvantage prevails even though the United States spends far more per person on health care than any other nation. To gain a better understanding of this problem, the National Institutes of Health (NIH) asked the National Research Council and the Institute of Medicine to convene a panel of experts to investigate potential reasons for the U.S. health disadvantage and to assess its larger implications. http://www.iom.edu/~/media/Files/Report%20Files/2013/US-Health-International-Perspective/USHealth_Intl_PerspectiveRB.pdf

4. http://www.fiercebiotech.com/slideshows/fda-approvals-2012

5. www.reiki.com

6. www.niddk.nih.gov/healt-information/health-topics/digestive-diseases/ibs/Pages/facts.aspx

7. James M Kinross, et. al., "Gut Microbiome-host interactions in health and disease," *Genome Medicine* 2011, 3:14

8. van Nood, et.al., "Duodenal Infusion of Donor Feces for Recurrent Clostridium difficile," *N Engl J Med.* Jan 2013. doi:10.1056/NEJMoa1205037

9. Rob Dunn, "Science Reveals Why Calorie Counts Are All Wrong," *Scientific American, The Food Issue: The Science of Feast, Fuel and Farm*, Volume 309, Issue 3

10. Gary Taubes, "What Makes You Fat: Too Many Calories, Or The Wrong Carbohydrates," *Scientific American, The Food Issue: The Science of Feast, Fuel and Farm*, Volume 309, Issue 3

11. Ross Greene, PhD, *The Explosive Child* (Harper Collins, 2005)

12. from sleepfoundation.org or www.cdc.gov/sleep/about_sleep/sleep_hygiene.htm

13. The Diagnostic and Statistical Manual of Mental Disorders, Fourth Edition.

14. The National Center for Complementary and Integrative Medicine (NCCAM), "Effect of Hypericum performatum (St. John's wort) in major depressive disorder: a randomized, controlled trial." *JAMA* 2002;287(14):1807-1814

15. Benedict Carey. The makers of antidepressants like Prozac and Paxil never published the results of about a third of the drug trials that they conducted to win government approval, misleading doctors and consumers about the drugs' true effectiveness, a new analysis has found. "In published trials, about 60 percent of people taking the drugs report significant relief from depression, compared with roughly 40 percent of those on placebo pills. But when the less positive, unpublished trials are included, the advantage shrinks: the drugs outperform placebos, but by a modest margin, concludes the new report, which appears Thursday in The New England Journal of Medicine. Previous research had found a similar bias toward reporting positive results for a variety of medications; and many researchers have questioned the reported effectiveness of antidepressants. But the new analysis, reviewing data from 74 trials involving 12 drugs, is the most thorough to date. And it documents a large difference: while 94 percent of the positive studies found their way into print, just 14 percent of those with disappointing or uncertain results did. The finding is likely to inflame a continuing debate about how drug trial data is reported. In 2004, after revelations that negative findings from antidepressant trials had not been published, a group of leading journals agreed to stop publishing clinical trials that were not registered in a public database. Trade groups representing the world's largest drug makers announced that members' companies would begin to release more data from trials more quickly, on their own database, clinicalstudyresults.org." The New York Times, January 17, 2008

16. Jay C. Fournier, MA et. al. "Antidepressant Drug effects and Depression Severity: A Patient-Level Meta-Analysis" *JAMA* 2010 Jan 6; 303(1): 47-53

17. Y. Osher and R. H. Belmaker, "Omega-3 Fatty Acids in Depression: A Review of Three Studies." *CNS Neuroscience & Therapeutics*, Volume 15,

Issue 2, pages 128-133 DOI: 10.1111/j.1755-5949.2008.00061.x

18. From the website www.methyl-life.com/symptoms-of-mthfr.html:

What kind of symptoms are associated with the MTHFR gene defects?

There are many different symptoms someone with one or both gene mutations might encounter. Not everyone has the same set of symptoms because there are many other genetic and environmental differences that complicate health. But if you boil it down, there is a key systemic problem that comes from low methylation and it causes three different symptom areas.

Systemic problem: Homocysteine levels are too high due to the fact that not enough Methylfolate is available to convert the Homocysteine into Methionine, SAMe and Glutathione. Think of Methylfolate (L-MTHF or 5-MTHF) as the wizard changing the bad guy (Homocysteine) into good guys (SAMe and Glutathione).

Three symptom areas:

1. Central Nervous System disorders - some of these come from Homocysteine not getting converted into SAMe. SAMe is responsible for creating Serotonin, Dopamine, and Norepinephrine (neurotransmitters responsible for mood, motivation, and to some degree energy levels - if these are low, then Depression is often the result, but even aggression and alcoholism are symptoms sometimes found in men). Pregnant women may encounter extreme *Post-partum depression*. Also, things like *Fibromyalgia, Chronic Fatigue Syndrome, Migraines, IBS* (Irritable Bowel Syndrome), *Memory loss* with *Alzheimer's* and *Dementia* and other psychiatric problems can be tied to this issue (*OCD, Bipolar, Schizophrenia*, and more). These challenges are typically more related to the 1298 gene mutation. A very recent clinical trial (not even published yet) was done by Dr. Fava (July, 2011) showed that giving L-Methylfolate (Metafolin) found in the prescription 'medical food', Deplin, was as effective as the top anti-depressant drugs available today (and without all the side effects).

2. Cardiovascular problems often occur when Homocysteine levels in the body are too high. *Heart attack, Stroke, Blood clots, Peripheral neuropathy, Anemia* even *Miscarriages* and *Congenital birth defects* can be related to this issue among others. These problems are typically more related to the 677 gene mutation, but the worst is for a person who has one 677 variant and one 1298 variant.

3. Environmental poisoning can increase when not enough Homocysteine gets converted into glutathione. Glutathione is responsible for detoxifying the body of the heavy metals we encounter in the environment - it is our body's most powerful antioxidant. When a body gets too *burdened by heavy metals and toxins,* a lot of unexpected health problems emerge. Some symptoms of this can be: nausea, diarrhea, abdominal pain, liver and kidney dysfunction, hypertension, tachycardia, pulmonary fibrosis, asthma, immune problems, hair loss, rashes and more.

Sometimes diseases/disorders fall under a 'two-pronged' cause, meaning the causes of it stem from both *genetic* and *environmental* problems). *Autism* is a big one that falls into this 'two-pronged' cause category *[American Journal of Biochemistry and Biotechnology, 2008]* along with *Fibromyalgia, Chronic Fatigue Syndrome* and more. MTHFR is at the top of a list of 16 genetic defects for autism. Another study showed 98% of children with autism had one or both of the MTHFR gene defects (677 and/or 1298). A recent clinical study indicated that mothers with MTHFR who didn't take folate during pregnancy were 7 times more likely to have an autistic child than mothers without the MTHFR gene defect *[Epidemiology, July 2011, Vol. 22, Issue 4, pgs 476-485].* Colon and gastric cancers also have key links to the MTHFR gene defects, just do an internet search on 'MTHFR and colon cancer' or 'MTHFR and gastric cancer' and you will find many clinical studies and articles on the subject

19. From the website www.enzymestuff.com

A "methyl" group is simply one carbon connected to three hydrogen atoms. It may be written as CH3 with the 3 being a subscript.

"Methylation" is not just one specific reaction. There are hundreds of "methylation" reactions in the body. Methylation is simply the adding or removal of the methyl group to a compound or other element.

So why do we care about methylation at all? In general, when some compounds receive a methyl group, this "starts" a reaction (such as turning a gene on or activating an enzyme). When the methyl group is "lost" or removed, the reaction stops (or a gene is turned off or the enzyme is deactivated). Some of the more relevant methylation reactions would be:

4. getting methyl groups "turns on" detox reactions that detox the body of chemicals, including phenols. So if you are phenol sensitive, and you increase your methylation, then theoretically your body can process

more phenols and you can eat fruits without enzymes!

5. getting methyl groups "turns on" serotonin, and thus melatonin, production. Therefore, if you are a under-methylator, you can increase your methylation and have higher more appropriate levels of serotonin and melatonin. This means you may not have to take SSRIs, or may have improved sleep.

6. if you are an over-methylator you can take certain supplements to decrease methylation and perhaps turn off reactions that need to be off. This may decrease aggression or hyperness, for example.

Amy Yasko, PhD is one of the foremost experts on the biochemistry of methylation cycles and the relevance to chronic illness. From the website www.dramyyasko.com:

Why is the Methylation Cycle Important?

The Methylation Cycle is a biochemical pathway that manages or contributes to a wide range of crucial bodily functions, including:

- Detoxification
- Immune function
- Maintaining DNA
- Energy production
- Mood balancing
- Controlling inflammation

All of these processes help the body respond to environmental stressors, to detoxify, and to adapt and rebuild. That's why lowered methylation function may contribute to many, major chronic conditions, including:

- Cardiovascular Disease
- Cancer
- Diabetes
- Adult neurological conditions
- Autism and other spectrum disorders
- Chronic Fatigue Syndrome
- Alzheimer's disease
- Miscarriages, fertility, and problems in pregnancy
- Allergies, immune system, and digestive problems
- Mood and psychiatric disorders

• Aging

Methylation is involved in almost every bodily biochemical reaction, and occurs billions of times *every second* in our cells. That's why figuring out where the Cycle can better perform its tasks contributes to health improvement, and reduce symptoms.

20. The Benson-Henry Institute for Mind Body Medicine at www.mass-general.org/bhi

21. Applied Behavior Analysis (ABA) principles and techniques can foster basic skills such as looking, listening and imitating, as well as complex skills such as reading, conversing and understanding another person's perspective.

22. From the website http://autism.about.com/od/autismterms/a/stimming.htm: "The term stimming is short for self-stimulatory behavior. In a person with autism, stimming usually refers to specific behaviors such as flapping, rocking, spinning, or repetition of words and phrases. Stimming is almost always a symptom of autism, but it's important to note that stimming is also a part of most people's behavior patterns. If you've ever tapped your pencil, bitten your nails, twirled your hair, or paced, you've engaged in stimming."

23. This summary is provided by a patient's mother and the names have been changed to maintain confidentiality.

24. From Dr. Amy Yasko's Simplified Road Map to Health, page 10, she recommends different forms of B12 based on a person's genetic test results. (These results can be obtained by using 23andme.com for raw DNA information and then another website like geneticgenie.com to provide the specific results in usable form. COMT = catechol-o-methyl transferase; VDR = vitamin D receptor; Taq is a site on the vitamin D receptor)

COMT V158M VDR Taq B12 types that should be tolerated

• —++ (TT) All three types of B12
• — +- (Tt) All three types with less methyl B12
• — — (tt) Hydroxy B12 and adenosyl B12
• +- ++ All three types with less methyl B12
• +- +- Hydroxy B12 and adenosyl B12
• +- — Hydroxy B12 and adenosyl B12

- ++ ++ Hydroxy B12 and adenosyl B12
- ++ +- Hydroxy B12 and adenosyl B12
- ++ — Mostly hydroxyl B12

25. Lindsay, et. al. "Risk Factors for Alzheimer's Disease: A Prospective Analysis from the Canadian Study of Health and Aging." *Am J Epidemiol* 2002 156(5):445-453

26. http://m.imdb.com/name/nm0080524/quotes

27. This summary is provided by a naturopath in British Colubia and his name have been changed to maintain confidentiality.

28. http://www.med.wisc.edu/news-events/study-shows-echinacea-may-reduce-cold-duration-by-only-one-day/30079

29. http://www.mayoclinic.org/diseases-conditions/common-cold/expert-answers/zinc-for-colds/faq-20057769

30. The Wikipedia entry summarizes: "[He] drank a Petri dish containing cultured *H. pylori*, expecting to develop, perhaps years later, an ulcer. He was surprised when, only three days later, he developed vague nausea and halitosis, (due to the achlorhydria, there was no acid to kill bacteria in the stomach, and their waste products manifested as bad breath), noticed only by his mother. On days 5–8, he developed achlorydric (no acid) vomiting. On day eight, he had a repeat endoscopy and biopsy, which showed massive inflammation (gastritis), and *H. pylori* was cultured. On the fourteenth day after ingestion, a third endoscopy was done, and Marshall began to take antibiotics. This story is related by Barry Marshall himself in his Nobel acceptance lecture Dec. 8, 2005, available for viewing on the Nobel website. [7] Interestingly, Marshall did not develop antibodies to *H. pylori*, suggesting that innate immunity can sometimes eradicate acute *H. pylori* infection. Marshall's illness and recovery, based on a culture of organisms extracted from a patient, fulfilled Koch's postulates for *H. pylori* and gastritis, but not for peptic ulcer."

31. Richard I. Horowitz, MD, *Why Can't I Get Better? Solving the Mystery of Lyme & Chronic Disease* (Printed in the United States of America: St. Martin's Press, 2013) pages 66-67.

32. Raphael B. Stricker, "Counterpoint: Long-Term Antibiotic Therapy Improves Persistent Symptoms Associated with Lyme Disease," *Clinical Infectious Disease* 2007; 45:149-57

33. Lisa Snider and Susan Swedo, "Post-streptococcal autoimmune disorders of the central nervous system," *Curr Opin Neurol* 16:359-365 and

Moretti, et.al., "What every psychiatrist should know about PANDAS: a review," *Clin Pract Epidemiol Ment Health.* 2008; 4:13.

34. http://www.ninds.nih.gov/disorders/disorder_index.htm

35. This summary is provided by a patient's mother and the names have been changed to maintain confidentiality.

36. http://www.theanalystmagazine.com

37. Teitelbaum, et al, "Effective Treatment of Chronic Fatigue Syndrome & Fibromyalgia—A Double-Blind, Randomized, Placebo-Controlled Study,"

J Chron Fat Syn. 2001; 8(2): 3-28). You can also check the website www.endfatigue.com or www.jacobteitelbaum.com.

38. Teitelbaum, et al, "The Use of D-Ribose in Chronic Fatigue Syndrome and Fibromyalgia: A Pilot Study," *Open Pain J.* 2012; 5: 32-37.

39. https://nccih.nih.gov/health/supplements/SAMe

40. Cordero, et.al., "Can coenzyme Q10 improve clinical and molecular parameters in fibromyalgia?" *Antioxid Redox Signal* 2013 Oct 20;19(12): 1356-1361.

41. F. Zeldan, et. al., "Brain Mechanisms Supporting the Modulation of Pain by Mindfulness Meditation," *The Journal of Neuroscience*, 6 April 2011, 31(14): 5540-5548.

42. http://ftp.cdc.gov/pub/Health_Statistics/NCHS/Dataset_Documentation/NAMCS/doc2010.pdf

43. M. Magill, MD, et. al, "New Developments in the Management of Hypertension," *Am Fam Physician.* 2003 Sep 1;68(5):853-858

44. http://rienstraclinic.com/health-info/systems/blood/rauwolfia/

45. This summary is provided by a naturopath in Washington state and his name have been changed to maintain confidentiality.

46. http://en.wikipedia.org/wiki/Reserpine

47. The AMA study has revealed that more than 42% of physicians across all specialties has at some time been sued for malpractice, and more than 20% have been sued two or more times. Based on a 2007-2008 survey of

a statistically valid sample (5285 physicians from 42 specialties randomly selected from the AMA physician masterfile) the survey asked whether the physician had ever been sued, and whether they had been named in a suit in the past year. The survey was jointly sponsored by the AMA, CMS, and 40 specialty societies, including ACEP.

48. http://www.hsph.harvard.edu/nutritionsource/what-should-you-eat/fats-and-cholesterol/

49. John Abramson, MD, *Over•ose• America: The Broken Promise of American Medicine* from Harper Perenniel, 2008

50. University of Pennsylvania School of Medicine, "Statin use not linked to a decline in cognitive function." *ScienceDaily* 18 November 2013.

51. From *J Assoc Physicians India* 1989 May;37(5)323-8: "Multicentric clinical trials of the efficacy of gugulipid conducted at Bombay, Bangalore, Delhi, Jaipur, Lucknow, Nagpur and Varanasi have been reported. Two hundred and five patients completed 12 week open trial with gugulipid in a dose of 500 mg tds after 8 week diet and placebo therapy. One patient showed gastrointestinal symptoms which did not necessitate withdrawal of the drug. A significant lowering of serum cholesterol (av. 23.6%) and serum triglycerides (av. 22.6%) was observed in 70-80% patients Double-blind, crossover study was completed in 125 patients with gugulipid therapy and in 108 patients with clofibrate therapy. Two patients had flu-like syndrome with clofibrate and opted out from the study. With gugulipid the average fall in serum cholesterol and triglycerides was 11 and 16.8% respectively and with clofibrate 10 and 21.6% respectively. The lipid lowering effect of both drugs became evident 3-4 week after starting the drug and had no relationship with age, sex, and concomitant drug intake. Hypercholesterolaemic patients responded better to gugulipid therapy than hypertriglyceridaemic patients who responded better to clofibrate therapy. In mixed hyperlipidaemic patients response to both drugs was comparable. HDL-cholesterol was increased in 60% cases who responded to gugulipid therapy. Clofibrate had no effect on HDL-cholesterol. A significant decrease in LDL-cholesterol was observed in the responder group to both drugs. "

52. Sahni, et. al., "Guggulipid Use in Hyperlipidemia," *American Journal of Health-System Pharmacy* 2005; 62(16):1690-1692

53. Myers, et.al., "Exercise Capacity and Mortality Among Men Referred for Exercise Testing," *NEJM*, Vol 346, No 11, March 14, 2002

54. Chan, et. al., "Water, other fluids, and fatal coronary disease: the Adventist Health Study," Am J Epidemiol 2002 May 1;155(9):827-33.

55. http://www.merriam-webster.com

56. Fowler, at. al., "Dynamic spread of happiness in a large social network: longitudinal analysis over 20 years in the Framingham Heart Study," BMJ. 2008; 337:a2338.

57. From www.sciencedaily.com: "Quantum entanglement is a quantum mechanical phenomenon in which the quantum states of two or more objects have to be described with reference to each other, even though the individual objects may be spatially separated."

58. http://www.brainyquote.com/quotes/quotes/j/johnupdike104128.html

59. This summary is provided by a patient of mine and his name have been changed to maintain confidentiality.

60. Altiner, et. al., "Sputum colour for diagnosis of a bacterial infection in patients with acute cough," Scand J Prim Health Care 2009; 27(20): 70-73

61. Miravitlles, et. al., "Sputum colour and bacteria in chronic bronchitis exacerbations: a pooled analysis," Europ Resp J 2011

62. Paul, Beiler, et.al., "Effect of Honey and Dextromethorphan on Nocturnal Cough and Sleep," Arch Pediatr Adolesc Med 2007 Dec;161(12):1140-6

Conclusion: In a comparison of honey, DM, and no treatment, parents rated honey most favorably for symptomatic relief of their child's nocturnal cough and sleep difficulty due to upper respiratory tract infection. Honey may be a preferable treatment for the cough and sleep difficulty associated with childhood upper respiratory tract infection.

63. Okada, et.al., "The 'hygiene hypothesis' for autoimmune and allergic diseases: an update," Clin Exp Immunol Apr 2010; 160(1):1-9.

64. Neil Pearce, Richard Beasley, Carl Burgess, and Julian Crane, Asthma Epi•emiology: Principles an• metho•s (New York, Oxford University Press, 1998)

65. Ben Goldacre, "Rusty Results," www.theguardian.com, Wednesday 1 September 2004 21.12 EDT

66. From Wikipedia: "Sarno's most notable (and controversial) achievement

is the development, diagnosis and treatment of TMS, which is not accepted by mainstream medicine. According to Sarno, TMS is a psychosomatic illness causing chronic back, neck, and limb pain which is not relieved by standard medical treatments. He includes other ailments, such as gastrointestinal problems, dermatological disorders and repetitive-strain injuries as TMS related. Sarno states that he has successfully treated over ten thousand patients at the Rusk Institute by educating them on his beliefs of a psychological and emotional basis to their pain and symptoms. Sarno's theory is, in part, that the pain or GI symptoms are an unconscious "distraction" to aid in the repression of deep unconscious emotional issues. Sarno believes that when patients think about what may be upsetting them in their unconscious, they can defeat their minds' strategy to repress these powerful emotions; when the symptoms are seen for what they are, the symptoms then serve no purpose, and they go away. Supporters of Sarno's work hypothesize an inherent difficulty in performing the clinical trials needed to prove or disprove the diagnosis, since it is difficult to use clinical trials with psychosomatic illnesses."

67. August West, "Helping Men Get Proactive About Health: A Conversation with John La Puma, MD," *Holistic Primary Care* Friday, 02 August 2013 21:01

68. David Brownstein, MD, *Io·ine: Why You Nee· It, Why You Can't Live Without It* ISBN: 9780966088274

69. Black, et.al., "Effects of Continuing or Stopping Alendronate After 5 Years of Treatment," *JAMA.* 2006; 296(24):2927-2938

70. Jehle, Hulter and Krapf, "Effect of potassium citrate on bone density, microarchitechture, and fracture risk in healthy older adults without osteoporosis: a randomized controlled trial," *J Clin Endocrinol Metab* 2013 Jan; 98(1): 207-17.

71. Marangella, et. al., "Effects of potassium citrate supplementation on bone metabolism," *Calfic Tissue Int* 2004 Apr;74(4):330-5

72. Julie Edgar, "Should Your Child Get the HPV Vaccine?" reviewed by Laura J. Martin, MD and From an Up-To-Date summary: Cancer of the uterine cervix is the third most common gynecologic cancer diagnosis and cause of death among gynecologic cancers in the United States [1]. Cervical cancer has lower rates than uterine corpus and ovarian cancer, as well as many other cancer sites. These rankings are similar to global estimates for

other developed countries [2]. Unfortunately, in countries that do not have access to cervical cancer screening and prevention programs, cervical cancer remains the second most common type of cancer (17.8 per 100,000 women) and cause of cancer deaths (9.8 per 100,000) among all types of cancer in women. Human papillomavirus (HPV) is central to the development of cervical neoplasia and can be detected in 99.7 percent of cervical cancers.

73. http://www.cancer.org/cancer/leukemiainchildren/index

74. Bleyer, Welch, "Effect of Three Decades of Screening Mammography on Breast-Cancer Incidence," *N Engl J Med* 2012; 367:1998-2005.

75. Rhodes, et. al., " Dedicated dual-head gamma imaging for breast cancer screening in women with mammographically dense breasts," *Radiology* 2011 Jan; 258(1):106-18

76. Donna Nazakawa, *The Autoimmune Epidemic* (New York: Touchstone, 2008), pages 72-75, 136

77. David Buchholz, MD, *Heal Your Headache* (Workman Publishing Company, 2002)

78. Robert M. Sapolsky, *Why Zebras Don't Get Ulcers* (Holt Paperbacks, 2004)

79. Donna Nazakawa, *The Autoimmune Epidemic* (New York: Touchstone, 2008), page 8

80. Donna Nazakawa, *The Autoimmune Epidemic* (New York: Touchstone, 2008), page 45

81. Donna Nazakawa, *The Autoimmune Epidemic* (New York: Touchstone, 2008), page 144

82. Gerber, Offit, "Vaccines and Autism: A Tale of Shifting Hypotheses," *Clin Infect Dis* 2009 48(4):456-461

83. Smith, et.al., "On-time Vaccine Receipt in the First Year Does Not Adversely Affect Neuropsychological Outcomes," *Pediatrics* 2010 June

84. "Immunization Safety Review: Multiple Immunizations and Immune Dysfunction," *Institute of Medicine* 2004 May

85. Kwok, " Vaccines: The real issues in vaccine safety," *Nature* 2011 May doi:10.1038/473436a

86. The Vaccine War on PBS show Frontline. Examining the emotionally

charged debate over medical risks vs. benefits and a parent's right to make choices about her child vs. a community's common good...

87. William Shaw, PhD, "Increased Acetaminophen Use Appears to be Major Cause of the Epidemics of Autism, AD(H)D and Asthma," *Journal of Restorative Medicine 2013* doi 10.14200/jrm.2013.2.0101

88. The Vaccine Book: Making the Right Decision for Your Child (Sears Parenting Library) by Robert W. Sears, MD

89. Heart and Stroke Foundation of Canada, "Influenza vaccine may reduce risk of heart disease and death: Flu shot may reduce risk of major cardiac event by 50 percent," *ScienceDaily*, 28 October 2012.

90. Michael Pollan, *The Omnivore's Dilemma* (New York, New York, Penguin Publishing, 2006)

91. http://www.fda.gov/AboutFDA/Transparency/Basics/ucm214868. htm What is the meaning of 'natural' on the label of food?

92. Andy Coghlan, "Is Opposition to Golden Rice "Wicked"?," online article from *NewScientist* http://www.slate.com/articles/health_and_science/new_scientist/2013/10/golden_rice_inventor_ingo_potrykus_green-peace_and_others_wicked_for_opposition.html and

Bjorn Lomborg, "The Deadly Opposition to Genetically Modified Food," online as http://www.slate.com/articles/health_and_science/project_syndicate0/2013/02/gm_food_golden_rice_will_save_millions_of_people_from_vitamin_a_deficiency. html

93. David H. Freedman, "The Truth About Genetically Modified Food," *Scientific American*, Volume 309, Issue 3

94. http://en.wikipedia.org/wiki/Norman_Borlaug

95. http://www.bastyr.edu/academics/areas-study/study-naturopathic-medicine/about-naturopathic-medicine

96. https://nccih.nih.gov/news/camstats/2007/camsurvey_fs1.htm

97. Brenda Watson, ND and Leonard Smith, MD, *Gut Solutions, Natural Solutions to Your Digestive Problems* (Renew Life, 2004)

98. http://www.mayoclinic.org/healthy-living/consumer-health/basics/alternative-medicine/hlv-20049491

99. http://www.uclh.nhs.uk/OurServices/OurHospitals/RLHIM/Pages/Home.aspx

100. Ben Goldacre TED: "Battling Bad Science," at www.ted.com/speakers/ben_goldacre

101. John Gray, PhD, *Men Are from Mars, Women Are from Venus* (Harper Publishing, 1992)

102. The iodine loading test involves the person taking 50mg of an iodine/iodide combination supplement after their first morning urine. They collect 24 hours of urine after that to include the first morning urine the next day. If the person has a systemic iodine deficiency, then most of the iodine will be utilized by the body and only a relatively small percentage will be excreted through the urine. From David Brownstein, MD, a normal result would be 45mg or more found in the 24 hour urine collection. Anything under 45mg would be considered iodine deficiency.

103. http://blog.gaiam.com/quotes/authors/esther-hicks?page=1

104. This summary is provided by a naturopath in Washington state and his name have been changed to maintain confidentiality.

105. This blog excerpt was provided by the mother of a patient of mine and their names have been changed to maintain confidentiality.

106. Dr. Shaw founded The Great Plains Laboratory, Inc., which I have found to be a solid resource for information and testing. Dr. Shaw worked for the Centers for Disease Control and Prevention (CDC), Children's Mercy Hospital, University of Missouri at Kansas City School of Medicine, and Smith Kline Laboratories. He is the author of *Biological Treatments for Autism and PDD*, originally published in 1998 and *Autism: Beyon• the Basics*, published in 2009. He notes in the cholesterol/autism article that "the brain is the most cholesterol rich organ in the body requiring a large amount to sustain the myelin sheath which coats nerve cells and helps conduct electrical impulses." He references later that, "individuals with cholesterol deficiency are more prone to aggressive behavior, lack of attention, increased number of infections and motor difficulty." There is a rare genetic condition called Smith-Lemli-Opitz Syndrome (SLOS) that causes cholesterol deficiency in the body and is associated with autistic features.

107. William Crook, MD, *The Yeast Connection, A Medical Breathrough* (Vintage Books, 1986)

108. *Conscious Eating* by Gabriel Cousens, MD p263-269

109. WellnessWatchersMD | Holistic Treatment for Candidiasis (Systemic Yeast Infections)

110. The Capital Steps is a performance group doing political satire out of Washington D.C.

111. Roger Dobson, "Cough medicines' effect is mainly placebo," *British Medical Journal* 2006 Jan 7; 332(7532): 8

112. Bent S, Kane C, Shinohara K, et al., "Saw palmetto for benign prostatic hypertrophy," *New England Journal of Medicine.* 2006; 354(6):557–566. "In the study, 225 men over age 49 who had moderate-to-severe symptoms of BPH were randomly assigned to receive either saw palmetto extract (a 160-mg capsule taken twice daily) or a placebo for 12 months." The conclusion: "The study found no significant differences between the saw palmetto and placebo groups in the two primary outcome measures (scores on the American Urological Association Symptom Index for BPH, and maximal urinary flow rate) or in secondary measures (prostate size, residual urinary volume after voiding, quality of life, and serum prostate-specific antigen levels)."

113. Clegg DO, Reda DJ, Harris CL, et al., "Glucosamine, chondroitin sulfate, and the two in combination for painful knee osteoarthritis," *New England Journal of Medicine* 2006; 354(8):795–808.

114. Richard I. Horowitz, MD, *Why Can't I Get Better? Solving the Mystery of Lyme & Chronic Disease* (Printed in the United States of America: St. Martin's Press, 2013) The case study is found in pages 99-105 and the specific excerpt is from page 105.